Concepts and Applications
WELLNESS

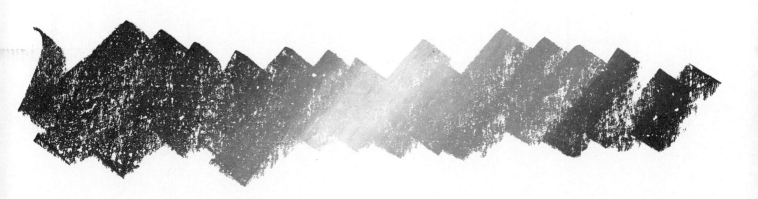

Concepts and Applications
WELLNESS

David J. Anspaugh, *P.E.D., Ed.D., CHES*
Professor of Health and Physical Education
Division Chairman of Fitness and Wellness
Memphis State University
Memphis, Tennessee

Michael H. Hamrick, *Ed.D., CHES*
Professor and Division Chairman
Health Science and Safety Education
Memphis State University
Memphis, Tennessee

Frank D. Rosato, *Ed.D.*
Professor of Health and Physical Education
Director of Fitness and Testing
Division of Fitness and Wellness
Memphis State University
Memphis, Tennessee

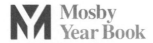
Mosby
Year Book

St. Louis Baltimore Boston Chicago London Philadelphia Sydney Toronto

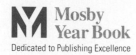
**Mosby
Year Book**
Dedicated to Publishing Excellence

Editor: Vicki Van Ry
Senior Developmental Editor: Michelle Turenne
Project Manager: Mark Spann
Production Editor: Christine M. Ripperda
Designer: Liz Fett
Illustrator: Tandy and Associates
Cover Illustration: ARTCO/by Jeff Cornell

Copyright © 1991 by Mosby–Year Book, Inc.
A Mosby imprint of Mosby–Year Book, Inc.

Mosby–Year Book, Inc.
11830 Westline Industrial Drive
St. Louis, MO 63146

Library of Congress Cataloging in Publication Data

Anspaugh, David J.
    Wellness: concepts and applications / by David J. Anspaugh,
Michael H. Hamrick, Frank D. Rosato.
       p.   cm.
    Includes bibliographical references and index.
    ISBN 0-8016-0034-0
    1. Health. 2. Self-care, Health. 3. Medicine, Preventive.
I. Hamrick, Michael H. II. Rosato, Frank D. III. Title.
RA776.A57 1991   *72974*
613—dc20   90-49845
                                       CIP

CL/CX/VH 9 8 7 6 5 4 3 2 1

Preface

Wellness: Concepts and Applications is unique because it assumes that health is not a destination but a journey. Wellness is not a static condition but a continual balancing of the different dimensions of human needs—spiritual, social, emotional, intellectual, and physical. Because we are all responsible for our own growth in these areas, this book strives to emphasize the importance of self-responsibility. And because we know that knowlege alone stimulates change for very few people, the reader is challenged to be actively involved in the learning process by constantly assessing how the information presented affects lifestyle from a personal perspective.

Wellness: Concepts and Applications is neither a fitness book nor a personal health text. Instead this text is designed to help students gain knowledge and understanding in a variety of areas, with the goal being to take that information and use it to make behavioral changes that will have a positive impact on their lives. In many cases these changes are necessary if people are to develop the skills, attitudes, beliefs, and habits that will ultimately result in the highest possible level of health and wellness.

Audience

When the fitness/wellness concept appears in university courses and programs, it is usually a scaled-down model of the traditional personal health course or an up-scale version of physical fitness courses. In some cases it is a hybrid of both personal health and fitness courses, with emphasis on self-participation in the medical marketplace. In terms of content, *Wellness: Concepts and Applications* is a hybrid because the physical components of wellness are blended with its many other components. However, caution will be exercised to avoid covering topics commonly found in personal health texts. The primary objectives of this text are to present cognitive health and wellness information appropriate for today's college students and to offer suggestions for their application. These suggestions consist of lifestyle behaviors over which people can exert some control. The emphasis is on self-responsibility, and this theme is implemented through a strong self-analysis and assessment component.

Content Highlights

Important features unique to *Wellness: Concepts and Applications* make it distinct from other texts.

Balanced approach: Unlike other approaches that emphasize only physical fitness as a major route to wellness, *Wellness: Concepts and Applications* provides a balanced presentation of the health benefits of exercise, diet, and cardiovascular wellness, along with the management of lifestyle change and consumer responsibility to achieve lifetime wellness.

Complete lifestyle decision-making information: Along with Assessment Activities that help apply the content, coverage of substance use, sexually transmitted diseases, and chronic health conditions is provided to enable and encourage responsible student decision-making.

Consumer-oriented: Chapter 11, Self-Responsibility in the Health-Care Market, offers information to help students become wise consumers.

Interdisciplinary author team: Two health ed-

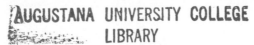

ucators and a fitness educator presently teaching wellness courses have combined their expertise to provide the most balanced presentation possible.

Full-Color: A full-color format is used throughout the photographs, line drawings, and design of the text to increase visual impact and to enhance the teaching-learning process.

Lifestyle Assessment Inventory: It is recommended that the Lifestyle Assessment Inventory in Appendix B be completed at both the beginning and the end of the course. It will provide a picture of how current lifestyle patterns are shaping students' lives, as well as provide a comparison to determine lifestyle improvements. Keep in mind that there are no right or wrong answers. The only useful answer is one that best reflects current practices.

Organization Highlights

Chapter 1, An Introduction to Health and Wellness: Presents the basic wellness model. This model includes the various components that constitute assumption of personal responsibility for enhancing one's quality of life. The benefits of high-level wellness are identified, and opportunities are provided to assess the point at which each individual is currently functioning in the quest for a higher level of wellness.

Chapter 2, Managing Lifestyle Change: Lists behaviors conducive to good health and provides an assessment to analyze one's own life to determine positive and negative behaviors. It includes steps to initiate lifestyle change and provides a contract for making the change. The plan allows for progress checks and follow-up.

Chapter 3, Forming a Plan for Good Nutrition: Presents nutrition concepts within the framework of the landmark document "Dietary Guidelines for Americans." The major misconceptions associated with vitamins, protein, fats, carbohydrates, and fiber are dispelled. Health practices that may improve common digestive problems are identified.

Chapter 4, Overcoming the Diet and Weight Obsession: Differentiates between body measurement by weight and by composition. Current theories associated with development of fat cells in human beings, weight gain, and obesity are discussed. Hazards associated with dieting in general and with certain popular diets are pointed out. The positive effects of exercise on body com-

position and weight management are stressed as the most healthful solution to weight control.

Chapter 5, Cardiovascular Health and Wellness: Describes the basic operation of the heart, selected heart diseases, and the methods currently employed in the treatment and prevention of these diseases. The risk factors associated with the development of heart disease are identified along with ways to reduce these risks.

Chapter 6, Exercise for Fitness and Leisure: Discusses components of health-related physical fitness and the principles of conditioning that contribute to total fitness. Methods for calculating target heart rate are provided. The problems associated with exercising in hot and cold weather are also covered.

Chapter 7, Coping With and Managing Stress: Examines the factors that cause stress and the psychological effects of stress on the body. The sources of stress and the long-term effects of stress on health are explored. Activities are used to assist students in identifying their personal stressors and determining an effective means of dealing with stress.

Chapter 8, Assuming Responsibility for Substance Use: Provides information on tobacco products, cocaine, marijuana, and other drugs, including the potential negative effects of each. The importance of taking individual responsibility for substance use is emphasized.

Chapter 9, Preventing Sexually Transmitted Diseases: Provides information on chlamydia, herpes, AIDS, and other diseases of concern. The importance of following safer sex practices is emphasized.

Chapter 10, Impact of Lifestyle on Common Conditions: Highlights conditions such as cancer, diabetes, arthritis, colds, influenza, and headaches. The chapter emphasizes the effects of a positive lifestyle to lessen and avoid the impact of these conditons.

Chapter 11, Self-Responsibility in the Health-Care Market: Discusses the importance of making wise decisions when entering the health-care market. The chapter provides guidelines for determining when, where, and how to choose health care wisely. Suggestions for learning how to identify information that can be trusted is included.

Chapter 12, Developing An Action Plan for Lifetime Wellness: Assessment Activities in the areas of medical history and personal wellness as well as an action plan are provided. Rather than include this information earlier in the text, this chapter provides a culminating, step-by-step guide for making behavioral change and a contract for making a specific commitment in a chosen area. For additional reinforcement, an evaluation form to help "get back on track" when encountering difficulty with a change is included.

Pedagogical Highlights

Wellness: Concepts and Applications uses a variety of learning aids to enhance student comprehension.

Key Terms: The most important terms for student retention have been boldfaced in the text for easy identification.

Chapter Objectives: These are introduced at the beginning of each chapter. They assist the student in identifying the chapter's key topics.

Chapter Summaries: These identify the major parts of the chapter and reinforce the chapter objectives.

Action Plan for Personal Wellness: These are provided at the end of the chapters to help students identify plans to implement change based on knowledge gained from the chapter.

Review Questions: Questions are provided to help students review and analyze material for overall understanding.

References: Accurate and current documentation is provided at the end of the chapters.

Annotated Readings: Additional current resources are provided for students to obtain further information.

Assessment Activities: Each chapter concludes with at least two Assessment Activities to help students apply the content learned in the chapter to their own personal decision-making. In addition, Chapter 12 is a culminating chapter of assessment activities. The text is perforated for easy removal of the Assessment Activities.

Appendixes:
- Lifestyle Assessment Inventory. Students complete the inventory at the beginning and end of the course to determine their lifestyle improvements.
- Nutritive Values of Foods. The nutritive values of common food items are provided. These values assist students in completing Assessment Activities in Chapter 3.
- Glossary: A comprehensive glossary is provided at the end of the text that includes all key terms as well as additional terms used

in the text. In addition, cross-references to the text are provided after each definition.

Supplements

An extensive package is available to the adopters of *Wellness: Concepts and Applications*. The package has been developed to assist the instructor in obtaining maximum benefit from the text. Each ancillary has been thoroughly reviewed to provide the highest quality possible. These features, which will enhance the appeal of the text, are:

Instructor's Manual and Test Bank: Each chapter begins with a brief overview of the content followed by a list of the objectives for that chapter. A detailed lecture outline and additional class activities have been developed for each chapter. Each chapter concludes with a resource section, including relevant media, software, and organization sources, and additional annotated readings. The Test Bank includes more than 1400 multiple choice, true-false, matching, and essay questions. All test items have been thoroughly checked for accuracy, clarity, and range of difficulty by instructors who also served as reviewers for the text. The manual concludes with 60 full-page transparency masters of helpful illustrations and charts.

Computerized Test Bank: Qualified adopters of this text may request a Diploma Computerized Test Bank package compatible with the IBM PC, Apple IIc, Apple IIe, and Macintosh microcomputers. This software is a unique combination of user-friendly computerized aids for the instructor. The following summarizes these software aids:
- Testing. A test generator allows the user to select items from the test bank either manually or randomly; to add, edit, or delete test items through a preset format that includes multiple choice, true-false, matching, or essay options; and to print exams with or without saving them for future use.
- Grading. A computerized record keeper saves student names (up to 250), assignments (up to 50), and related grades in a format similar to that used in manual grade books. Statistics on individual or class performance, test weighting, and push-button grade curving are features of this software.
- Tutoring. A tutorial package uses separate items from the test bank for student review.

Student scores can be merged into the grading records.
• Scheduling. A computerized data book makes class planning and schedule management quick and convenient.

Overhead Transparency Acetates: Forty-eight of the text's most important illustrations, diagrams, tables, and charts are available as acetate transparencies. Attractively designed in full-color, these useful tools facilitate learning and classroom discussion and were chosen specifically to help explain difficult concepts. This package is also available to qualified adopters of the text.

Acknowledgments

The authors with to express their heartfelt thanks to Susan Bingham and Susan Hunter for their support, research, and typing of the manuscript. Although unstated at times, their patience and perseverance have always been appreciated.

We also wish to thank the reviewers, whose contributions have added significantly to the text. To the following, a grateful acknowledgment of their expertise and assistance:

Pat Barrett
Radford University

Wilson Campbell
Northeast Louisiana University

Arlene Crosman
Linn-Benton Community College

Betty Edgley
Oklahoma State University

Mary Mahan
Miami-Dade Community College

Eva W. McGahee
North Georgia College

Brenda Obert
University of Maine-Farmington

Glen J. Peterson
Lakewood Community College

Russell F. Smiley
Normandale Community College

John G. Smith
Long Beach City College

Rod Smith
Clark College

James A. Streater, Jr.
Armstrong State College

Michael L. Teague
University of Iowa

Luke E. Thomas
Northeast Louisiana University

Gary L. Wilson
The Citadel

A sincere word of thanks to Ed Murphy and Donna Sokolowski for their help in ensuring that the conceptualization of this project became a reality. Sincere appreciation must also be expressed to the excellent production staff at Mosby-Year Book: Christine Ripperda, Liz Fett, and Mark Spann. Finally, a special tribute is due to Michelle Turenne for caring so much that the ultimate product be the best product possible. Her judgment, creativity, and refining of the text have added immeasurably to the project.

David J. Anspaugh
Michael H. Hamrick
Frank D. Rosato

Student Preface

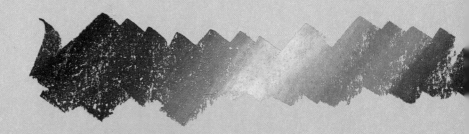

Wellness is a balance of all areas of health. It involves more than physical fitness and proper nutrition. It involves a higher quality of life and a state of well-being. Wellness is a lifestyle choice.

Wellness: Concepts and Applications combines the important elements of fitness with today's relevant health issues in nutrition and weight management, stress management, substance use, sexually transmitted diseases, and the health care market to help you make lifestyle decisions that will positively affect your wellness.

Features

We have included features in *Wellness: Concepts and Applications* that you will find to be helpful in achieving lifetime wellness:

Consumer-Oriented. Chapter 11, Self-Responsibility in the Health Care Market, provides factual and helpful information such as choosing a physician. Using this chapter will enable you to make wise consumer decisions.

Lifetime Wellness. *Wellness: Concepts and Applications* is packed with Assessment Activities, Action Plans for Personal Wellness, and a Lifestyle Assessment Inventory to help you apply the chapter content to your own lifestyle. These activities will help you progress to final Chapter 12 that will enable you to develop an action plan for a lifetime of wellness.

Full-color presentation. The use of full-color throughout *Wellness: Concepts and Applications* provides a presentation that is both instructional and visually exciting.

Pedagogy

Wellness: Concepts and Applications includes important tools called *pedagogy* to help you learn. The next few pages graphically illustrate how to use these study aids to your advantage.

The chapters open with a list of key terms and objectives. These reinforce the important terms to become familiar with while reading the chapter and the objectives to be accomplished after completing each chapter.

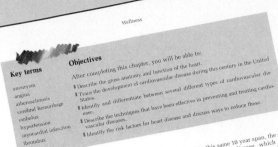

Wellness

4

Key terms

aneurysm
angina
atherosclerosis
cerebral hemorrhage
embolus
hypertension
myocardial infarction
thrombus

Objectives

After completing this chapter, you will be able to:

▌ Describe the gross anatomy and function of the heart.

▌ Trace the development of cardiovascular disease during this century in the United States.

▌ Identify and differentiate between several different types of cardiovascular disease.

▌ Describe the techniques that have been effective in preventing and treating cardiovascular diseases.

▌ Identify the risk factors for heart disease and discuss ways to reduce these.

Cardiovascular disease includes a constellation of diseases that affect the heart and blood vessels. The 5 major forms of cardiovascular disease as classified by the American Heart Association are coronary heart disease, hypertensive disease, rheumatic heart disease, strokes, and congenital heart defects. Cardiovascular disease-the leading cause of death in the United States-accounts for 47% of all deaths. Twenty-five percent of Americans (approximately 66 million people) have one or more forms of heart or blood vessel disease. There have been approximately 1,500,000 heart attacks in each of the last few years and more than 500,000 of these result in death. Three hundred thousand or 60% of these deaths occur before the victim reaches a hospital emergency room. This is a tragedy that is even more tragic because a significant number of these premature deaths could have been circumvented with early and proper treatment.

Fifty percent of the victims wait an average of 2 hours before seeking medical attention. Denying the possibility that a heart attack may be in progress is the primary reason for the delay. Denial is reinforced because the symptoms of a heart attack are similar to those of other physical ailments and we are more prone to believe that it is one of the other problems rather than a heart attack.

Although the figures are foreboding, and while there is much that remains to be done in the battle against cardiovascular disease, substantial progress has occurred during the last 3 decades. The death rate for all cardiovascular diseases declined by approximately 23% from 1976 to 1986. During this same 10 year span, the death rate from coronary heart disease, which is responsible for the majority of heart attack deaths, declined by 28%. Deaths from strokes declined by 4% during the same period. The downward trend in the death rate from cardiovascular disease has been attributed to lifestyle changes and more sophisticated medical diagnosis and treatment.

The Fundamentals of Circulation

The Heart and Blood Vessels

Circulation is better understood if one is familiar with the basic anatomy and function of the heart. The heart consists of cardiac muscle and weighs between 8 and 10 ounces. It is about the size of a fist and lies in the center of the chest. The heart is divided into 2 halves or pumps by a wall (the septum) and each half is subdivided into an upper chamber (the atrium) and a lower

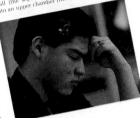

Key terms are set in boldface type throughout each chapter to help you become more familiar with them.

Full-color artwork is used throughout the text to enhance learning.

Chapter 7

Cardiovascular Health and Wellness

5

The Development of Adiposity

At this point, it may be productive to discuss some basic information regarding the growth and development of **adipose cells** (fat cells). Adipose cells grow by **hypertrophy** (an increase in size) and **hyperplasia** (an increase in number). Fat cells increase significantly in size during the first six months of **postnatal** life (after birth) and by one year of age they are similar in size to those of adolescents. From one year of age to puberty, the size of fat cells remains essentially stable but they proliferate in number so that growth is in the form of hyperplasia during this period. In puberty, both size and number increase substantially.

Gender differences in the deposition of subcutaneous fat become noticeable during and after puberty. Males distribute fat primarily in the upper half of the body while females deposit it in the lower half. The percentage of fat reaches peak values early in adolescence for males and then declines during the remainder of adolescent growth. Females experience a continuous increase in the percentage of fat from the onset of puberty to age 18. Fig. 6-6 shows how fat is manufactured in the body. From approximately two years of age, obese children develop a greater number of fat cells than children of normal weight. Some evidence suggests that overfeeding in infancy stimulates the development of excess fat cells and predisposes affected children to later obesity. However, newer evidence indicates that obesity later in life is unaffected by overfeeding in early life. Underfeeding in early life does not guarantee the prevention of obesity in later life. Neonatal adiposity is not a good predictor of adult obesity. Studies have shown that most infants who are obese during the first year of life tend to slim down to normal weight by the age of 9.

Genetic Considerations

Obesity is a complex eating disorder with multiple causes. It was formally declared a disease a few years ago by the National Institutes of Health Development Conference.

The genetic influence in weight control is becoming more clearly established. Researchers at the University of Pennsylvania examined the relative fatness and the body type of adults who had been adopted childhood. They classified 540 adoptees into one of the following categories: thin; median weight; overweight; and obese. They found that the subjects resembled their bio-

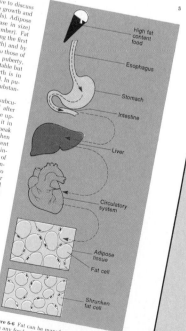

High fat content food

Esophagus

Stomach

Intestine

Liver

Circulatory system

Adipose tissue

Fat cell

Shrunken fat cell

Figure 6-6 Fat can be manufactured in the body from any food when intake exceeds need. Fat droplets travel to the liver from the stomach and intestines and then enter the circulatory where they are delivered to the cells and organs. When more energy is stored in adipose tissue. Excess fats are needed, fats are released from adipose cells. If the energy needs continue, the cells will shrink.

Assessment Activities conclude the chapters and contain inventories, activities, and exercises. These help you apply the chapter content to your personal lifestyle and your own decision-making.

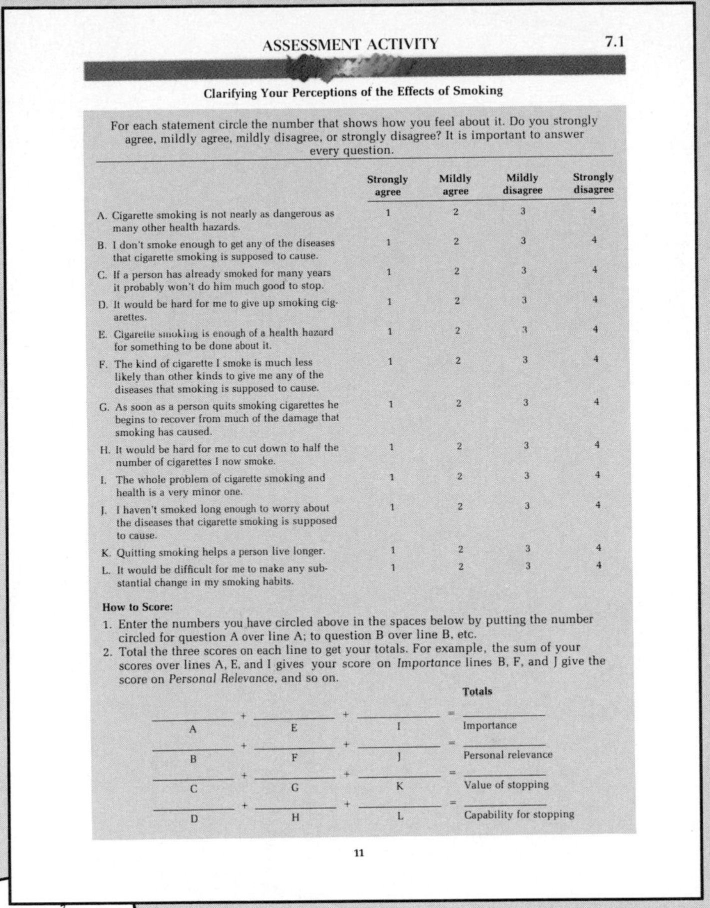

ASSESSMENT ACTIVITY   7.1

Clarifying Your Perceptions of the Effects of Smoking

For each statement circle the number that shows how you feel about it. Do you strongly agree, mildly agree, mildly disagree, or strongly disagree? It is important to answer every question.

	Strongly agree	Mildly agree	Mildly disagree	Strongly disagree
A. Cigarette smoking is not nearly as dangerous as many other health hazards.	1	2	3	4
B. I don't smoke enough to get any of the diseases that cigarette smoking is supposed to cause.	1	2	3	4
C. If a person has already smoked for many years it probably won't do him much good to stop.	1	2	3	4
D. It would be hard for me to give up smoking cigarettes.	1	2	3	4
E. Cigarette smoking is enough of a health hazard for something to be done about it.	1	2	3	4
F. The kind of cigarette I smoke is much less likely than other kinds to give me any of the diseases that smoking is supposed to cause.	1	2	3	4
G. As soon as a person quits smoking cigarettes he begins to recover from much of the damage that smoking has caused.	1	2	3	4
H. It would be hard for me to cut down to half the number of cigarettes I now smoke.	1	2	3	4
I. The whole problem of cigarette smoking and health is a very minor one.	1	2	3	4
J. I haven't smoked long enough to worry about the diseases that cigarette smoking is supposed to cause.	1	2	3	4
K. Quitting smoking helps a person live longer.	1	2	3	4
L. It would be difficult for me to make any substantial change in my smoking habits.	1	2	3	4

How to Score:
1. Enter the numbers you have circled above in the spaces below by putting the number circled for question A over line A; to question B over line B, etc.
2. Total the three scores on each line to get your totals. For example, the sum of your scores over lines A, E, and I gives your score on *Importance* lines B, F, and J give the score on *Personal Relevance*, and so on.

Totals

___A___ + ___E___ + ___I___ = _____			Importance
___B___ + ___F___ + ___J___ = _____			Personal relevance
___C___ + ___G___ + ___K___ = _____			Value of stopping
___D___ + ___H___ + ___L___ = _____			Capability for stopping

11

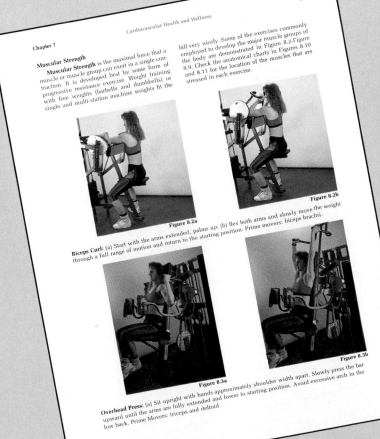

Cardiovascular Health and Wellness

Muscular Strength

Muscular Strength is the maximal force that a muscle or muscle group can exert in a single contraction. It is developed best by some form of progressive resistance exercise. Weight training with free weights (barbells and dumbbells) or single and multi-station machine weights fit the bill very nicely. Some of the exercises commonly employed to develop the major muscle groups of the body are demonstrated in Figure 8.2-Figure 8.9. Check the anatomical charts in Figures 8.10 and 8.11 for the location of the muscles that are stressed in each exercise.

Figure 8.2b

Figure 8.2a

Biceps Curl: (a) Start with the arms extended, palms up: (b) flex both arms and slowly move the weight through a full range of motion and return to the starting position. Prime movers: biceps brachii.

Figure 8.3b

Figure 8.3a

Overhead Press: (a) Sit upright with hands approximately shoulder width apart. Slowly press the bar upward until the arms are fully extended and lower to starting position. Avoid excessive arch in the low back. Prime Movers: triceps and deltoid.

An abundant use of instructional full-color photographs are included.

The chapters include *Action Plans for Personal Wellness* that enable you to determine an action plan to enhance your lifestyle.

These provide an ideal review for studying for exams.
The chapters end with a list of summary points that include the major points of the chapter.

Review questions quiz you on your understanding of chapter content and help you in test preparation.

Detailed references identify research used in preparing each chapter. The research cited is from the latest available publications.

Additional annotated readings are provided to obtain further information about specific topics.

Wellness

8

Action plan for personal wellness

An important consideration in assuming responsibility for one's own quality of life is utilizing information. After reading this chapter, answer the following questions and determine an action plan for enhancing your own lifestyle.

1 Based on the information presented in this chapter, along with what I know about my family's health history, the health problems/issues that I need to be most concerned about are:

2 Of those health concerns listed in #1, the one I most need to act on is:

3 The possible actions that I can take to improve my level of wellness are (try to be as specific as possible):

4 Of those actions listed in #3, the one that I most need to include in an action plan is:

Summary

■ People use drugs for a variety of reasons including recreational/social, sensation seeking, religious/spiritual, to achieve altered states, as a sign of rebellion and alienation, or as a result of peer pressure. Usage usually involves a combination of reasons.
■ Caffeine is probably the most used drug in America. It is a stimulant that speeds heart rate, increases blood pressure, and can cause insomnia.
■ Nicotine is an addictive agent found in tobacco. The tars found in tobaccos are carcinogenic agents.
■ Cocaine use has become epidemic in the US. Cocaine can be snorted, injected, or freebased (smoked).
■ Chlamydia is a bacteria and the most common STD in the U.S. Untreated, it can cause arthritis, damage the heart and blood vessels, and sterility. Pelvic inflammatory disease (PID) may result in ectopic pregnancies. Treatment is available.
■ Herpes is caused by the herpes simplex virus. In humans, lesions are usually located either around the mouth or the genital area. Herpes does not go away, but remains dormant in the human body and can recur at any time. While men do not experience major long-term complications, women may develop cancer of the cervix or infect newborns during the birth process. There is no cure for herpes.

■ Viral hepatitis is an injury to the liver. Hepatitis has several types of viruses associated with it.
■ The second leading STD is gonorrhea. Gonorrhea can lead to sterility in males and females and PID in women. Symptoms are often unnoticed by women but can cause serious problems if untreated. While there is no immunity developed to the disease, treatment is available.
■ Syphilis is caused by bacteria. There are four stages of syphilis and the full effects may not be experienced for 10 to 20 years after infection occurs.
■ AIDS is the result of the human immunodeficiency virus (HIV) that attacks the immune system. AIDS can be transmitted if an individual has symptoms or not. Deadly diseases associated with AIDS are Pneumocystis carinii pneumonia and Kaposi's sarcoma.
■ AIDS is only spread through intimate sexual contact, the sharing of needles, or from mother to child. There is no cure for AIDS and over 50% of the cases diagnosed since 1981 have died.
■ The only positive way to prevent acquiring a STD is through abstinence or monogamy. Use of condoms is associated with decreased risk when there are a number of sexual partners.

Chapter 7   *Cardiovascular Health and Wellness*

Review Questions

9

1. List reasons why people might choose to use drugs.
2. List and define the five classifications of drugs.
3. Discuss the risks associated with smoking and list the steps when attempting to quit.
4. Discuss why cocaine and its derivatives represent an extreme danger to anyone using the drug.
5. How can people accept responsibility for their sexual behavior?
6. Why does chlamydia represent a serious problem?

7. Discuss why HPV is more dangerous for females than for males.
8. What are the various kinds of viral hepatitis and how are they spread?
9. List and explain the 4 stages of syphilis.
10. What are precautions that can be taken to protect against the spread of AIDS?
11. Why, if one STD is present, may it be necessary to get treatment for more than one disease?

References

1. Schlaadt, R.G., and Shannon, P.T., Drugs of Choice: Current Perspectives on Drug Use. Englewood Cliffs: Prentice Hall, 1986.
2. Mermelstein, N.H. Caffeine, Contemporary Nutrition, 9:1-2, 1984.
3. Carroll, C.R. Drugs in Modern Society. Dubuque, Iowa, 2nd edition: Wm. C. Brown, 1989.
4. LeMonick, M. Should women drink less?, Time, May, 1987, 129:6, P. 66.
5. Witters, W.L., and Venturelli, P.J. Drugs and Society. Boston, MA: Jones and Bartlett, 1988.
6. Waldinger, R.J. Fundamentals of Psychiatry. Washington D.C.: American Psychiatric Press, 1986.
7. Felding, J.E. Smoking: Health Effects and Control. Professional Education Publication, New York: American Cancer Society, 1986.
8. The Health Consequences of Involuntary Smoking: A Report of the Surgeon General. Department of Health and Human Services, DHHS (CDC), Washington, D.C.: U.S. Government Printing Office, 1986.
9. Smoking Cessation-here's how to stop, The Mayo Clinic Health Letter, August, 1987. p. 2-3.
10. Nicotine addiction, The Mayo Clinic Health Letter, March, 1989, p. 6.
11. Hour by hour crack, Newsweek. November 1988, p. 64-75.
12. Morganthau, T., Crack and crime, Newsweek, June, 1986, p. 78.
13. Wilbur, R., Drugs that fight coke, American Health, 6%, p. 44-47, 1987.

14. Witters, W. and Venturelli, P. Drugs and Society. Boston: Jones and Bartlett Publishers, 1988.
15. Mann, Peggy. Marijuana Alert. New York. McGraw-Hill Book Company, 1985.
16. Gerald, M. Pharmacology: An Introduction to Drugs, Englewood Cliffs, N.Y.: Prentice Hall 1981.
17. The Nightmare Drugs, A Medical Essay-Mayo Clinic Health Letter, November 1989.
18. Genital Warts and Cancer: The Health Letter, 32:8, P. 4. October 1988.
19. Symptoms of HPV Commonly Missed. The Commercial Appeal, August 20, 1989, p. 5E.
20. Chlamydia: Cloak and Dagger, Harvard Medical School Health Letter, 13:12, p. 7. October 1988.
21. Chlamydia Trachomatis Infection: Mortality and Morbidity Weekly Report, 33:805-807, 1985.
22. Braude, A.I., Davis, C.E. and Fierer, J., editors. Infectious Diseases and Medical Microbiology, ed. 2, Philadelphia: W.B. Saunders Co., 1986.
23. Crowly, L.V.: Introduction to Human Disease, ed. 2. Boston, 1988. Jones and Bartlett Publishers.
24. Haseltine, W.A. and Wong-Staal, F., The Molecular Biology of the AIDS Virus, Scientific American, 259:4, p. 52-64, October, 1988.
25. Yarber, W.L., AIDS: What Young Adults Should Know. Reston, VA: AAHPERD, 1987.

Annotated Readings

Gallup, George, Jr. and Gallup, Alec. AIDS-We worry about the wrong things. American Health, June, 1988, pp. 50-52.
A worldwide special report that seeks answers to what people know and the common fears concerning the AIDS epidemic.

Hall, Stephen, S.: Gadfly in the ointment, Hippocrates, September/October, 1988, p. 76-82.
A controversial article that discuss a molecular biologist's Peter Duesberg view that AIDS is NOT caused by the HIV virus. His views have generally won him the scorn of colleagues. Right or wrong, the articles point out how little is actually known about the disease.

Pekkanen, John: Confessions of doctors on drugs, Hippocrates, November/December, 1988, p. 92-94.
Doctors, nurses, and other health professionals abuse drugs. No one knows exactly how broad the problem is, but estimates are that up to 15% of all doctors will be dependent on alcohol or other mind-altering drugs.

Tierney, John: The nicorette generation, Hippocrates, May/June, 1989, p. 32-33.
A humorous look at the use of nicorette to break the smoking addiction.

Whelan, Elizabeth M.: To your health, Across the Board, January, 1988, p. 49-53.
Moderate drinking may aid in prolonging life. Determining the right amount and if the statistics really apply to each person is unknown at this time.

Brief Contents

Detailed Contents

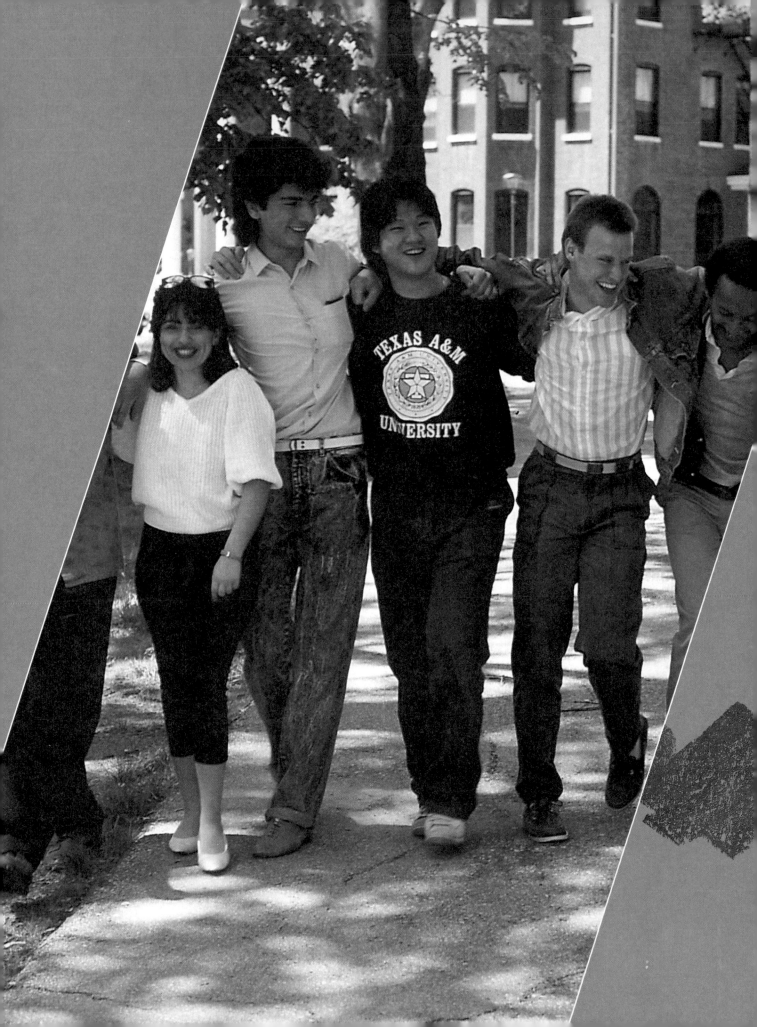

Chapter 1

An Introduction to Health and Wellness

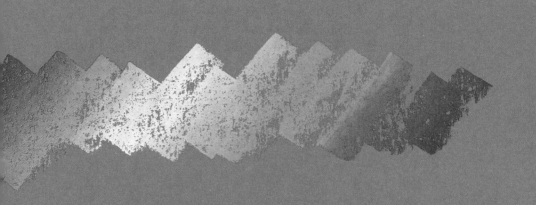

Objectives

After completing this chapter you will be able to:

▌ Define health and wellness
▌ Discuss the components of wellness
▌ List the factors that contribute to wellness behavior
▌ Describe the concepts associated with making wellness decisions

Today the five leading causes of death in the United States are cardiovascular disease, cancer, cerebrovascular disease, accidents, and chronic obstructive pulmonary disease. These five conditions accounted for 76% of the total number of deaths in the United States in 1988.[1] All of these conditions or occurrences illustrate the dangers associated with making negative lifestyle choices. Traditionally, if an individual displayed no disease symptoms, that individual was considered "healthy." A departure from this concept first came in the 1940s, when the World Health Organization (WHO) proposed that health was "a state of physical, mental, and social well-being and not merely the absence of disease or infirmity."[2] Though this definition was an expansion of previous concepts, it still viewed health as a primarily static condition and continued to limit the human potential to affect health.

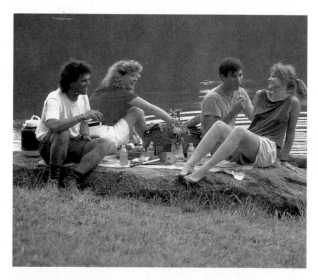

There are many activities that enhance the quality of life.

A more current and possibly better definition of **health** is "a continuous balancing of the physical, emotional, social, intellectual, and spiritual components of an individual in such a fashion as to produce happiness and a higher quality of existence." This definition of health indicates that health is not static and that the potential for change is always present. In fact, health moves along a continuum from optimal health to premature death (Figure 1-1). An individual's position on this continuum is subject to change at any time and is affected by many factors, including physical health, activity level, nutritional patterns, personal demands, career goals, time of year, and effectiveness in managing stress.

Implicit in Figure 1-1 is the idea that the direction an individual moves on the continuum is largely determined by the activities he or she pursues and the individual's attitudes toward these activities. These activities/behaviors and attitudes can prevent illness and promote health, or they can diminish or destroy peace of mind and physical well-being. Because individual behaviors are intrinsic to health, people must learn to assume responsibility for their health by developing the skills necessary to improve it.

Wellness means engaging in attitudes and behaviors that enhance quality of life and maximize personal potential. Although the concept of wellness implies working toward a highly developed level of health, it does not mean that an individual will make the best choice in every situation or even that "perfect wellness" is achievable. Wellness emphasizes the need to take responsibility for engaging in behaviors that develop optimal health. Health is affected by human behavior, and the responsibility for engaging in health-promoting behavior rests with each individual. Everyone can participate in behaviors that promote disease prevention and well-being and that

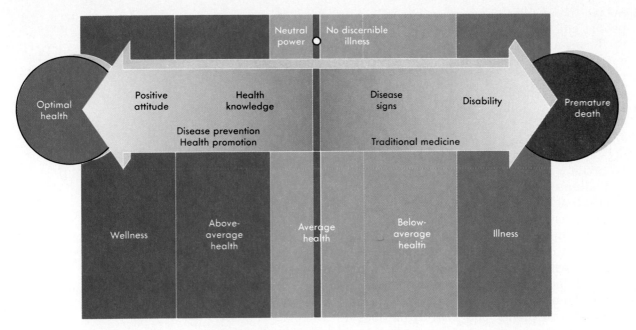

Figure 1-1 The health continuum.

help the individual look and feel better. The dynamic, ongoing process of wellness requires daily decision-making in the areas of nutrition, stress management, physical fitness, preventive health care, emotional health, and other aspects of health.

Traditional medicine has approached health from a different perspective. It has neither encouraged participation in activities that educate people about or protect them from chronic conditions or lifestyle diseases nor reduced the incidence of these diseases. Instead, it has attempted to repair damage after it has been done without eliminating its causes. **Health promotion** is the art and science of helping people change their lifestyle and thereby move toward a higher state of wellness.[3] Wellness is the goal that requires individuals to work to prevent, delay, or diminish the effects of chronic or disabling conditions. Each person can choose to develop a sound diet, a sufficient exercise program, methods of managing stress, and a regular schedule of medical check-ups and to reduce or eliminate the use of drugs, tobacco, and alcohol. The rest of this text will provide information and suggest health-promoting activities to help people accept the personal challenge of wellness.

Components of Wellness

Achieving a high level of wellness requires the individual to constantly balance and main-

tain the following components (Figure 1-2). Within each component are factors that must be dealt with if optimal health is to be enjoyed.

▋ **Spiritual:** the belief in some force that serves to unite human beings. This force can include nature, science, religion, or a higher power. It also includes a person's own morals, values, and ethics. Everyone has a personal perception of spirituality. It is the spiritual component that provides meaning and direction in life and enables each person to grow, learn, and meet new challenges. Optimal spirituality is a person's ability to discover, articulate, and act on his or her basic purpose in life.[4]

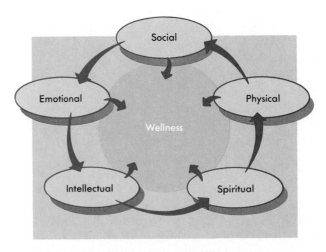

Figure 1-2 The dimensions of wellness.

- **Social:** the ability to interact successfully with people and within the environment of which each person is a part. It is the ability to develop and maintain intimacy with specific others and respect and tolerance for those with different opinions and beliefs.
- **Emotional:** the ability to control stress and to express emotions appropriately and comfortably. Emotional health is the ability to recognize and accept feelings and express them appropriately and not to be defeated by setbacks and failures.
- **Intellectual:** the ability to learn and use information effectively for personal, family, and career development. Intellectual wellness means striving for continued growth and being able to learn to deal with new challenges effectively.
- **Physical:** the ability to carry out daily tasks, develop cardiovascular fitness, maintain adequate nutrition and proper body fat, avoid abusing drugs and alcohol or using tobacco products, and generally invest in positive lifestyle habits.

Personal environment, though not a direct component of wellness, does influence quality of life. The five primary components of wellness can be enhanced or diminished according to a person's immediate environment. For example, people who know that when they are in their own homes, they are subject to physical or verbal abuse need their energy to protect themselves—energy that could otherwise be used to develop a wellness lifestyle. Although environment can have a negative effect on wellness in cases like this, personal environment can also contribute to total wellness. People who feel loved and cared for at home can direct this energy into developing themselves to their highest potential. For a person to achieve his or her highest potential, the individual must feel safe and at ease. Personal environment includes everything that a person learns and/or perceives. Only genetic factors are excluded from personal environment.

Obviously, each of the five components of wellness overlap to a certain extent, and factors in one component often directly affect the factors in another. Some of the factors in each component are under the individual's direct control, and some are not. For example, it has been reported that 53% of the factors influencing quality of life can be influenced by the lifestyle of the individual (Figure 1-3). Of the factors affecting quality of life, 10% are environmental, meaning they involve relationships and interaction with family, friends, and the community, and 16% are affected by the physicians and health-care facili-

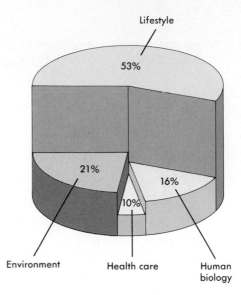

Figure 1-3 Influences on determining quality of life.

ties that are available.[5]

Hypothetically 21% of the factors affecting health are beyond the individual's control. This 21% consists of the genes and hereditary tendencies received from the parents. However, it is important to remember that if medical history indicates a family predisposition toward a particular disease, such as heart disease, the health decisions that an individual makes can affect the course of the disease, delay the onset, minimize the effects, or possibly prevent the disease from developing at all.

For example, the effects of a genetic predisposition to heart disease can be minimized significantly if the individual chooses to exercise, to follow proper nutrition guidelines, and not to smoke. It is not always possible to prevent disease from occurring, but the choices a person makes do affect health and quality of life.

Wellness involves working on all aspects of the model, not emphasizing only one or two areas. If the more obvious issues are handled in a positive manner, less overt issues also will be handled in a healthier manner. For example, learning to control daily stress levels from a physiological perspective helps to maintain the emotional stamina needed to handle a crisis situation.

Several lifestyle habits have been associated with good health and longevity[6]:
1. Sleeping 7 to 8 hours a night
2. Eating breakfast regularly
3. Never or rarely eating between meals
4. Staying at or near the ideal weight for an individual's height

5. Never smoking
6. Using alcohol moderately or not using alcohol at all
7. Exercising regularly

The preceding list is far from all-inclusive; for example, medical services, physical environment, and social interactions include many factors that also affect quality of life, but everyday activities form the basis for the other decisions an individual makes. The greater the effort and the more extensively wellness activities are engaged in (unless obsessive behaviors begin to occur), the more positive are the results.

There are no guarantees, but it is known that the chance of premature death can be reduced significantly by following a wellness lifestyle. For example, deaths associated with heart disease have been reduced by 30% in the last 15 years. This decline has been attributed directly to the reduction of smoking among men, decreased intake of dietary fat, increased exercise, and control of body weight. All of these adjustments represent the incorporation of healthy lifestyle changes.[7]

Why Wellness?

Assuming responsibility for a person's own health requires forethought and effort. *Why* should a person undertake this effort? First, a look at the 10 leading causes of death readily reveals that the big killers are lifestyle-related diseases (Table 1-1). People in the United States have become victims of high-fat, high-salt, high-sugar, low-fiber diets. This situation has been complicated by stress, lack of exercise, smoking, and use of alcohol and drugs. Among younger Americans accidents remain the leading killer. Particularly disturbing about this fact is that so many of the accidents are alcohol and drug related. Clearly the decisions that people make affect the chances of an accident or even death occurring.

The number one killer for men and women remains heart disease. The American Heart Association (AHA) reports that more than 1.5 million people suffer heart attacks each year. More than 500,000 of these people die. In approximately half of these cases, the first evidence of heart disease is the heart attack. About half of the people who die from heart disease are men in the most productive years of their lives—ages 40 to 65. Another 5% of heart attacks occur in people under 40. The American Heart Association estimates that $700 million is spent each year replac-

TABLE 1-1 Estimated number of deaths from the 15 leading causes

1. Heart disease	767,400
2. Cancer	488,240
3. Cerebrovascular diseases	150,300
4. Accidents	97,500
5. Chronic obstructive lung disease	81,960
6. Pneumonia and influenza	77,330
7. Diabetes mellitus	39,610
8. Suicide	30,260
9. Chronic liver disease, such as cirrhosis	26,080
10. Atherosclerosis	23,700
11. Homicide	22,190
12. Nephritis (inflammation of the kidneys)	21,890
13. Septicemia (pathogenic bacteria in the blood)	20,850
14. Conditions originating in the perinatal period	18,510
15. Infection with the human immunodeficiency virus	16,210

ing employees who have suffered heart attacks. Furthermore, the total annual cost of cardiovascular disease is projected to be $88.2 billion in 1989.[8]

The AHA reports that 66 million Americans have some form of cardiovascular disease. Strokes afflict 500,000 Americans, and more than 60 million adults suffer from hypertension.[9] It is important to note that many of the risk factors for cardiovascular disease are reversible (see Chapter 5) and can be changed through positive wellness activities.

The second leading cause of death in the United States is cancer, a disease that knows no age limits. Cancer is responsible for the death of more children, ages 3 to 14, than any other disease. It has been estimated that in 1988 more than 985,000 people were diagnosed as having cancer and that approximately 494,000 people died from the disease. This figure represents a death every 64 seconds from cancer or one out of every five deaths in the United States. Medical costs for cancer were estimated to be $71.5 billion in 1985.[10] Once again the lifestyle choices of avoiding tobacco products, following a low-fat diet, increasing intake of foods high in vitamin A (such as yellow and green vegetables), preventing obesity, eating a high-fiber diet, avoiding salt-cured or nitrate-cured foods, and keeping alcohol consumption to a moderate level provide excellent protection against cancer. Another important

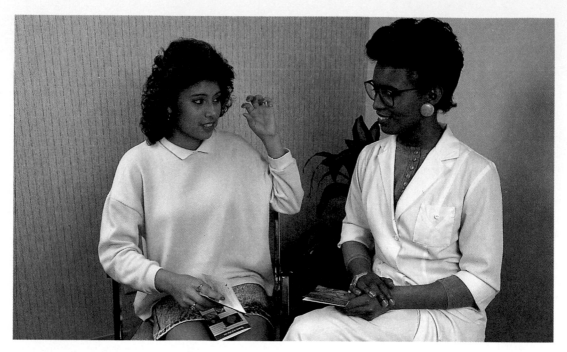

Wise use of medical services available is one aspect of accepting responsibility for health.

factor in prevention is doing self-screening examinations. For men self-examination of the testicles is important. Women need to self-examine their breasts and at age 35 have a baseline mammogram (an x-ray that can identify cancers too small to be felt).

Aside from the risk of disease, it is estimated that 15% of the Gross National Product (GNP) will be spent on health care by the early 1990s.[11] These costs reflect lost productivity and an increase in the cost of doing business, which is passed on to the consumer. The overall annual cost of health care in the United States has skyrocketed from $50 billion to $500 billion in the last 20 years. In some states the cost of insurance for a family of four has risen by 400% since 1980.[12]

In an attempt to contain costs, some businesses have stopped hiring smokers or overweight individuals. Businesses and corporations have begun to offer health-promotion programs in nutrition education, weight management, stress reduction, and exercise.[12] These measures also represent business and corporate attempts to help employees reach their potential while cutting health-care costs.

Engaging in activities that enhance quality of life is a priority for the United States. Since 1987 the Public Health Service of the Department of Health and Human Services has lead an effort to formulate the national disease-prevention and health-promotion objectives for the year 2000. These objectives are still being developed, but several objectives intended to increase the quality of life of the nation's people are included. Figure 1-4 contains a list of these proposed objectives.[13]

Benefits of High-level Wellness

Many people diminish the quality of their lives without realizing it. They may "do death" (become involved in activities that contribute directly to decreased lifespan or quality of life) by abusing drugs and/or alcohol or by feeling so badly about themselves that they allow others to treat them abusively. "Doing death" includes any form of action or inaction that diminishes an individual's function as a human being. Wellness is a looking toward life; it is the opposite of "doing death."

Since wellness is a daily striving toward being the best that a person is capable of being, it demands commitment and involves regular exercise, proper nutrition, maintenance of optimal body composition, awareness of personal needs

Figure 1-4: Proposed health objectives for the United States for the year 2000

The following objectives are intended to improve the quality of life for all Americans:

- Increase to at least 60% the proportion of people age 6 and older who participate in moderate physical activities three or more days per week for 20 or more minutes per session
- Increase to at least 30% the proportion of people age 6 and older who participate in vigorous physical activities that promote the development and maintenance of cardiorespiratory fitness three or more days per week for 20 or more minutes per session
- Increase to at least 50% the proportion of people age 6 and older who regularly perform physical activities that maintain muscular strength, muscular endurance, and flexibility
- Reduce overweight among people ages 20 to 74 to a prevalence of less than 20%
- Reduce overweight among adolescents (ages 12 to 17) to a prevalence of less than 15%
- Increase to at least 75% the proportion of overweight people age 12 and older who have adopted sound dietary practices combined with physical activity to achieve weight reduction
- Increase to at least 80% the proportion of people age 6 and older who know that regular exercise reduces the risk of heart disease, helps maintain appropriate body weight, reduces the symptoms of depression and anxiety, and enhances self-esteem
- Increase to at least 25% the proportion of people age 6 and older who can identify correctly the frequency and duration of exercise thought to promote cardiorespiratory fitness most effectively
- Increase to at least 65% the proportion of primary-care providers who assess and counsel their patients on the frequency, duration, type, and intensity of each patient's physical activity as part of a thorough evaluation and treatment program
- Increase to at least 45% the proportion of children and adolescents in grades 1 through 12 who participate in daily physical-education programs in school
- Increase to at least 70% the proportion of physical education teachers who spend 30% or more of class time on skills and activities that promote lifetime participation in physical activity
- Increase the proportion of companies offering employer-sponsored fitness programs as follows:
  Companies with 50 to 99 employees: 25%
  Companies with 100 to 249 employees: 35%
  Companies with 250 to 749 employees: 45%
  Companies with 750 or more employees: 65%
- Increase to at least 40% the proportion of people age 6 and older who participated in the physical-activity programs of at least one community organization within the past year
- Increase the number of community swimming pools, hiking, biking, and fitness-trail miles, and park and recreation open-space acres to at least one pool per 25,000 people, one trail mile per 10,000 people, and four acres of developed open space per 1,000 people (or one managed acre per 250 people)
- Increase to at least 30% the proportion of life insurers that offer lower individual premiums to people who exercise regularly and maintain a physically active lifestyle

and effort to fulfill these needs in a positive manner, and overall healthy behavior. Superficially, living a wellness lifestyle appears difficult. In fact, not living a wellness lifestyle is more difficult because it results in more illness, depression, premature death, decreased quality of life, diminished sense of fulfillment, and diminished satisfaction with life. But wellness improves each of the above situations. In addition, it improves how a person looks and feels while on the jour-

ney toward wellness. Wellness can be beneficial in the following areas:

- Improved cardiovascular system
- Increased muscle tone, strength, flexibility, and endurance, resulting in improved physical appearance
- Decreased risk of developing or dying from chronic diseases and accidents
- Decreased recovery time after injury, illness, and childbirth

■ Regulation and improvement of overall body function
■ Increased ability to emphasize the positive
■ Increased ability to cope with stress and resist depression
■ Increased energy level and job productivity and decreased absenteeism
■ Delay of the aging process
■ Improved awareness of personal needs and how to meet them
■ Increased ability to communicate emotions to others and to act assertively rather than aggressively or passively
■ Supplying the body with proper nutrition
■ Expansion and development of intellectual abilities from a cognitive base and application of these abilities to their fullest extent in society
■ Acting from an internal locus of control
■ Learning to view life's difficulties as challenges and opportunities rather than overwhelming threats
■ Development of the self-confidence and ability to reach out to, understand, and care about others

Although attempting to lead a wellness lifestyle does not guarantee a "happily-ever-after" existence, it helps provide the tools for a *happier* ever after. The biggest payoff of wellness may be the attitude that helps each person to see life's possibilities and work toward the ones that are the most personally fulfilling.

Accepting the Challenge to Strive for Wellness

The key to accepting the challenge to strive for high-level wellness is motivation. No single principle or incident can provide the stimulus necessary to institute change and maintain positive lifestyle habits. When people perceive themselves as healthy, their motivation for changing lifestyle may not be very high. The stimuli for change increase when people perceive in their lives some impetus for change, such as being overweight, tiring too easily, or smoking too much. Any number of needs, motives, or fears may affect decision making at any one time. Fear may be a powerful motivator. A man who has suffered a heart attack may be highly motivated to stop smoking, start exercising, and change his eating habits, but a heart attack may not affect another person at all. Fear may even prevent some people from seeking information or checkups

necessary for minimal health. A woman who discovers a lump in her breast may become too paralyzed by fear to seek medical attention.

To make beneficial changes, people need to understand the many influences that create individual behavior. Certainly the *family* initiates a person's initial health habits and outlooks. Children don't begin to brush their teeth because of a concern for dental care but because their parents insist on it. *Social pressure* becomes increasingly important as children age. All people are influenced by the desire and need to belong or to act like someone they admire. Adolescents and teenagers are especially susceptible to wanting to "fit in," sometimes in a way that harms their health. For example, a friend or family member who smokes may influence a youngster's decision to begin to smoke.

A significant contribution to acceptance of the challenge of wellness is the knowledge and attitudes that are assimilated during a lifetime. If people are to change their health habits, information must be internalized and considered valuable. Unfortunately knowledge alone is not enough to bring about change. People know that they should wear their seat belts or that they should not smoke, yet they don't buckle up and continue to use tobacco products. For change to occur, the person's belief system must be affected.

By definition an *attitude* is a predisposition for action; that is, what people believe and value as having importance is what they are most likely to pursue. It is important to build a sound and accurate knowledge base, but information must also be weighed in relation to the following factors:

1. Based on the information, is the person at risk for negative lifestyle consequences?
2. How high a risk exists if a decision is made NOT to institute change?
3. If a lifestyle change is made, what are the benefits or advantages?

By personalizing information, people are motivated by what they value. For some people, motivation comes in the form of attitudes (values) concerning the desire to look better, feel better, or be more self-reliant. The more highly a health benefit is valued, the greater the chance of making and adhering to the change. Support in the form of compliments from friends and family certainly helps to provide motivation and reinforcement. However, if the challenge of wellness is to be accepted for a lifetime, eventually changes

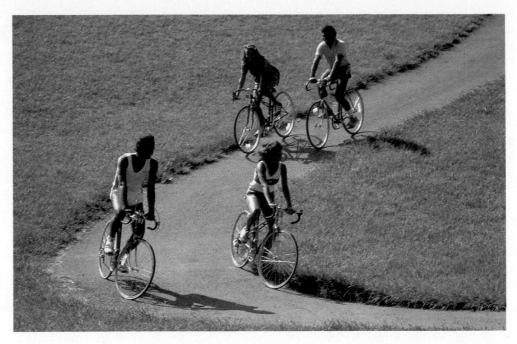

Lifestyles and beliefs are influenced by a variety of factors.

must be made based on an internalized desire to make that difference. Beginning an exercise program is a noble undertaking, but doing it because a friend wants to almost certainly dooms the effort to failure. The ability to achieve any health change must result from a personal, ongoing, and ultimately permanent goal and not from a desire to please or impress another person. If people engage in wellness activities because the activities are important to *them*, the wellness challenge has been accepted.

Concepts Influencing Acceptance of the Wellness Challenge

To be successful in the quest for improved quality of life, it is important to understand the concept of **locus of control.** An individual's locus of control may be either internal or external. When people view problems concerning their health or any other part of their lives as generally "out of their control"; that is, they view themselves as being at the mercy of other people, places, and events, they are said to have an *external locus of control*. On the other hand, people who view their own behaviors as having a major effect on the course of their lives and certainly on their health, people who feel that they are at least

partially the "masters of their fate" and recognize that they can change the course of their health, are said to have an *internal locus of control*. To increase success in wellness activities, people who have an internal locus of control are more likely to assume the necessary responsibility.

Another vital concept in a wellness lifestyle is **self-efficacy.**[14,15] Self-efficacy refers to people's belief in their ability to accomplish a specific task or behavior. This theory suggests that people's belief in their ability to perform specific behaviors influences all of the following:

1. Their choice of behavior and the situations that will be avoided or attempted, such as attempts to reduce use of drugs, alcohol, or cigarettes, to initiate an exercise regimen, or to practice relaxation.
2. The effort they will expend participating in a specific task. Often, more energy is devoted to a task, such as brushing and flossing teeth, when the individual perceives that it will be successful.
3. How long a person will persist with a task, such as maintaining an exercise program, even when facing difficulties.
4. Emotional reactions, such as anxiety. Negative emotions may be aroused when an individual is confronted with the threat of failure.[16]

There are four ways in which people define their ability to succeed at various tasks:

1. By actually performing or accomplishing the task
2. By seeing others perform or accomplish the task without adverse effects
3. Through verbal persuasion
4. Through stressful or taxing experiences or circumstances that arouse the emotions

Information from one or all of these sources must be interpreted and internalized by each person before the sources will affect efficacy expectations.

A strong sense of efficacy for behaving in a healthy fashion is central to self-regulation of a person's life.[17] If high-level wellness is to be achieved, the individual must see himself as successful and believe that he can accomplish a task. Just as locus of control helps determine mind-set, self-efficacy establishes behavior leading toward achievement of high-level wellness. Self-efficacy is the link between knowing what to do and actually accomplishing the task.

Wellness—Your Decision

Individuals must choose among many different lifestyles. Some of these lifestyle choices will help to develop and maintain optimal wellness, but some will not. Wellness is not a moral issue. It is a matter of intelligent decision making. Decisions should be based on the most reliable and comprehensive information available on the effects of behavior on health and lifestyle.

The younger an individual is, the less apparent are the effects of lifestyle. However, as people age, lifestyle habits and patterns affect and alter the body, and physical, spiritual, emotional, social, and intellectual capabilities are shaped and molded accordingly. The effects of lifestyle on wellness are cumulative. Every day of every year, the behaviors people engage in determine the form, composition, and functional capabilities of their bodies and minds. Living a wellness lifestyle can help retain or even improve the appearance, vitality, and fitness of youth. Wellness can be a way of life for anyone who chooses it. This decision is yours.

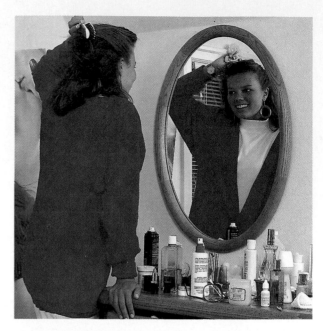

The ultimate decision on lifestyle depends upon the individual.

Appraising An Individual's Own Wellness

One method of assessing the current status of individual health is a questionnaire called a Lifestyle Inventory (LI). Such an assessment is included in Appendix A. The LI should be viewed as an indication of where to begin to make lifestyle changes. The individual should keep in mind that lifestyle change is a gradual process that continually evolves throughout a person's lifetime. It is not an overnight, magical solution that happens without work or effort. The LI also should not be viewed as a rigid diagnostic instrument that mandates particular solutions to each problem. It is a guide to help isolate problem areas that can then be targeted gradually for change.

After the assessment has been taken and scored, it is time to examine the aspects of life that are creating barriers to change (See Assessment Activity 1-1). The individual may need to consider increasing control over his own life to make positive changes.

Summary

▌ Health is a constantly changing state of being that moves along a continuum from optimal health to premature death and is affected by an individual's attitudes and activities.

▌ Wellness means to engage in activities and behaviors that enhance quality of life and maximize personal potential by consistent balancing of physical, emotional, spiritual, intellectual, and social health.

▌ Personal motivation is the only way a person will adopt and maintain a wellness lifestyle. This motivation can be affected by family members and social pressure.

▌ For change to occur, knowledge alone is insufficient. Attitudes and beliefs are the catalysts of behavior change because the more highly a health benefit is valued, the greater the chance of making a change and adhering to it.

▌ An external locus of control is a belief that the factors controlling people's lives are outside the people themselves, thus beyond their control. An internal locus of control is a belief in which the individual views himself as being in control.

▌ Self-efficacy refers to the beliefs people have in their ability to accomplish a specific task or behavior. These beliefs specifically affect ability to perform or achieve. A strong sense of self-efficacy is central to self-regulation of an individual's life.

 ## Action plan for personal wellness

An important consideration in assuming responsibility for the individual's own quality of life is using information. After reading this chapter and analyzing the various assessment activities, answer the following questions and determine an action plan for enhancing your own lifestyle.

1 Based on the information presented in this chapter and what I know about my family's health history, the health problems or issues that I need to be most concerned about are:_____

_____

_____

2 Of the health concerns listed in no. 1, the one I most need to act on is:_____

_____

_____

3 Possible actions that I can take to improve my level of wellness are (try to be as specific as possible):_____

_____

_____

4 Of the actions listed in no. 3, the one that I most need to include in an action plan is:_____

_____

_____

5 Factors I need to keep in mind to be successful in my action plan are:_____

_____

_____

Review Questions

1. What are the relationships between the components of wellness and personal health? (Define and explain them.)
2. What are some of the beneficial results of engaging in a wellness lifestyle? What is the key to accepting the challenge of such a lifestyle?
3. When changing behavior, information must be weighed in relation to what factors?
4. What is the difference between internal and external locus of control?
5. What is self-efficacy? What does it influence?
6. What are the ways in which people define their ability to succeed at a given task?

References

1. National Center for Health Statistics, US Public Health Service, Department of Health and Human Services, Washington, DC, 1987.
2. World Health Organization: Constitution of the World Health Organization, Chronicle of the World Health Organization 1:29-43, 1947.
3. O'Donnell MP: Definition of health promotion, Am J Health Prom, premier issue, 1(1):4-5, 1986.
4. Chapman LS: Developing a useful perspective on spiritual health: love, joy, peace and fulfillment, Am J Health Prom 2(22):12-17, fall 1987.
5. Murphy TA and Murphy D: The wellness for life workbook, ed 4, San Diego, 1987, Fitness Publications.
6. Breslow L and Enstrom JE: Persistence of health habits and their relationship to mortality, Prev Med 9:469-483, 1980.
7. Whelan EM: The truth about America's health, USA Today Magazine Society for the Advancement of Education 55-58, May 1987.
8. Heart facts: 1989, Dallas, 1989, American Heart Association.
9. Leiman TL, editor: Building a healthy America: conquering disease and disability, New York, 1987, Mary Ann Liebert Publishers.
10. Cancer facts and figures: 1988, New York, 1989, American Cancer Society.
11. Califano JA: America's health care revolution: who lives? who dies? who pays? New York, 1986, Random House, Inc.
12. Miller A: Can you afford to get sick? Newsweek, p 45-46, Jan 30, 1989.
13. US Department of Health and Human Services, Public Health Service: Promoting health/preventing disease, draft of year 2000 objectives for the nation, Washington, DC, 1989, The Department.
14. Koenig R: HMOs shed socialized image gaining acceptance on Wall Street, The Wall Street Journal, p 27, Aug 16, 1984.
15. Bandura A: Self-efficacy: toward a unifying theory of behavior change, Psychol Rev 84:191-215, 1977.
16. Lyn L and McLeroy KR: Self-efficacy and health education 56(2):317-321, Oct 1986.
17. Schunck DH and Carbonari JP: Self-efficacy models. In Malarazzo JD et al, editors: Behavioral health: a handbook of health enhancement and disease prevention, New York, 1984, 230-247, John Wiley & Sons, Inc.
18. Noland MP: The efficacy of a new model to explain leisure exercise behavior, doctoral dissertation, College Park, 1981, University of Maryland.
19. Greenberg JS: Comprehensive stress management, Dubuque, Iowa, 1987, 232-233, Wm C Brown Group.

Annotated Readings

Chapman LS: Developing a useful perspective on spiritual health: well-being, spiritual potential and the search for meaning, Am J Health Prom 31-39, winter 1987.
Spiritual health is one component of total wellness. The author defines spiritual wellness, reasons for less emphasis on spirituality in today's society, and a spiritual wellness inventory.

Flieger K: Why do we age? FDA Consumer 22(8):20-25, Oct 1988.
There are reasons why people grow old. This article discusses the hows and whys of aging as they are currently understood.

Folkenberg J: The mouth as the body's mirror, FDA Consumer, Dec 1989 to Jan 1990.
Surprisingly the mouth offers many clues to both the physical and the mental health of the individual.

Gurin J, editor: Doing better, feeling worse, Am Health 105-110, July/Aug 1988.
Dr. Arthur Barsky, a psychiatrist, states that while health in the United States has vastly improved in the last 20 years, people often perceive themselves as being less healthy than they actually are.

Perry P: Can this man beat the odds? Am Health 48-56, April 1987.
After suffering a heart attack, Bob Finnell began to adapt to a different lifestyle to improve his health. Suggestions for improving health that are applicable to everyone are provided.

Scott HD and Cabral RM: Predicting hazardous lifestyles among adolescents based on health-risk assessment data, Am J Health Prom 2(4):23-28, spring 1988.
Health-risk appraisals can be used as predictive instruments in the areas of health and emotional wellness.

Siegal BS: Love, medicine, and miracles, New York, 1986, Harper & Row, Publishers, Inc.
As a surgeon dealing with cancer patients, Dr. Siegal found many "exceptional" patients who often became survivors. These people frequently exhibit an internal locus of control and other positive attitudes.

Tierney, J: "Buying time," In Health (Formerly Hippocrates), January, February 1990, pp. 35-44.
Various individuals claim that they can keep people young. This article examines the claims that are made offering hope for the young and the maturing.

ASSESSMENT ACTIVITY   1-1

Barriers to Change

Most of us have changes we would like to make in our lives or things we say we would like to accomplish, but we have so many "reasons" why we cannot make the desired changes. When we say we are "too busy" or "too tired" or the change is "too difficult," we are making excuses. Another way to view excuses is as *barriers* to change.

Directions: Below is a rating scale that will help you to recognize the barriers you may find when you try to make a change. Decide on a health or lifestyle change you would like to make, and check it against each of the barriers listed by circling the appropriate rating. For example, you may want to start an exercise program. Is the cost of joining a spa or fitness club a major barrier to you in starting the program? If you circle 5, 6, or 7, you are encountering a major obstacle.

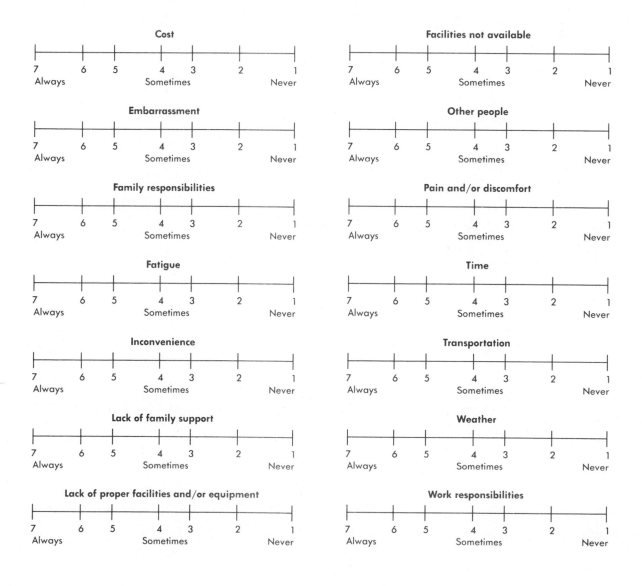

After completing the rating scale, review the barriers to the change(s) you want to make in your life that you have identified. What are some possible solutions or strategies for dealing with the barriers you identified?

Barrier   **Solution(s)**

_____   _____

                               _____

                               _____

                               _____

_____   _____

                               _____

                               _____

                               _____

_____   _____

                               _____

                               _____

_____   _____

                               _____

                               _____

                               _____

_____   _____

                               _____

                               _____

_____   _____

                               _____

                               _____

                               _____

Health Locus of Control

Locus of control is an important component of individual wellness. This activity will assist you in identifying your locus of control and your ability to affect your health. This rating scale is an adaptation of the Multidimensional Health Locus of Control Scales. The test is composed of three subscales:

1. The *Internal Health Locus of Control Scale (I)* measures whether you feel that you have control over your own health.
2. The *Powerful Others Health Locus of Control Scale (P)* measures whether you feel that powerful individuals, such as physicians or other health professionals, control your health.
3. The *Chance Health Locus of Control Scale (C)* measures whether you feel your health is due to luck, fate, or chance.

Directions: For each answer, choose a number from 1-5 that best describes your feelings.

5 = Strongly agree	2 = Disagree
4 = Agree	1 = Strongly disagree
3 = Neither agree nor disagree	

Internal health locus of control

_____ If I get sick, it is my own behavior that determines how soon I get well.
_____ I am in control of my health.
_____ When I get sick, I am to blame.
_____ If I take care of myself, I can avoid illness.
_____ If I take the right actions, I can stay healthy.

Powerful others health locus of control

_____ Having regular contact with my physician is the best way for me to avoid illness.
_____ Whenever I don't feel well, I should consult a medically trained professional.
_____ My family has a lot to do with my becoming sick or staying healthy.
_____ Health professionals control my health.
_____ When I recover from an illness, it's usually because other people such as doctors, nurses, family, and friends, have been taking good care of me.
_____ Regarding my health, I can only do what my doctor tells me to do.

Chance health locus of control

_____ No matter what I do, if I am going to get sick, I will get sick.
_____ Most things that affect my health happen to me accidentally.
_____ Luck plays a big part in determining how soon I will recover from an illness.
_____ My good health is largely a matter of good fortune.
_____ No matter what I do, I am likely to get sick.
_____ If it is meant to be, I will stay healthy.

To obtain your score for a subscale, add the numbers you chose in that subscale.

1. A score of 23 to 30 on any subscale means you have a strong inclination toward that particular dimension. For example, a high "C" score indicates you hold strong beliefs that your health is a matter of chance.
2. A score of 15 to 22 means you are moderate on that particular dimension. For example, a moderate "P" score indicates you have moderate belief that your health is due to powerful others.
3. A score of 6 to 14 means you are low on that particular dimension. For example, a low "I" score means you generally do not believe that you control your own health.

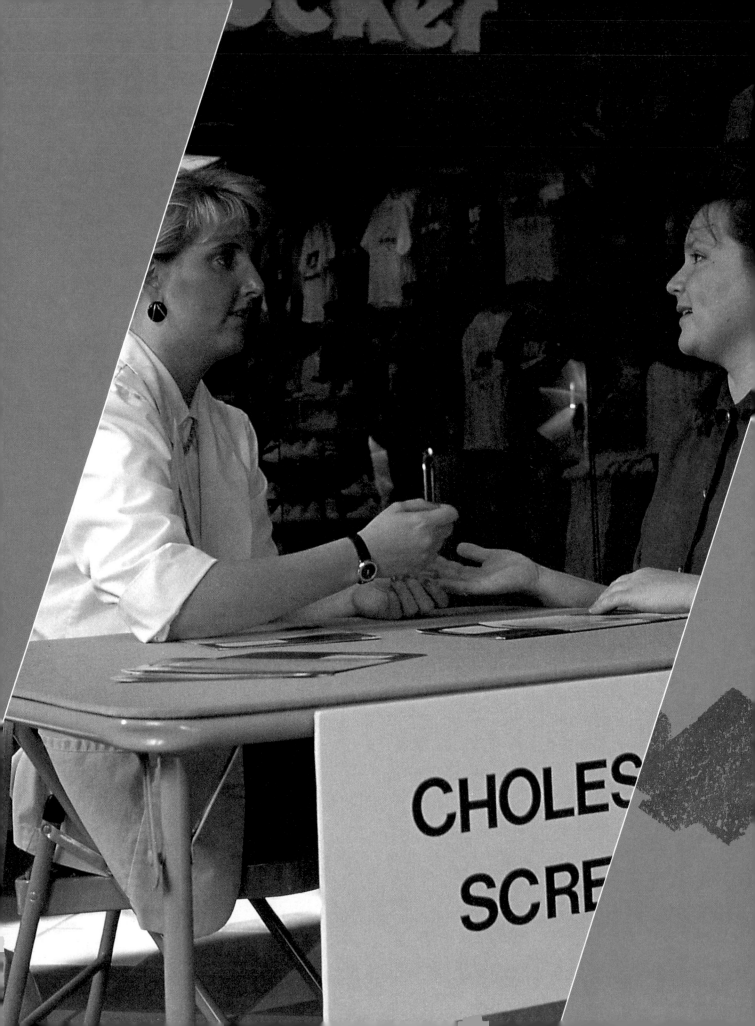

Chapter 2

Managing Lifestyle Change

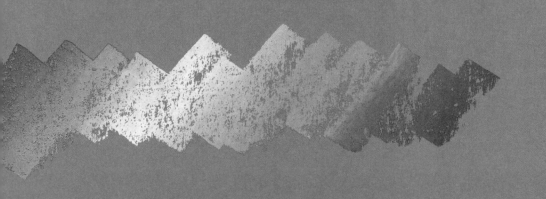

Key terms

behavior assessment

behavioral contract

health-behavior gap

health-promoting be-
haviors

preventive health
behaviors

self-help

Objectives

After completing this chapter, you will be able to:

❚ Discuss some of the underlying assumptions of lifestyle change

❚ Identify influences on behavior

❚ Explain the advantages and disadvantages of various approaches to lifestyle change

❚ Describe basic principles of lifestyle management

❚ Formulate a self-help plan for lifestyle change

Throughout Chapter 1 you read about specific areas of wellness over which you can exercise some control. Whether managing your diet, choosing health care products, coping with stress, or reducing the risk of developing chronic diseases, you have experienced many opportunities to improve both the quantity and the quality of your life. However, many of these opportunities are likely to require some change in lifestyle. In this chapter you will be asked to take an inventory of your health practices and to consider ways to change those practices that may be detrimental to your health.

Lifestyle Change: A Matter of Choice

Most Americans today know that they can exercise control over their lifestyle. Included in this belief is the idea that *morbidity,* the incidence of disease, and *mortality,* the incidence of death, are influenced substantially by the way we choose to live. According to a Gallup survey conducted for *American Health*[1] magazine, almost three fourths of the people polled believed that if they eat right, don't smoke, and get regular checkups, they have a good chance of preventing cancer. An even larger number, more than 80%, believed that they can significantly reduce their chances of having a heart attack by watching their weight and blood-fat level.

More than ever, people are putting these beliefs into action. Americans seem to be motivated by an unprecedented quest for improved health and well-being (Figure 2-1). This is especially true for older Americans, who are more likely than their younger peers to engage in **preventive health behaviors,** health practices that promote

wellness and prevent or reduce morbidity and/or mortality.

The trend toward healthy living and the added belief that people can be assertive in the health field are encouraging signs of a change in both attitudes and behaviors concerning health. Still, there is much room for improvement. A serious discrepancy remains between knowing what is good for health and doing it. Health professionals often refer to this discrepancy as the **health-behavior gap.** Americans are still far short of achieving the original 226 objectives established in the landmark 1979 publication *Healthy People: the Surgeon General's Report on Health Promotion and Disease Prevention.*[2] In a midcourse review of the progress made toward accomplishing these objectives, as many as 60 of the objectives, or more than 25%, had not been achieved by the 1990 target date.[3] Objectives related to weight control, illicit drug use, control of violent behavior, teenage pregnancy, and control of sexually transmitted diseases seem to be beyond reach. Furthermore, the health-behavior gap appears to be most serious for college-age students. In a recent study, comparisons of health behaviors by age groups led to the following conclusion: "While those aged 65 or more have the best overall records for practicing good health and safety behavior, change for the better is being led by those in the middle years. And we still have not found the way to motivate young adults to start good health behavior."[4] If the past turns out to be a good predictor of the future, there is good reason for concern, especially among college-age adults, about the extent to which new national health objectives (see Chapter 1) for the year 2000 will be attained.

Figure 2-1 Improvements in preventive health behaviors

According to a survey on preventive health behaviors conducted by Louis Harris and Associates, Americans showed improvement in several important areas:

▌ The proportion of adults who say they smoke cigarettes has fallen to 26%. This is the lowest smoking rate ever registered in a Harris survey measuring this trend. This smoking rate is 15% lower than it was in the 1970s.

▌ Five percent of adults admit they use recreational drugs. This rate represents a 4% decrease from 1984. The biggest drop in drug use is among young adults.

▌ The majority of people who have tried to lose weight have resorted to measures such as gaining more self-control (77%), cutting down on sugar (75%), and cutting down on red meat (67%).

▌ Many people have made progress in avoiding a high-cholesterol diet. Forty-eight percent of adults, up 6% from 1983 and 1987, say they "try a lot" to avoid eating too many high-cholesterol foods.

▌ The proportion of American adults who frequently walk for exercise has increased. Fifty-two percent say they had walked at least several times a week during the month before the survey.

Underlying Assumptions in Lifestyle Change

The following four assumptions can form a basis for appreciating the difficulty of successfully completing a lifestyle change:

▌ Lifestyle change is one of the most pervasive human endeavors.

▌ Health habits and practices are learned.

▌ Lifestyle habits and practices can be changed.

▌ A successful lifestyle-change program requires a plan.

Lifestyle change: A pervasive human endeavor. Perhaps the most obvious observation that can be made about people's lifestyles is that few if any of us are so satisfied with the way we manage our lives that we don't contemplate some sort of change at some point. Whether it is improving study habits, coping with loneliness, managing personal finances, dealing with test anxiety, or losing weight, many of us either spend an inordinate amount of time trying to alter some aspect of our health or waste time worrying about it. The fact that we usually fail does not diminish the fact that we try, sometimes over and over. Lifestyle change is so pervasive that for many people, making New Year's resolutions to change health practices has become as much of an American tradition as exchanging holiday gifts.

Health habits and practices: Learned behaviors. A fundamental assumption underlying lifestyle-change programs is that behavior is a learned response. For example, we are not born with a taste for some foods and a dislike for others. And using seat belts is not a function of heredity. Like most other behaviors, health behav-

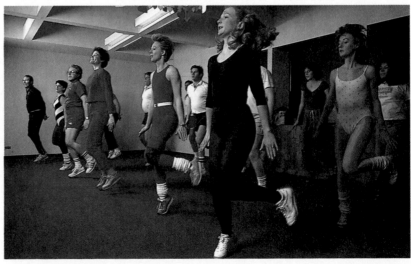

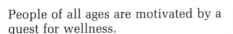
People of all ages are motivated by a quest for wellness.

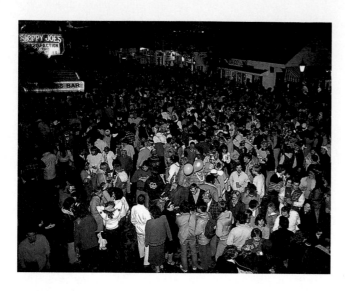

Making New Year's resolutions to change health practices is an American tradition.

iors are learned responses to both obvious and subtle stimuli. This learning begins the day we are born and continues throughout life. It is important to remember that this is just as true for behaviors that promote good health as for behaviors that diminish it.

Examples of direct stimuli that help to shape behavior include parents and family, role models, advertising, and social norms. In many instances these influences are combined to form a single powerful influence on behavior, such as an advertisement for cigarettes using "ideal" masculine and/or feminine models, depending on the brand of cigarettes and the target population. Advertisers are successful not only at marketing products but also at influencing people to think they need various products.

Subtle forces also shape behavior. A good example is *subliminal advertising*, a technique in which messages, words, and symbols are embedded or hidden in the pictures, sounds, or words used in advertisements. Theoretically these messages, though not directly observable, can be perceived by the subconscious mind in such a way as to influence behavior.

Much of our behavior is also motivated by psychological needs. An infant whose main source of attention and stimulation comes during feeding time may learn to associate food with the deeper psychological needs of love and affection. A parent who consistently uses food to appease an unhappy child may be inadvertently establishing a preoccupation with food that endures far beyond childhood.

The above examples help not only to explain the myriad complex forces that contribute to behavior but also to illustrate why successful lifestyle change is so difficult to achieve.

Lifestyle habits and practices: They can be changed. Although easier said than done, the hope and promise of any lifestyle-change program is that bad habits can be unlearned and new habits can be learned. However, to be successful it is helpful to understand three errors in thinking that are almost universal:

1. Lifestyle change is a temporary goal rather than a lifelong change. This belief is especially common for some behaviors, like losing weight. When they hold this belief, people often reach their goal, then revert to their original behaviors and subsequently find themselves right back where they started. Perhaps more than anything else, this attitude accounts for the high *recidivism* (the tendency to revert to the original behavior) rate of many programs. Recidivism is high for most lifestyle programs. The real test of a program's success is not so much how many people reach their goal as how many people successfully maintain that goal for at least 2 years. In other words, the lower the recidivism rate, the more successful the program.

2. All behaviors are equally difficult or easy to change. This attitude could be expressed in the following way: "If I can stop biting my fingernails, you should be able to stop smoking." It is incorrect to assume that all behaviors are equally changeable. For most people, using seat belts is not the same as controlling drug dependency.

Lifestyle changes vary considerably in complexity. The more complex a lifestyle change is, the more difficult it will be to change.

3. Lifestyle change requires only a good dose of willpower. This is an oversimplification of the truth; willpower does not work for most behaviors. Even the few behaviors, such as cigarette smoking and alcoholism, which can be treated using determination and willpower as preferred treatments, have been only partially successful. This observation has given rise to two recent innovative approaches, one in which people learn controlled drinking,[5] as opposed to *abstinence* (complete avoidance), and another in which people learn how to use willpower.[6] Although the success of these approaches has yet to stand the test of time, they do demonstrate the emergence of nontraditional thinking about age-old problems.

Planning: a prerequisite to success. Several approaches to behavior change are available. *Psychotherapy* is an approach in which patients try to identify innermost sources of conflict dating back to early childhood experiences. Theoretically therapy provides insight into troublesome behaviors. The problem with psychotherapy is that knowledge and insight are not sufficient motivators for change for many people.

Cold turkey is an approach in which people use willpower to achieve total abstinence. The limitations of this approach are (1) it seldom works, (2) it ignores the reasons for the undesirable behavior, (3) it provides little learning, and (4) it encourages an obsession with the behavior, often leading to a "rebound effect," in which the undesired behavior actually gets worse.

Reactance motivation is another theory that explains why cold-turkey approaches don't work. Reactance motivation, which was recently associated with drinking among college students,[7] suggests that telling people to abstain completely from doing something often produces the opposite reaction. For many people it isn't difficult to recall instances in their own lives in which they behaved a certain way primarily because they were told that they could not or should not behave that way. Coercion in particular leads to the arousal of reactance, which in turn tends to reduce *compliance*. The theory suggests that high reactance motivation is associated with high recidivism.

Rather than psychotherapy and cold-turkey approaches, we recommend an approach that puts you in control of your health, requires your involvement, and permits you to determine what you do and how and when you do it. This approach, called a *self-help* approach to lifestyle change, is discussed in detail in the following section.

Developing a Self-Help Plan for Lifestyle Change

A **self-help** approach assumes that individuals can manage their lifestyle change and can learn to control those features in their environment that are detrimental to health. In other words, expensive, long-term, professional help is

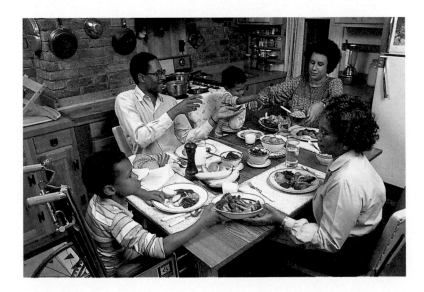

Parents are powerful role models for health promoting behaviors.

Figure 2-2 Examples of health-promoting behaviors

Specific Behaviors Conducive to Good Health

- I avoid the extremes of too much or too little exercise.
- I get an adequate amount of sleep.
- I avoid adding sugar and salt to my food.
- I include 15 to 20 grams of fiber in my diet each day.
- I plan my diet to ensure consumption of an adequate amount of vitamins and minerals.
- I brush and floss my teeth after eating.
- I avoid driving under the influence of alcohol or drugs.
- I drive within the speed limit.
- I wear my seat belt whenever travelling in an automobile.
- I avoid the use of tobacco.
- I consume fewer than two alcoholic drinks per day.
- I know the instructions provided with any drug I take.
- I do my part to promote a clean and safe environment.
- I feel positive about my life.
- I feel enthusiastic about my life.
- I can express my feelings of anger.
- I can say "no" without feeling guilty.
- I engage in activities that promote a feeling of relaxation.
- I am able to develop close, intimate relationships.
- I am interested in the views of others.
- I am satisfied with my study habits.
- I am satisfied with my spiritual life.
- I am tolerant of the values and beliefs of others.

not a prerequisite for everyone trying to make a lifestyle change. Instead, change is within the grasp of each individual. But a self-help approach comes with a price: the time and thought devoted to planning. Successful lifestyle change is almost impossible to achieve without a plan. Just as a research paper requires considerable planning, so does lifestyle change. The self-help plan that follows applies principles of behavior management and should facilitate your efforts to turn your health goals into reality.

First, Take an Inventory

The first step in any lifestyle-change program is to evaluate personal health habits and practices. A good way to start is simply to make a list of your **health-promoting behaviors,** things you do to maintain and/or improve your level of wellness. If you have a difficult time getting started, you can refer to the list of health-promoting behaviors in Figure 2-2. Make another list of *health-inhibiting behaviors,* things you do that may be detrimental to your health (see Assessment Activity 2-1: Assessing Your Health Behavior). If your lists are specific and if they identify behaviors that relate to wellness in its broadest sense (that is, the physical, social, emotional, and psychological aspects of health), it should be possible to make comparisons between the two lists that give insight and information about your lifestyle.

Detailed, comprehensive lifestyle questionnaires, such as the one that accompanies this text (see Appendix), can provide even more information about specific health practices and behavioral tendencies that can be targeted for change. Many of these questionnaires are similar to those you might complete for your physician or even purchase in the form of computer software. Regardless of the tool you use, remember that the goal is to learn more about yourself.

Two reasonable questions to ask at this point might be "which behaviors present the greatest threat to my health?" and "which behaviors should be targeted first for change?"

The answer to the second question is strictly an individual matter depending on the frequency and intensity of various behaviors, genetic predisposition to certain health problems, overall health profile, personal motivation, and perhaps the answer to the first question.

The first question can be answered by referring to the Prevention Index (Figure 2-3), which lists 21 key health-promoting activities in order of increasing importance as rated by a panel of public health experts.[8] Each activity has an assigned weighted score based on a 10-point scale indicating its importance in preventing disease and promoting health. Therefore smoking, with a score of 9.78, is viewed as having the greatest effect on health. Getting 7 to 8 hours of sleep each night, with a score of 6.71, has the least effect on health. However, it is important to note that a low score on the prevention index does not minimize the importance of an activity. It only means that the activity has less of an effect on health than the other activities. All of the activities are viewed as having a significant influence on health.

Second, Start with the Right Attitude

There are very few limits to what we can do for ourselves if we have the right attitude. This is especially true when it comes to planning a change in the way we live. Answering the questions in Assessment Activity 2-2 may shed some light on your attitude and help determine if you are ready to start a lifestyle-change program.

Most of us make two serious mistakes when starting a lifestyle change. First, we expect miracles by setting unrealistic goals. There is no better way to guarantee failure than to set goals that are far too ambitious. Such goals doom us to failure, and failure is the worst enemy of any lifestyle-change program. For many people the emotional baggage that comes with failure and/or the fear of failure easily discourages future efforts at lifestyle change.

Second, we often view lifestyle change as a temporary goal rather than a lifetime change. Nowhere is this more true than it is for weight-loss programs, in which people set a goal, go on a diet until they reach their goal, and then revert to their original eating habits. Invariably they regain the lost weight. The proper attitude would be to change eating habits in such a way that they will endure for a lifetime. Of course, this is a difficult attitude to accept because lifestyle change by its very nature puts us at war with ourselves. When we try to change some aspect of behavior, we are denying ourselves something that feels comfortable or that provides some source of enjoyment or pleasure. Denial is a powerful psychological force that often triggers a preoccupation that worsens the health behavior being changed. This is why dieters often become more obsessive-compulsive about food during a diet than they were before the diet. The same is true for many other lifestyle-change programs.

It may be more reasonable to strive for moderation than to set goals that require abstinence or a complete reversal of behavior. For example, rather than giving up ice cream completely, it may be more realistic for a dieter to limit ice cream to smaller portions or to substitute low-fat ice cream. Rather than starting a fitness program with a 5-mile jog, it may be more appropriate to start with a 1-mile walk. For many people moderation requires a higher level of learning and/or adjustment than abstinence does. In moderation

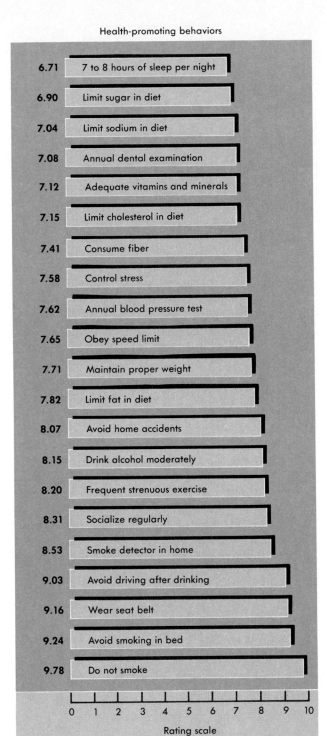

Health-promoting behaviors

Rating	Behavior
6.71	7 to 8 hours of sleep per night
6.90	Limit sugar in diet
7.04	Limit sodium in diet
7.08	Annual dental examination
7.12	Adequate vitamins and minerals
7.15	Limit cholesterol in diet
7.41	Consume fiber
7.58	Control stress
7.62	Annual blood pressure test
7.65	Obey speed limit
7.71	Maintain proper weight
7.82	Limit fat in diet
8.07	Avoid home accidents
8.15	Drink alcohol moderately
8.20	Frequent strenuous exercise
8.31	Socialize regularly
8.53	Smoke detector in home
9.03	Avoid driving after drinking
9.16	Wear seat belt
9.24	Avoid smoking in bed
9.78	Do not smoke

Rating scale: 0 1 2 3 4 5 6 7 8 9 10

Figure 2-3 The prevention index.

success depends on being able to control behavior, learning to live with certain stimuli, and still having the discipline to break the behavioral cycle. In abstinence success depends on complete avoidance, usually by removing the stimulus, such as when a smoker throws away all of his or her cigarettes. A key factor in choosing either

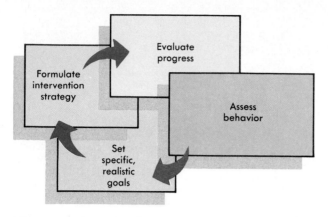

Figure 2-4 Steps in planning lifestyle change.

moderation or abstinence when changing health-inhibiting behaviors is the amount of control a person has over his or her environment. For example, it may be difficult to improve study habits in a college dormitory because it is not likely that one person can control the noise and distractions from other students in the dormitory. In this case it may be more desirable to try to improve study habits in a controlled environment, such as a library.

No single strategy for lifestyle change is right for everybody. The key is to get involved in planning your personal program and not to be afraid to use your imagination. You know yourself better than anyone else does. Remember, your attitude has the power to spur you on to success or doom you to failure. There is no substitute for the power of positive thinking. If you find yourself thinking about failure, practice a technique called *thought stopping*, in which the negative thought ("I can't improve my study habits; I've always failed in the past") is replaced with a positive one ("I will do better," or "I am doing better").

Third, Develop a Plan of Action

When structuring a plan of action, it is helpful to follow basic principles of lifestyle management. These principles include (1) assessing behavior, (2) setting specific, realistic goals, (3) formulating intervention strategies for lifestyle change, and (4) evaluating progress (Figure 2-4).

Assess behavior. Behavior assessment, the collection of data on target behaviors, is the lifeline of any lifestyle-change plan. It involves the process of counting, recording, measuring, observing, and describing. Anything that can be quantified is subject to assessment. Behaviors are

scrutinized as if under a microscope. In this sense, the individual becomes his or her own psychologist.

Assessment tools are usually in the form of daily logs, journals, and diaries for recording behaviors. It is essential that data be collected long enough to note behavioral trends and tendencies, usually a minimum of 1 to 2 weeks.

Sometimes a behavior assessment will prompt a change in behavior without any other action. In most lifestyle-change programs a plan of action is not started until it is clear that assessment alone will not be enough to alter the behavior completely. Bootzin[9] illustrates this point by citing the experience of a friend: "A friend of mine discovered that he was interspersing the phrase 'you know' in almost every sentence he spoke. He decided to try to suppress that behavior. The first step he took—as it turned out, the only step that was required—was to record the number of times he said 'you know.' Each day that he recorded, his frequency of emitting that phrase decreased. Recording served as a sufficient intervention to bring that verbal behavior under control."

An added benefit of the assessment phase is that it provides clues to a person's commitment to making a change in his or her life. A thorough, detailed log is a good sign that the individual has enough motivation to carry on the plan even when its novelty wears off.

When the assessment phase is finished, there should be sufficient information to form a behavioral profile, state specific goals, and customize an intervention program that matches goals and strategies to a person's unique circumstances and personality.

Set specific, realistic goals. Setting "specific" goals means setting goals that focus on concrete, observable, measurable behaviors. There is a big difference between a behavioral goal to overcome shyness and a goal that requires a person to initiate a conversation with a different person each day for the next week or between a goal to "act safely" and a goal to make a point to fasten seat belts when travelling in a car. If goals are specific, we know precisely what it is we are trying to accomplish and where, when, and how often it will take place. The real payoff of using precise language is that we get instant, specific feedback on our progress. We know if our plan is succeeding or if it needs to be revised.

Another way to increase specificity is to establish a timetable for achieving goals. A timeta-

Figure 2-5 Sample behavioral contract for lifestyle change

I, _____, pledge that within the next 12 weeks, beginning September 1 and ending November 30, I will accomplish the goals listed below.

_____   _____
              Signature   Witness

My health goal is to improve my physical fitness by participating in an activity program 3 days a week for a minimum of 30 minutes a day.

My intermediate goals are to
- Assess my physical fitness using the Rockport Walking Fitness Test*—September 1
- Start a walking program—September 3
- Start a walking/jogging program—September 17
- Progress to a jogging program—October 15

Intervention strategies:
- Work out after classes and before dinner
- Involve roommate

Rewards:
- Buy a pair of expensive jogging/walking shoes
- Buy a jogging suit

Penalty:
- Buy jogging shoes and/or jogging suit for my roommate

*See Chapter 6 for information on the Rockport Walking Fitness Test.

ble adds structure to the plan and provides a bench mark for evaluating progress.

"Realistic" behavioral goals are reasonable and relate to our personal circumstances. Setting realistic goals also means forming them in the context of correct information. For example, an informed dieter would know that it is not reasonable or wise to set a goal to lose 10 pounds in a week. A more reasonable, achievable goal would be 1 to 2 pounds. It also would not make sense for a college student to begin a physical fitness program that requires university facilities just before going home for the Christmas holidays.

When setting goals, it is best to start off small. Setting a modest goal initially facilitates some degree of success, which is good for confidence. For complex lifestyle changes, behavioral psychologists recommend breaking down an ambitious, long-range goal into a set of intermediate goals, beginning with the easier ones then moving gradually and progressively to more difficult ones. As a rule goals should be structured around

the theme of moderation. Extreme goals promote the erroneous attitude that lifestyle change is temporary. They create a strong sense of denial, encourage preoccupation with target behaviors, and invariably lead to failure. Exceptions include cigarette smoking, alcoholism, and drug dependence, for which abstinence is still the primary treatment.

Formulate intervention strategies. No single strategy is right for all behaviors and all people. What works for one person may fail miserably for another person. This makes it extremely important for an individual to get involved personally in individualizing intervention strategies that fit his or her behavioral profile and behavioral goals. Some of the more common types of strategies include use of behavioral contracts, stimulus control, positive and negative reinforcers, and behavior substitution.

A **behavioral contract** is a written agreement between people in a lifestyle-change program (Figure 2-5). Although they vary in style and

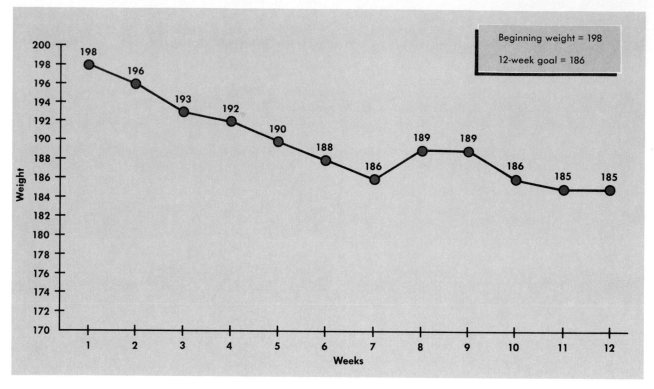

Figure 2-6 Example of graphic display of behavioral contract to lose weight.

form, most contracts include a statement of long-range and intermediate health goals, target dates for completion of each goal, rewards and punishments, intervention strategies, and signatures of witnesses. They are not legal documents, so simplicity and creativity are encouraged.

After you have drafted a contract, work out a method of graphing your progress (Figure 2-6). Display the contract and graph where you and others can see them. This way, they become tangible affirmations of your commitment to the agreement.

Stimulus control is a behavioral technique that involves elimination or manipulation of the circumstances associated with the undesirable behavior. One way to change a behavior is to eliminate altogether the stimulus causing it. A smoker can't smoke if there are no cigarettes, an ice cream binge isn't possible if a trip to the ice cream parlor is refused, and loud music cannot interfere with studying if the radio is put away.

Another way to alter a behavior is to modify the stimulus. This is sometimes referred to as *behavior shaping*. Instead of eliminating the stimulus, the situation is modified to prompt, or "shape," desirable behavior. For example, a student who finds that it is virtually impossible to

study in a dormitory might try to study in a different environment, such as the library. Another student might try to improve the quality of his or her studying by setting a study schedule that starts with a 30-minute session and progressively increases over time to several hours a day. When doing so, the student might record the amount of time spent on-task, that is, studying. When on-task studying occurs on 3 consecutive days, study time is increased in increments of 30 minutes.

The use of *positive* and *negative reinforcers* is fundamental to stimulus-control strategies (Figure 2-7). Positive reinforcers are rewards earned for achieving lifestyle goals; negative reinforcers are usually thought of as penalties. Although the use of positive and/or negative reinforcers is strictly an individual matter, most lifestyle-change programs emphasize the positive. Many people like to treat themselves to rewards, which vary according to their financial resources. Rewards can include special treats, the purchase of a desired item, or participation in an enjoyable activity. Rewards may range from a book to an expensive, week-long vacation at a resort. You might find it interesting and helpful to think of a list of rewards that would be suitable for you. Of

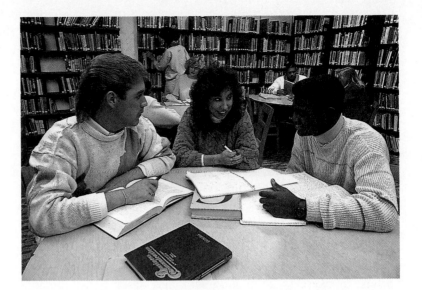

Improving some health habits may require a change in the environment.

course, there is no substitute for success. The actual achievement of a stated lifestyle goal is the strongest positive reinforcement for most of us. It provides the best incentive for continuing with a lifestyle-change program.

For many people negative reinforcers serve as powerful motivators for change. For example, a student who cuts most classes and is chronically late for those that he does attend could write a contract that requires him to deposit $200 with a counselor. The contract might further stipulate that the counselor is to return $20 to him each week he does not miss class or go to class late. But for each week he does not fulfill his contract, he would forfeit $20 to a charitable organization.

Another good stimulus-control strategy is formation of a *support group*, which might include a roommate, family, friends, classmates, or someone else who can identify with your lifestyle goal. Such a group not only provides a source of encouragement but also holds you accountable for your goals. Involving someone else in the process will make it easier for you to stick to your plan. Some people enjoy exercise more if they do it with a partner. Others benefit from the discipline of having another person available for reinforcement.

When you join a support group, you are publicly affirming what you plan to do and how and when you plan to do it. We all value the opinions of other people and want to appear successful in their eyes. An added bonus of a support group is that often friendships are formed that last a lifetime. Many people feel that the formation of support groups is the key to success for many of the more popular and visible health-change programs.

Behavior substitution, in which a new behavior is substituted for the undesirable one, is the most common technique used by people trying to

Figure 2-7 Examples of stimulus-control strategies for losing weight

- Eat in a certain place—not all over the house.
- Eliminate from your immediate environment all food that can be eaten without careful preparation.
- Always sit down to a carefully set place at the table and eat only one helping of planned foods.
- Prepare only enough for one meal at a time.
- Eat slowly.
- Chew each bite 25 to 50 times.
- Put down utensils after every mouthful.
- Partway through the meal, stop and relax without eating for 2 to 3 minutes.
- Leave some food on your plate at each meal.
- Plan to eat some meals alone (there is a tendency to overeat in social situations).
- Put your weight record where a friend can see it.
- Eat a carefully balanced diet so that you are not deprived of a particular food element.

change some aspect of their lifestyle without professional help. When this technique is applied, the goal is to think of a behavior that is incompatible with the one being altered. Examples include chewing gum to suppress the urge to smoke, substituting diet colas for sweetened colas, and playing a game of racketball instead of watching television.

A word of warning about behavior substitution is worth heeding: Be careful that the behavior being substituted does not create a new problem while solving the old one. For example, some smokers initiate their cigarette habit as a way to control eating. In other words, they trade compulsive eating for compulsive smoking. The result is a new health habit that is more detrimental than the original habit. Therefore it is important to exercise good judgment and observe sound principles of healthy living when choosing to substitute behaviors.

Evaluate progress. There is no way of knowing if a lifestyle-change plan is working without constant monitoring. This means assessing each goal according to the conditions and timetable specified at the beginning of the program. Consistent monitoring makes it possible to get immediate feedback about progress. This feedback in turn can then provide a basis for continuing with the program as it is or for making adjustments. However, avoid the temptation to overmonitor progress. Plan evaluation checkpoints at time intervals that are short enough to provide sufficient time to achieve goals but not so short that they promote preoccupation with target behaviors. Depending on the nature and complexity of the problem behavior, the timing of evaluations could range from a weekly basis for a weight-loss program to a daily basis for a plan to improve study habits.

Regardless of the results, it is important to maintain the proper perspective about success and/or failure. Many people succumb to the attitude trap that we either succeed or fail completely. This is a serious error in thinking and can be devastating to a person's motivation. When goals are not fully realized, the proper attitude is to view the shortcoming as justification for making adjustments in the lifestyle-change program. Maybe the goals were too general or too unrealistic. Maybe the intervention strategies lacked relevance. Maybe the program didn't include enough time. It may be necessary to reshape goals, set a more realistic schedule, change the rewards and/or penalties, or formulate different intervention strategies.

Above all, maintain a healthy perspective about yourself. Don't burden yourself with guilt if you fall short of your goals. Simply admit your shortfall and make adjustments. What seems important now often pales in significance when viewed within a broader context. You might consider how significant this event is likely to be to you 2 years from now. Doing this will help establish the right perspective on your progress and the larger scale of your life. More important are the answers to the following questions: "What did you learn from this experience?" "What did you learn about yourself?" "What can you do differently?" Lifestyle change is a lifelong project that requires insight into yourself, skillful planning, and plenty of practice.

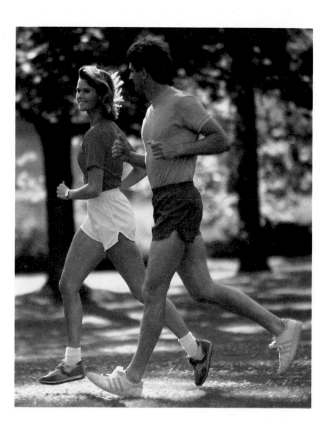

Involving another person in a lifestyle change program makes it easier to stick to a plan.

Summary

- Many Americans now believe that it is possible to exercise control over many health-promoting and health-inhibiting behaviors.
- The discrepancy between health knowledge and health behavior is greatest among young adults.
- Lifestyle change is one of the most pervasive human endeavors.
- A fundamental belief in lifestyle-change programs is that health behavior is a learned response and therefore can be changed.
- Health behavior is influenced by many complex forces, including family, role models, social pressure, advertising, and psychological needs.

- The four steps in a lifestyle-change program are assessing behavior, setting specific and realistic goals, formulating intervention strategies, and evaluating progress.
- Intervention strategies used in lifestyle change include behavioral contracts, stimulus control, positive and negative reinforcers, support groups, and behavior substitution.
- Lifestyle change should be viewed as a learning experience rather than a test of willpower.

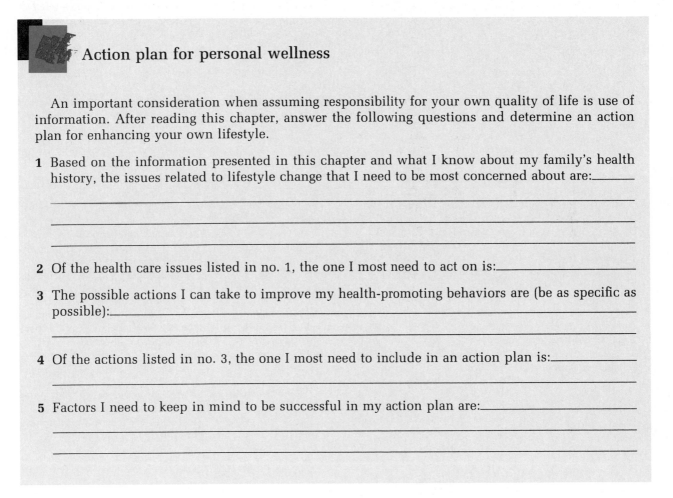

Action plan for personal wellness

An important consideration when assuming responsibility for your own quality of life is use of information. After reading this chapter, answer the following questions and determine an action plan for enhancing your own lifestyle.

1 Based on the information presented in this chapter and what I know about my family's health history, the issues related to lifestyle change that I need to be most concerned about are:_____

_____

_____

_____

2 Of the health care issues listed in no. 1, the one I most need to act on is:_____

3 The possible actions I can take to improve my health-promoting behaviors are (be as specific as possible):_____

_____

4 Of the actions listed in no. 3, the one I most need to include in an action plan is:_____

_____

5 Factors I need to keep in mind to be successful in my action plan are:_____

_____

_____

Review Questions

1. What are the five specific health practices that illustrate the generalization that health habits are learned?

2. What are the differences between health-promoting behaviors and health-inhibiting behaviors? Give two examples of each.

3. What are the reasons for the high recidivism rate in many if not most lifestyle-change programs? Discuss all three.

4. What are the similarities and differences among the psychotherapy, cold-turkey, and self-help approaches to lifestyle change?

5. What are five criteria for determining a person's readiness for a lifestyle-change program?

6. If a college student wants to use the principles of behavior assessment to asses his or her study habits, what specific things can be measured, recorded, and/or observed?

7. What is an example of a lifestyle goal that is stated both specifically and realistically?

References

1. Guerin J, editor: Beating the big ones, Am Health 6(3):41, 1987.
2. US Department of Health, Education, and Welfare: Healthy people: the surgeon general's report on health promotion and disease prevention objectives, Washington, DC, 1979, US Government Printing Office.
3. Office of Disease Prevention and Health Promotion: The 1990 health objectives for the nation: a midcourse review, US Public Health Service, Washington, DC, 1986, US Government Printing Office.
4. Survey highlights: the prevention index '89, summary report, a report card on the nation's health, Emmaus, Pa, 1989, Rodale Press, Inc.
5. Gallagher W: If you can't teetotal, Am Health 8(5):48, 1988.
6. Associated Press: Bad habits need work to resolve: willpower is challenge, Commercial Appeal 150(115): B1, 1989.
7. Engs R and Hanson D: Reactance theory: a test with collegiate drinking, Psychol Rep 64:1083, April 1989.
8. Survey highlights: The prevention index '89, summary report, a report card on the nation's health, Emmaus, Pa, 1989, Rodale Press, Inc.
9. Bootzin R: Behavior modification as therapy: an introduction, Cambridge, Mass, 1975, Winthrop Publishers.

Annotated Readings

1. Amler R and Dull H: Closing the gap: the burden of unnecessary illness, New York, 1987, Oxford University Press, Inc.
Documentation and intervention strategies resulting from the Health Policy Consultation of the Carter Center of Emory University. Public health experts identify the major risks to good health in the United States and outline the preventive actions that can reduce these risks.
2. Barsky A: Worried sick: our troubled quest for wellness, Boston, Mass, 1988, Little, Brown & Company, Inc.
Written for people who find that health is on their minds more and more and for people who want to look after their own health without the effort becoming too burdensome and worrisome. Emphasizes how health is affected by perception and attitude.
3. Carter-Scott C: Negaholics, New York, 1989, Villard Books.
"Negaholics"—a term used to describe the addiction to negative thinking and self-doubt that affects the health of many people. The individual becomes aware of his or her own negativity and then learns a 12-step program for steady, permanent recovery.
4. Lierman T: Building a healthy America: conquering disease and disability, Washington, DC, 1987, Capitol Associates, Inc.
Presents facts, figures, and information to help people become effective advocates for health and explains how the federal government works for health, how to lobby for health, the status of various diseases, and where to get more information and help.
5. Office of Disease Prevention and Health Promotion: Disease prevention/health promotion: the facts, Palo Alto, Calif, 1988, Bull Publishing Co.
Compilation of facts, figures, and statistics for priority areas in health as identified in the 1990 Health Objectives for the Nation.
6. Ornstein R and Sobel D: Healthy pleasures, Reading, Mass, 1989, Addison-Wesley Publishing Co, Inc.
Presents numerous practical suggestions on how to live life in a way that enriches rather than just maintains health, such as ways to mobilize positive beliefs, expectations, and emotions—from cognitive therapy, relaxation training, and successful behavior modification practices.
7. Robbins A: Unlimited power, New York, 1987, Ballantine/Del Rey/Fawcett Books.
Shows how mind power determines what you can and cannot do and how you can harness your mind power to attain personal goals.

ASSESSMENT ACTIVITY   2-1

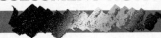

Assessing Your Health Behavior

Before planning a lifestyle-change program, you will find it helpful to take an inventory of your health behaviors. Doing this should reveal important information about your lifestyle and should also help you identify areas in need of improvement.

Directions: In this assessment you are asked to make two lists. In the left column list the things you do to maintain and/or improve your level of health. These things represent your health-promoting behaviors. In the right column list the things you do that may be detrimental to your health. These are your health-inhibiting behaviors. Try to be specific. Include the things that affect your mental, emotional, social, spiritual, and physical health. If you have a hard time thinking of specific activities, you might refer to Figure 2-2 or the Lifestyle Inventory, located in the Appendix.

Health-Promoting Behaviors

1. _____
2. _____
3. _____
4. _____
5. _____
6. _____
7. _____
8. _____
9. _____
10. _____
11. _____
12. _____
13. _____
14. _____
15. _____

Health-Inhibiting Behaviors

1. _____
2. _____
3. _____
4. _____
5. _____
6. _____
7. _____
8. _____
9. _____
10. _____
11. _____
12. _____
13. _____
14. _____
15. _____

Which health-inhibiting behavior would you be willing to change right now?_____
_____
_____

ASSESSMENT ACTIVITY

2-2

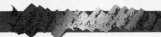

Assessment of Readiness For Lifestyle Change

Directions: Indicate "yes" or "no" to each of the following questions by placing a check mark in the appropriate column. If you can answer "yes" to the following questions, you are ready to begin a lifestyle-change program.

Questions	Yes	No
1. Do you view lifestyle change as a lifetime goal rather than a temporary, short-term goal?	_____	_____
2. Are you willing to get personally involved in planning a lifestyle-change program?	_____	_____
3. Are you prepared for some disappointments?	_____	_____
4. Are you willing to experiment with different ideas?	_____	_____
5. Do you have the patience to accept success in small increments stretched over a long period?	_____	_____
6. Are you willing to set modest, realistic goals?	_____	_____
7. Are you willing to make some changes in the way you live?	_____	_____

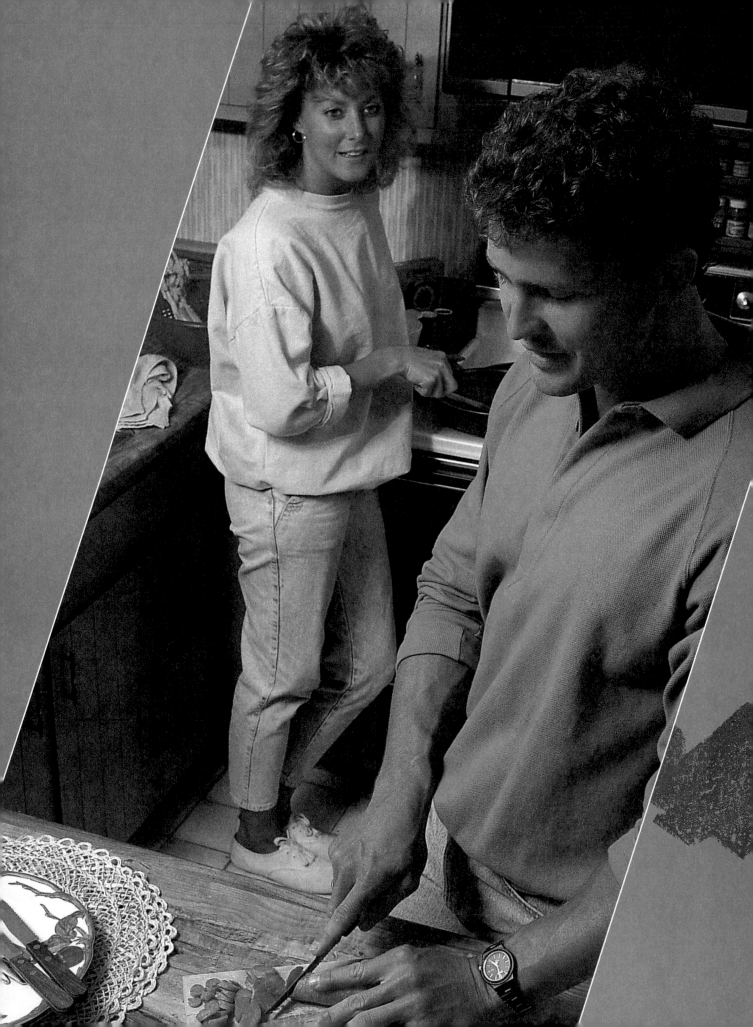

Chapter 3

Forming a Plan for Good Nutrition

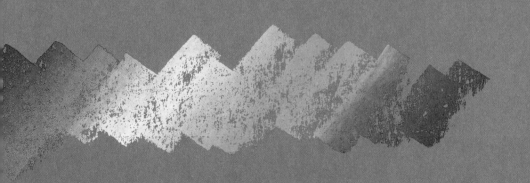

Key terms

amino acids

calorie

cholesterol

complex carbohy-
drates

essential nutrients

fiber

minerals

nutrient density

recommended di-
etary allowances

saturated fats

tropical oils

vitamins

Objectives

After completing this chapter, you will be able to:

▌ Discuss the dietary guidelines for Americans

▌ Identify the major nutrition deficiencies and problems in the typical American diet

▌ Describe the principles behind planning a nutritionally balanced diet

▌ Identify health practices that may help prevent common digestive problems

Nutrition has captured the interest and curiosity of Americans perhaps more than any other topic related to fitness and wellness. Whether it is cholesterol or sodium, fat or fiber, or sugar or vitamins, nutrition issues make headlines in both scientific journals and popular magazines. And everybody seems to be an expert. So much is written by so many that it is difficult to know what and whom to believe.

In this chapter basic concepts of the science of *nutrition*, the study of nutrients and the way the body processes them, are presented to guide you through the maze of nutrition information. The concepts presented here within the framework of the now-familiar *Dietary Guidelines for Americans* should provide a basis for sound nutritional planning that can serve you throughout your lifetime.

Dietary Guidelines for Americans

The relationship between nutrition and health has changed dramatically during the past 50 years. Until as recently as the 1940s, diseases such as rickets, pellagra, scurvy, beriberi, xerophthalmia, and goiter (caused by a lack of or deficiency in vitamin D, niacin, vitamin C, thiamin, vitamin A, and iodine, respectively) were common in the United States and throughout the world. Today, thanks to an abundant food supply, fortification of some foods with critical trace

nutrients, and better methods of improving the quality of foods, such deficiency diseases have virtually been eliminated in developed countries. Nutrition deficiencies are rarely reported in the United States, and when they do occur, they are usually associated with poverty, high-risk conditions (such as premature birth or alcoholism), and conditions related to prolonged chronic illnesses.[1]

The deficiency diseases of the past have been replaced by diseases of dietary excess and imbalance. For most Americans the problem has become one of overeating—too many calories for our activity levels and an imbalance in the nutrients consumed with the calories. Six of the top ten causes of death in the United States are associated with diet (heart disease, some types of cancer, stroke, non-insulin–dependent diabetes mellitus, atherosclerosis, and chronic liver disease). The association between diet and health is so convincing that nutrition was designated as one of the key target areas in the 1979 landmark publication *Healthy People: the Surgeon General's Report on Health Promotion and Disease Prevention.* Also in the late 1970s the U.S. Senate commissioned a huge study on nutrition that eventually concluded that overconsumption of certain dietary components is now a major concern for Americans. Chief among these concerns is the disproportionate consumption of foods high in fats, often at the expense of foods high in

Figure 3-1 Nutrition objectives for Americans[2]

Fats and cholesterol

Reduce consumption of fat (especially saturated fat) and cholesterol. Choose foods relatively low in fat and cholesterol, such as vegetables, fruits, whole-grain foods, fish, poultry, lean meats, and low-fat dairy products. Prepare food using methods that add little or no fat.

Energy and weight control

Achieve and maintain a desirable body weight. To do this, choose a dietary pattern in which energy (caloric) intake is consistent with energy expenditure. To reduce energy intake, limit consumption of foods high in calories, fats, and sugars and minimize alcohol consumption. Increase energy expenditure through regular participation in sustained physical activity.

Complex carbohydrates and fiber

Increase consumption of whole-grain cereal products and other foods, vegetables (including dried beans and peas), and fruits.

Sodium

Reduce sodium intake by choosing foods low in sodium and limiting the amount of salt added during food preparation and at the table.

Alcohol

To reduce the risk of developing chronic disease, drink alcohol in moderation (no more than two drinks per day) if at all. Avoid drinking alcohol before or while driving, operating machinery, taking medication, or engaging in any other activity requiring the use of judgment. Avoid drinking alcohol during pregnancy.

Fluoride

Community water systems should contain fluoride at levels necessary to prevent tooth decay. If such water is not available, use other sources of fluoride.

Sugars

Persons who are particularly vulnerable to dental caries, especially children, should limit the amount and frequency of consumption of foods high in sugar.

Calcium

Adolescent girls and adult women should increase consumption of foods high in calcium, including low-fat dairy products.

Iron

Children, adolescents, and women of childbearing age should be sure to consume foods that are good sources of iron, such as lean meats, fish, certain beans, and iron-enriched cereals and whole-grain products. (This issue is of special concern for low-income families.)

complex carbohydrates and fiber that may be more conducive to health.[2] A list of the key nutrition objectives is given in Figure 3-1. These recommendations provide the basis for the federal nutrition policy stated in the *Dietary Guidelines for Americans*[3]:

- Eat a variety of foods.
- Maintain desirable weight.
- Avoid too much saturated fat and other fats and cholesterol.
- Eat foods containing adequate starch and fiber.
- Avoid too much sugar.
- Avoid too much salt.
- If you drink alcoholic beverages, do so in moderation.

▉ TABLE 3-1 The four food groups in a daily plan for good nutrition

Food group	Servings per day	Sample foods	Main nutrients provided
Milk and cheese products	2*	Cheese, milk, yogurt, pudding or custard, cottage cheese, and ice cream	Calcium, protein, zinc, riboflavin, vitamin B_{12}, and thiamin
Meat, fish, poultry, and beans	2†	Beef, pork, poultry, fish, eggs, dried beans, peas, nuts, peanut butter, sunflower seeds, tofu, cheese, and tuna	Protein, iron, niacin, riboflavin, zinc, vitamin B_{12}, and thiamin
Fruits and vegetables	4	Fruits, vegetables, juices, and salads	Vitamin A, folacin, vitamin C, iron, thiamin, fiber, and riboflavin
Breads and cereals (grains)	4	Bread, crackers, dry cereal, cooked cereal, muffins, pasta, rice, and tortillas	Niacin, iron, magnesium, thiamin, zinc, riboflavin, and fiber
Fats, sweets, and alcohol		Foods from this group should not replace any foods from the main four groups. Amounts consumed should be determined by the energy needs of the individual.	

*Two to three servings for children and three to four servings for teens, adults less than 24 years old, and pregnant or lactating women.

†Three servings for pregnant or lactating women.

▉ TABLE 3-2A National research council recommended dietary allowances, revised 1989

Category	Age (years) or condition	Weight* (kg)	Weight* (lb)	Height* (cm)	Height* (in)	Protein (g)	Fat-soluble vitamins Vitamin A (µg RE)†	Vitamin D (µg)‡	Vitamin E (mg α-TE)§	Vitamin K (µg)
Males	15-18	66	145	176	69	59	1,000	10	10	65
	19-24	72	160	177	70	58	1,000	10	10	70
	25-50	79	174	176	70	63	1,000	5	10	80
	51+	77	170	173	68	63	1,000	5	10	80
Females	15-18	55	120	163	64	44	800	10	8	55
	19-24	58	128	164	65	48	800	10	8	60
	25-50	63	138	163	64	50	800	5	8	65
	51+	65	143	160	63	50	800	5	8	65
Pregnant						60	800	10	10	65
Lactating	1st 6 Months					65	1,300	10	12	65
	2nd 6 Months					62	1,200	10	11	65

The allowances, expressed as average daily intakes over time, are intended to provide for individual variations among most normal persons as they live in the United States under usual environmental stresses. Diets should be based on a variety of common foods in order to provide other nutrients for which human requirements have been less well defined. See text for detailed discussion of allowances and of nutrients not tabulated.

*Weights and heights of Reference Adults are actual medians for the U.S. population of the designated age, as reported by NHANES II. The use of these figures does not imply that the height-to-weight ratios are ideal.

Eat a Variety of Foods

The best way to plan a nutritionally balanced diet is to eat a variety of foods from the four basic food groups (Table 3-1). Eating a variety of foods helps to ensure that the **Recommended Dietary Allowances (RDA)** of **essential nutrients**—substances that cannot be made by the body and therefore must be supplied through the diet—are provided. RDAs serve as important nutritional bench marks in that they represent the minimum level of intake of essential nutrients necessary to meet the needs of healthy people (Table 3-2). A helpful guide for remembering how many servings from each food group to include in the diet to ensure consumption of the RDA of essential nutrients for adults is to use the 2:2:4:4 formula: two servings from the meat group, two servings from the milk group, four servings from the fruits and vegetables group, and four servings from the grain group. Although this formula may not be a cure-all for everyone, it serves as a suitable foundation for planning a diet that provides sufficient amounts of the more than 50 nutrients that people need each day.

Seek the right balance. Food is made up of six classes of nutrients: carbohydrates, fat, protein, vitamins, minerals, and water. Some experts list fiber as a seventh nutrient though it is technically a carbohydrate. Three of these nutrients—carbohydrates, fat, and protein—are called energy nutrients because they provide energy for the body. Food energy is expressed in the form of kilocalories. A **calorie** is defined as the amount of heat required to raise the temperature of a gram of water 1° C. A kilocalorie equals 1,000 calories of heat energy. Common reference to calories usually excludes the prefix "kilo," mainly for convenience. A gram of carbohydrates provides 4 calories (kilocalories) of energy, a gram of protein also provides 4 calories, a gram of fat provides 9 calories, and alcohol (which is in a category separate from these main groups) provides 7 calories per gram.

The recommended diet for Americans calls for an emphasis on complex carbohydrates as the major source of energy. Forty-eight percent of our calories should come from complex carbohydrates. This percentage is more than double the present amount in the typical American diet, which consists of 42% fat, 12% protein, 24%

■   **TABLE 3-2A—cont'd**

Water-soluble vitamins							Minerals						
Vita-min C (mg)	Thia-min (mg)	Ribo-flavin (mg)	Niacin (mg NE)¶	Vita-min B$_6$ (mg)	Fo-late (μg)	Vita-min B$_{12}$ (μg)	Cal-cium (mg)	Phos-phorus (mg)	Mag-nesium (mg)	Iron (mg)	Zinc (mg)	Iodine (μg)	Sele-nium (μg)
60	1.5	1.8	20	2.0	200	2.0	1,200	1,200	400	12	15	150	50
60	1.5	1.7	19	2.0	200	2.0	1,200	1,200	350	10	15	150	70
60	1.5	1.7	19	2.0	200	2.0	800	800	350	10	15	150	70
60	1.2	1.4	15	2.0	200	2.0	800	800	350	10	15	150	70
60	1.1	1.3	15	1.5	180	2.0	1,200	1,200	300	15	12	150	50
60	1.1	1.3	15	1.6	180	2.0	1,200	1,200	280	15	12	150	55
60	1.1	1.3	15	1.6	180	2.0	800	800	280	15	12	150	55
60	1.0	1.2	13	1.6	180	2.0	800	800	280	10	12	150	55
70	1.5	1.6	17	2.2	400	2.2	1,200	1,200	320	30	15	175	65
95	1.6	1.8	20	2.1	280	2.6	1,200	1,200	355	15	19	200	75
90	1.6	1.7	20	2.1	260	2.6	1,200	1,200	340	15	16	200	75

†Retinol equivalents. 1 retinol equivalent = 1 μg retinol or 6 μg β-carotene.
‡As cholecalciferol. 10 μg cholecalciferol = 400 IU of vitamin D.
§α-tocopherol equivalents. 1 mg d-α tocopherol = 1 α-TE.
¶1 NE (niacin equivalent) is equal to 1 mg of niacin or 60 mg of dietary tryptophan.

TABLE 3-2B Estimated sodium, chloride and potassium minimum requirements of healthy adults*

Age	Weight (kg)*	Sodium (mg)*,†	Chloride (mg)*,†	Potassium (mg)‡
>18§	70.0	500	750	2,000

*No allowance has been included for large, prolonged losses from the skin through sweat.
†There is no evidence that higher intakes confer any health benefit.
‡Desirable intakes of potassium may considerably exceed these values (~3,500 mg for adults).
§No allowance included for growth. Values for those below 18 years assume a growth rate at the 50th percentile reported by the National Center for Health Statistics and averaged for males and females.

TABLE 3-2C Estimated safe and adequate daily dietary intakes of selected vitamins and minerals for adults*

Vitamins	
Biotin (µg)	Pantothenic acid (mg)
30-100	4-7

Trace Elements†				
Copper (mg)	Manganese (mg)	Fluoride (mg)	Chromium (µg)	Molybdenum (µg)
1.5-3.0	2.0-5.0	1.5-4.0	50-200	75-250

*Because there is less information on which to base allowances, these figures are not given in the main table of RDA and are provided here in the form of ranges of recommended intakes.
†Since the toxic levels for many trace elements may be only several times usual intakes, the upper levels for the trace elements given in this table should not be habitually exceeded.

sugar, and only 22% complex carbohydrates (Figure 3-2). Changing the diet to emphasize complex carbohydrates means eating significantly more fruits and vegetables, grain products, bread, spaghetti and other pasta, beans and peas, rice, and potatoes and significantly less fat and sugar.

Avoid protein excess. One of the main reasons Americans have so much trouble maintaining the right balance in their dietary habits is the mistaken notion that if a modest amount of protein is good for you, then large amounts must be even better. Because protein is a "body builder," people believe that it makes you strong and that it is better for you than carbohydrates. This is a myth. Protein consumed in excess of the body's requirement is not converted to muscle; rather, it

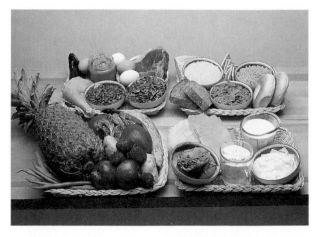

We should eat a variety of foods from the four food groups.

is converted to energy or stored as fat as are surplus carbohydrates.

Protein is an essential nutrient. It is different from carbohydrates and fats, the other nutrients that supply energy, in that it contains nitrogen in addition to carbon, hydrogen, and oxygen. Because of their unique chemical structures, proteins contain the basic materials for cell growth and repair. They also help the body form antibodies to fight disease and produce substances such as insulin, enzymes, and hemoglobin.

Protein is made up of small chemical structures called **amino acids.** Both animal and plant proteins are made up of approximately 20 amino acids. Eleven of these amino acids can be produced in the body; nine of them cannot be made by the body and therefore must be supplied by the diet.[4] These nine are called *essential amino acids.* A *complete protein* is one that contains all of the essential amino acids. A *high-quality protein* is one that not only is complete but also contains the essential amino acids in amounts proportional to the body's need for them. Protein sources from animals, including meat, fish, poultry, eggs, milk, and cheese are examples of high-quality, complete proteins.

A *low-quality protein,* or *incomplete protein,* is one that does not contain all of the essential amino acids in the proportions needed by the body. Examples include nuts, beans, seeds, wheat, rice, oats, and whole grains. Before a low-quality protein can be converted into a complete protein, it must be matched with another source of low-quality protein. This is because the body cannot make partial proteins, only complete ones; protein synthesis operates by the "all-or-none law." If an amino acid is supplied by one source in an amount smaller than is needed, the total amount of protein that can be made from the other amino acids will be limited. Therefore if a diet does not include sources of complete protein, as might occur in a *vegetarian* diet, it is important to include the right mix of foods. Some vegetarians *(lacto-ovo-vegetarians)* omit meat, fish, and poultry from their diets but eat eggs and dairy products. Others *(lactovegetarians)* exclude eggs and consume only dairy products. Both of these types of vegetarians consume high-quality proteins and do not need to worry about protein deficiency. *Strict vegetarians,* people who eat an all-plant diet, may need to be discriminating in their food selections because plant proteins are low-quality proteins. To obtain all of the essential amino acids from plant sources, strict vege-

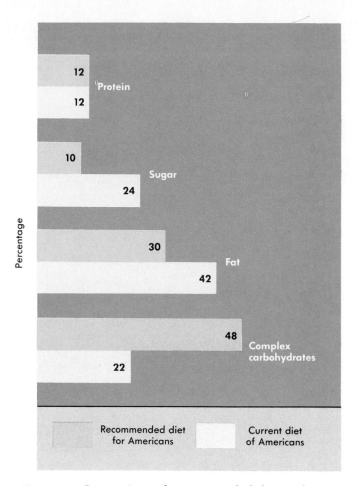

Figure 3-2 Comparison of recommended diet and current diet of Americans.

tarians are advised to eat a variety of foods from the legume groups, beans, peas, and peanuts, combined with foods from the cereal and whole-grain group, including pasta, wheat, rice, oats, and corn. The practice of combining protein sources from cereal and grains with legumes is called *protein complement.* It permits the deficiencies in essential amino acids in one group to be compensated for by the essential amino acid content of the other group.

Recommended protein intake. The recommended dietary allowance for protein is 0.8 grams per kilogram of body weight per day (see Assessment Activity 3-1). The average 19 to 22-year-old man weighs 154 pounds and requires 56 grams of protein per day. The average woman weighs 120 pounds and needs 44 grams of protein per day. Women who are pregnant or lactating require an additional 30 and 20 grams of protein respectively.

■ **Figure 3-3 Facts about vitamins**

Vitamin	Food sources	Benefits to wellness	Deficiency signs and symptoms
Water-soluble vitamins			
B-complex	Meat products (beef, pork, poultry, eggs, fish), milk, cheese, grains, dried beans, nuts, starchy vegetables	Facilitates release of energy from other nutrients Aids in formation of red blood cells, growth and function of the nervous system, and the formation of hormones Contributes to good vision and healthy skin Assists in the metabolism of proteins, fats, and carbohydrates	Fatigue, nausea, weakness, irritability, depression, weight loss, inflamed skin, cracked lips, muscle pain, cramps, or twitching, low blood sugar, decreased resistance to disease, nerve dysfunction
C (ascorbic acid)	Citrus fruits, strawberries, cantaloupe, honeydew melons, broccoli, brussels sprouts, green peppers, cauliflower, spinach	Contributes to production of collagen Aids in protection against infection Contributes to tooth and bone formation and repair, as well as wound healing Aids in absorption of iron and calcium	Dry, rough, and scaly skin, bleeding gums, slowly healing wounds, listlessness, fatigue, low glucose tolerance

In terms of calories, it is recommended that protein make up 12% of the diet. For most Americans this means cutting down on protein intake. Average levels of protein consumption of 60 grams per day for women and 90 grams per day for men are well above the RDA.[2] According to a nationwide study[1] of protein consumption among Americans, meat, fish, and poultry provide 47% of protein intake; milk, cream, and cheese provide 19%; grains provide 17%; vegetables provide 5%; and fruit provides 2% (10% was unaccounted for).

When more protein is consumed than is needed by the body, it is converted into energy or stored as fat. The body is less efficient at converting protein to energy than it is at converting carbohydrates to energy. This is just as true for active people as it is for sedentary people. Exercise and other physical activities do not change the body's need for protein. What active people need is food that is readily converted to energy: carbohydrates. This fact is finally being observed by people who plan training meals for athletes that consist of a large proportion of complex carbohydrates. Loading up on complex carbohydrates before a race is a common practice among marathon runners.

A common misconception among weight lifters and body builders is that consumption of large quantities of *protein supplements*, usually in the form of commercially made protein powder, enhances muscle development. But protein supplements are not needed to increase muscle mass during strength training. Extra protein is not converted to muscle; as stated previously, excess protein is converted to extra energy or stored as fat.

It is possible for some people to consume too much protein. Excess protein may cause the body to excrete calcium, the mineral that strengthens bones and teeth. There is also concern that high protein intake may put excessive strain on the kidneys to excrete the excess nitrogen supplied by the protein into the urine. Although the kid-

Figure 3-3—cont'd

Vitamin	Food sources	Benefits to wellness	Deficiency signs and symptoms
Fat-soluble vitamins			
A	Milk, cheese, butter, fat, eggs, liver, dark-green leafy vegetables, carrots, cantaloupe, yellow squash, sweet potatoes	Essential for growth of epithelial cells, such as hair, skin, and mucous membranes Aids in vision in dim light Contributes to bone growth and tooth development Plays a role in reproduction (sperm production and estrogen synthesis) Increases resistance to infection	Decreased resistance to infection, skin changes, alteration of tooth enamel, night blindness, corneal deterioration
D	Milk (fortified), butter, cheese, eggs, clams, fish, salmon, tuna. Also, sunlight stimulates vitamin D production	Essential for bones and teeth Contributes to calcium and phosphorus absorption	Bone softening and fractures, muscle spasms, tooth malformation
E	Vegetable oils, green leafy vegetables, liver, eggs, whole-grain cereals and breads	Assists in formation of red blood cells and muscle tissue Aids in absorption of vitamin A Serves as an antioxidant, which preserves vitamins and unsaturated fatty acids	Destruction of cell membrane of red blood cells
K	Green leafy vegetables, liver, cabbage, cauliflower, eggs, tomatoes, peas, potatoes, milk	Aids in normal formation of the liver Contributes to normal blood clotting	Severe bleeding, prolonged coagulation, bruising

neys of most normal, healthy people can handle a nitrogen excess without difficulty,[4] the job of excreting unneeded nitrogen can be burdensome if the kidneys are under strain. This is why people with kidney failure are placed on low-protein diets. It also explains why people who go on high-protein diets to lose weight (not a good idea—see Chapter 4) are encouraged to drink large quantities of water to flush out the kidneys.

Protein in food. The foods that supply plenty of complete proteins are those in the milk and meat groups. Foods in the vegetable and bread groups contribute small amounts of protein to the diet, but these amounts become significant when several servings are consumed.

Vitamins. **Vitamins** are organic compounds found in food that are necessary in small amounts for good health. Unlike carbohydrates, fats, and proteins, vitamins yield no energy. Instead, they serve as catalysts that enable energy nutrients to be digested, absorbed, and metabolized. Diets deficient in the RDA of vitamins may impair the physiological processes of the body and lead to deficiency diseases. One of the major advantages of a varied diet is that it helps to ensure consumption of the right amount and balance of vitamins.

Vitamins are grouped into two categories: water-soluble vitamins and fat-soluble vitamins. Water-soluble vitamins include the vitamin B complex and vitamin C (Figure 3-3). They are present in the watery components of food, distributed in the fluid components of the body, excreted in the urine, needed in frequent small doses, and unlikely to be toxic, except when taken in *megadoses* (very large quantities).

Fat-soluble vitamins include vitamins A, D, E, and K and are found in the fat and oily parts of food. Because they cannot be dissolved and absorbed in the bloodstream, vitamins must be absorbed into the lymph with fat and transported by proteins by way of the lymph. When consumed in excess of the body's need, fat-soluble vitamins are stored in the liver and fat cells. Their storage makes it possible to survive for days, weeks, or even months or years without consuming them. At least three of the fat-soluble vitamins (A, D, and K) may even accumulate to toxic levels. Megadoses of these vitamins should be avoided.

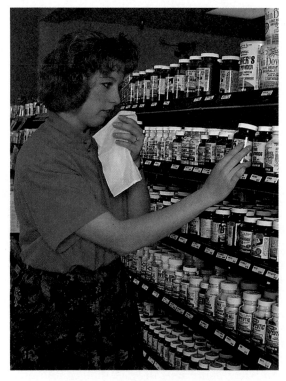

The common cold is a contagious, infectious disease, not a nutritional disease.

Vitamin supplements. Advertising has people believing that vitamins provide energy and prevent disease and that taking more vitamins means more energy and better health. Consequently, 40% of all Americans take one or more vitamin supplements in multiple and single doses, in natural and synthetic formulations, and in amounts 10 or more times higher than recommended.[5] Vitamins do *facilitate* the release of energy from carbohydrates, fats, and proteins, but they don't *provide* energy. If they did, they would be classified as an energy nutrient. It is not possible to survive on water and vitamins.

One of the most common misconceptions about vitamins concerns vitamin C and the common cold. Colds are contagious, infectious diseases and are not nutritional diseases. Despite all the claims, the common cold cannot be prevented or cured by consuming vitamin C. Carefully controlled studies have failed to show that large doses of vitamin C prevent colds. In fact, large doses of vitamin C (more than 200 mg per day) will fully saturate body tissues and will be excreted in the urine.

An amusing example of how people can be fooled by Mother Nature into thinking that a specific measure can prevent certain illnesses occurred during a study conducted at the University of Minnesota and was recently reported in a health newsletter[6]: One group of students was given vitamin C. The control group was given a placebo. To show that vitamin C has any effect, it must have produced better results than the placebo. One student wrote to the university the following year, even though he was no longer enrolled, to ask if he could have the cold medicine again because he had not had a single cold all winter. The problem was that he had received the placebo, not the vitamin C. The study failed to show any link between cold prevention and vitamin C consumption. The point is that if a person has been convinced that vitamin C helps and he or she wants to take reasonable amounts, it is not likely to cause any harm. But the individual should not expect any benefits.

The consensus among medical scientists is that healthy adults who eat a variety of foods do not need vitamin supplements. Taking large amounts of vitamins of any kind provides no known benefit and can instead cause harm. With a varied diet, even a multiple vitamin is rarely necessary. Several exceptions are infants, who may need dietary supplements at given times, and pregnant and lactating women. Occasionally vitamin supplements are needed by people with irregular diets or unusual lifestyles or by people following certain weight-reduction regimens or strict vegetarian diets.[5] When taken as supplements, vitamins should be viewed as medicine and therefore should be recommended by a physician.

Natural vs. synthetic vitamins. Many people mistakenly believe that the vitamins present in food are somehow better than the vitamins made in the laboratory. But a vitamin has the same chemical structure regardless of its source, and the body cannot distinguish between natural and synthetic vitamins. Of course, few people would argue that individuals who meet the RDA of vitamins through food sources enjoy better nutritional health.

Nor is it true that foods grown with natural, organic fertilizers are more nutritious or have more vitamins than food grown with chemical fertilizers. Plants cannot make a distinction in fertilizers. In fact, natural fertilizers cannot be used directly on the plants. They must first be broken down into the same compounds found in chemical fertilizers. Vitamins do not come from the soil, but are manufactured by genetically controlled processes within the plants themselves. (This is not true for some minerals such as iron.)

Minerals. **Minerals** are simple but important nutrients. They are simple because as inorganic compounds they lack the complexity of vitamins, and they are important because they fulfill a variety of functions. For example, sodium and potassium affect shifts in body fluids, calcium and phosphorus support the body's structural framework, iron is the core of hemoglobin (an oxygen-carrying compound in the blood), and iodine facilitates production of thyroxine (a hormone that influences metabolic rate).

There are 20 to 30 important nutritional minerals. Compared with other nutrients, minerals should be consumed in small amounts. Minerals that are present in the body and are required in large amounts, greater than 5 grams (1 teaspoon) per day, are called *major minerals* or *macrominerals*. They include, in descending order of prominence, calcium, phosphorus, potassium, sulfur, sodium, chloride, and magnesium. Major minerals contribute from 60% to 80% of all inorganic material in the human body.

Minerals that are required in small amounts, less than 5 grams per day, are called *trace minerals* or *microminerals*. There are more than a dozen trace minerals, with the best-known ones being iron, zinc, and iodine (Figure 3-4).

Some minerals are similar to water-soluble vitamins in that they are readily excreted by the

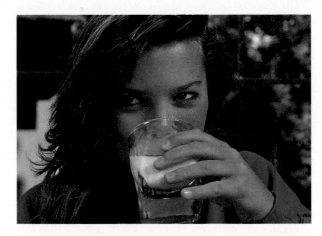

According to the Surgeon General, the majority of adolescent girls and adult women need to increase their consumption of high calcium foods.

kidneys, do not accumulate in the body, and rarely become toxic. Others are like fat-soluble vitamins in that they are stored and are toxic if taken in excess.

Minerals are different from vitamins in that they are indestructible and require no special handling during food preparation. The only precautions are to avoid soaking minerals out of food and throwing them away in cooking water. As long as they are kept in food, minerals may be handled in any way without fear of losing them.

Major minerals are abundant in the diet; therefore deficiencies are highly unlikely, especially if a variety of foods is included. If a deficiency does occur, it is most likely to be a calcium deficiency. About 80% of women over the age of 18 who were surveyed by the National Academy of Sciences reported having diets deficient in calcium.[1] During adolescence and early adulthood calcium deficiency can jeopardize bone development. In postmenopausal women, calcium deficiency is one factor thought to cause osteoporosis (see Chapter 6). Consequently, the Surgeon General's report on nutrition established a dietary goal for adolescent girls and adult women to increase consumption of foods high in calcium, including low-fat dairy products. Dark-green leafy vegetables are also good sources of calcium.

Of the various trace minerals, iron is the most abundant. It is also the one of most concern to

Figure 3-4 Facts about minerals

Major (macro) minerals
Calcium, phosphorus, potassium, sulfur, sodium chloride, and magnesium

Trace (micro) minerals
Iron, iodine, zinc, selenium, manganese, copper, molybdenum, cobalt, chromium, fluorine, silicon, vanadium, nickel, tin, cadmium

Minerals of special concern*

Calcium

Wellness benefits: Contributes to bone and tooth formation, general body growth, maintenance of good muscle tone, nerve function, cell membrane function, and regulation of normal heart beat
Food sources: Dairy products, dark-green vegetables, dried beans, shellfish
Deficiency signs and symptoms: Bone pain and fractures, muscle cramps, osteoporosis

Iron

Wellness benefits: Facilitates oxygen and carbon dioxide transport, formation of red blood cells, production of antibodies, synthesis of collagen, and use of energy
Food sources: Red meat (lean), seafoods, eggs, dried beans, nuts, grains, green leafy vegetables
Deficiency signs and symptoms: Fatigue, weakness

Sodium

Wellness benefits: Essential for maintenance of proper acid-base balance and body fluid regulation, aids in formation of digestive secretions, assists in nerve transmission
Food sources: Processed foods, meats, table salt
Deficiency signs and symptoms: Rarely seen. Vomiting in children or profuse sweating may reduce sodium. Sodium is of special concern because of its overconsumption among Americans. Large dietary intake is associated with hypertension in some people.

*Calcium and iron are of special concern because deficiencies are likely to exist, especially among women and children.

nutritionists. Iron deficiency in the diet is responsible for the most prevalent form of anemia in the United States. Iron deficiency hampers the body's ability to produce *hemoglobin*, a substance needed to carry oxygen in the blood. A lack of hemoglobin can cause fatigue and weakness and can even have an effect on behavior and intellectual function. Individuals at high risk of developing anemia are children from low-income families, adolescents, and women of childbearing age. Proper infant feeding through use of iron-fortified milk or breastfeeding is the best safeguard against iron deficiency in infants. Among adolescents and adults iron intake can be improved by increasing consumption of iron-rich foods, such as lean red meats, fish, certain kinds of beans, and iron-enriched cereals and whole-grain products. In some cases, especially premenopausal women with inconsistent diets, iron supplements may be justified. Also, consuming foods that contain vitamin C enhances the body's ability to absorb iron.

Water. Next to air, water is the substance most necessary for survival. Everything in the body occurs in a water medium. Although people can live without vitamins and minerals for extended periods, without water, death is likely to result in a few days.

Water makes up about 60% of the body's weight. Every cell in the body is bathed in water of the exact composition that is best for it. Even tissues that are not thought of as "watery" contain large amounts of water. For example, water makes up about 75% of brain and muscle tissues. Even bone tissue is more than 20% water. As a rule the bodies of men contain more water than the bodies of women because they have more muscle tissue, and muscle tissue holds more water than fat tissue, which is more prominent in the bodies of women.

Water plays many roles and performs many functions. It is vital to digestion and metabolism because it acts as a medium for chemical reactions in the body. It carries oxygen and nutrients to the cells through blood, regulates body temperature through perspiration, lubricates the joints, removes waste through sweat and urine, protects an unborn child, and even assists in respiration by moistening the lungs to facilitate intake of oxygen and excretion of carbon dioxide.

The average adult consumes and excretes about 96 ounces of water a day. People exposed to high temperatures, hot climates, or strenuous physical activity need considerably more water. Although most of our water intake comes from beverages, solid foods also make a significant contribution. Most fruits are more than 80% water, meats are 50% water, bread is 33% water, and butter is approximately 15% water.

Some beverages and foods can increase our need for water. Alcoholic beverages, tea, and coffee contain water but can actually have a contradictory effect on the body. An ounce of pure alcohol requires 8 ounces of water to be metabolized. Caffeinated beverages stimulate the adrenal glands and serve as *diuretics*, increasing water output and raising the need for water. The sugar and sodium found in many beverages and foods place an extra burden on the body because they require water to be dissolved, used, and excreted.

How much water should you drink? People are advised to drink six to eight 8-ounce glasses of fluids per day, whether or not they are thirsty.[7] Although thirst is usually a good indicator of the body's need to replenish its water supply, it is possible for a person to drink just enough fluid to quench his or her thirst but not enough to satisfy the body's needs. People who exercise a lot or live in a hot climate require more water. Also, people on high-protein diets need more water than they thirst for to provide the kidneys with enough water to flush out the

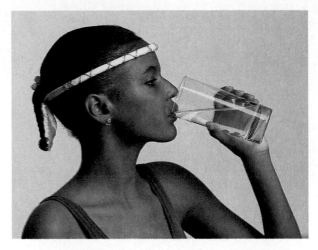

We should drink six to eight 8-ounce glasses of water daily.

waste products of protein metabolism. Under normal circumstances it is unlikely that too much water can be consumed because the body is efficient at getting rid of what it doesn't need. However, there is a correct way to take in fluids. It is important to spread water consumption throughout the day. A sudden drinking binge in a short period early in the day will not satisfy the body's needs later on in the day. Instead, it will be excreted by the kidneys.

Maintain Desirable Weight

The achievement and maintenance of a desirable weight is a complex issue and is treated separately in this text. For a thorough and complete discussion of principles for maintaining desirable weight, refer to Chapter 4.

Avoid Too Much Fat, Saturated Fat, and Cholesterol

Perhaps the greatest shortcoming of the American diet is the abundance of fat. The *Dietary Guidelines* call for no more than 30% of total daily calories in fat. However, fat intake is much higher than that for most people. The good news is that fat consumption is decreasing. According to a 1985 survey[1] fat consumption dropped to 37% for women and 36% for men, compared with 42% for both groups 10 years earlier. Although this downward trend in fat consumption is a source of encouragement, it remains far short of the intended goal of a maximum 30%.

Basic facts on fats. *Fat*, also called *lipid*, is a compound made by chemically bonding fatty acids to glycerol to form *glycerides*. When three fatty acids are hooked to glycerol, the fat com-

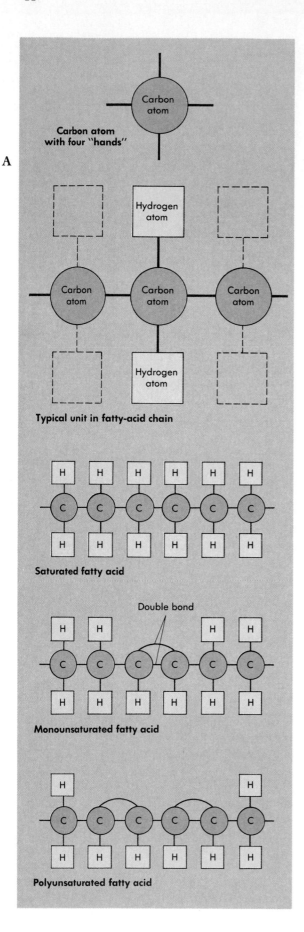

A

Carbon atom with four "hands"

Typical unit in fatty-acid chain

Saturated fatty acid

Monounsaturated fatty acid

Polyunsaturated fatty acid

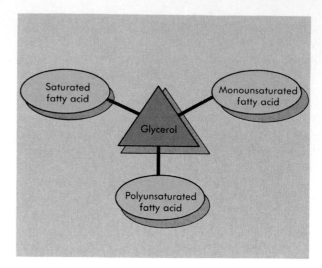

B

Figure 3-5 The basic fat facts. **A,** Fatty acids vary according to their chemical structure: (1) saturated fats have all of their carbon atoms occupied with hydrogen; (2) monounsaturated fats have one point in the carbon chain unoccupied with hydrogen; and (3) polyunsaturated fats have at least two points in the carbon chain unoccupied with hydrogen. **B,** Triglycerides are usually a mixture of different fatty acids.

pound is called *triglyceride.* Almost 95% of fat stored in the body is triglyceride, with the remaining 5% consisting of other glycerides and cholesterol. When reference is made in literature to fat, it is usually in reference to triglycerides. The fatty acids that make up triglycerides can be saturated, monounsaturated, or polyunsaturated.

Chemically, fats are chains of carbon atoms strung together with hydrogen atoms. If it is a **saturated fat,** virtually all of the fatty acids are saturated. That is, the carbon chain carries all the hydrogen atoms it can handle (see Figure 3-5, The Basic Fat Facts). If it is *unsaturated,* there is room in the carbon chain for more hydrogen. If the chain is *monounsaturated,* there is room for one hydrogen atom. If it is *polyunsaturated,* there is room for more than one hydrogen atom. If it is *highly polyunsaturated,* there is room for many more hydrogen atoms.

The saturated/unsaturated ratio of food also may be affected by food-processing techniques. Because unsaturated fats are less stable than their saturated counterparts, they are prone to spoilage. Consequently, for many foods, manufacturers employ a chemical process called *hydrogenation,* in which hydrogen atoms are added to the unsaturated or polyunsaturated fats to make them more saturated and more resistant to spoil-

Figure 3-5 Basic fat facts

Fat is a compound made by chemically bonding fatty acids to glycerol. These fat compounds are called glycerides. When three fatty acids are bonded to glycerol, the compound is known as a *triglyceride*. If there is only one fatty acid, the fat is a *monoglyceride*, and if there are two fatty acids, it is a *diglyceride*. These terms are commonly seen on the ingredient lists for food products. The fatty acids are the important part of the compound. They can be saturated, monounsaturated, or polyunsaturated.

Fatty acids are made by forming a chain of carbon atoms. You can think of each carbon atom as having four "hands" to "hold hands," or bond, with other atoms. A typical unit in a fatty-acid chain has one four-handed carbon atom holding hands with two other carbon atoms and the other two hands holding with two hydrogen atoms. A *saturated fat* exists when two hands of every carbon atom are holding hands with two hydrogen atoms. There is no room to hold hands with any more hydrogen atoms. An *unsaturated fatty* exists when there are one or more spots on the chain where two hands of one carbon atom are holding two hands of another carbon atom—called a double bond. If this double bond occurs in only one place, the chain is called a *monounsaturated fatty acid*. When two or more spots are involved, it is called a *polyunsaturated fatty acid*.

The fish oils that have many spots with double bonds are called *highly polyunsaturated fatty acids*. If a food label says *hydrogenated*, it means hydrogen has been added to some of the unsaturated carbon atoms to make the fatty acid more saturated. This is often done to make the fatty acid more solid or to improve the shelf life of the product.

Triglycerides are usually a mixture of fatty acids. One of the three fatty acids attached to glycerol may be saturated, another monounsaturated, and the third polyunsaturated. Almost any combination can occur. So the fat in your food is not just saturated or unsaturated, but a mixture.

age. This is important to remember because many people mistakenly assume that the word "polyunsaturated" on a food label means that the fat in the food is not saturated. This is not necessarily true. The only way to be sure is to check the small print on the label. If the words "hydrogenated" or "partially hydrogenated" can be found, the food contains varying amounts of saturated fats.

Saturated and unsaturated fats can be differentiated by their appearance. Saturated fat is solid at room temperature. Lard, fat marbled in meat, and hardened grease left from a skillet of sausage are good examples. Polyunsaturated fats are liquid at room temperature. Examples include safflower and corn oil. Solid vegetable shortenings are partially hydrogenated and have a soft consistency. Coconut oil, palm kernel oil, and palm oil are exceptions. They are vegetable oils and are liquid at room temperature, yet they are among the most saturated of all fats.

Fish oils are among the most unsaturated fats available. They are roughly twice as unsaturated as vegetable oils. They do not harden even at low temperatures. Their unsaturation has created special interest in relation to seafood and heart dis-

ease. Fatty acids in cold-water seafood consist of *omega-3 fatty acids*, which are powerful at lowering cholesterol and triglyceride levels and reducing clot-forming rates, thereby reducing the risk of heart disease.

Of all the blood fats, **cholesterol,** a waxy substance that is technically a steroid alcohol found only in animal foods, is probably the most famous and surely the most researched one. High levels of cholesterol are usually discussed as one of the major risk factors of cardiovascular disease, as in this text. For information on cholesterol, refer to Chapter 5: Cardiovascular Health and Wellness.

Health effects of fat. Fats are an essential part of every cell. They maintain the health of the skin and hair, provide insulation and protection for body organs, help transport and absorb vitamins A, D, E, and K, and provide a concentrated source of energy. But in excess, fats are associated with several health conditions.

Health studies usually report the health risks associated with dietary fat within the context of total intake of fat and saturated fat. Although it is likely that a diet high in total fat is linked closely with a diet high in saturated fat and vice versa, it

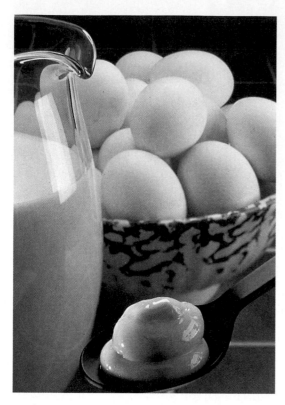

Recommendations by the medical community to reduce fat in our diets has resulted in the development of Simplesse, a new fat substitute.

is possible to have a diet low in one and still high in the other. This in turn can alter the risks of developing various health conditions.

Because very little energy is used to transfer fat from foods to fat storage (the body requires only 3 calories to store 100 calories of fat as fat, but it takes 23 to 27 calories to digest 100 calories of carbohydrates and store it as fat) and because fat contributes more than twice as many calories as protein and carbohydrates, it is not surprising that a high intake of total dietary fat is associated with obesity. Obesity in turn increases the risk of developing high blood pressure and consequently increases the risk of stroke and non-insulin–dependent diabetes mellitus. In addition, total dietary fat increases the risk of developing some types of cancer, especially cancer of the breast, colon and uterus. There is also an association between dietary fat and gallbladder disease.

Consumption of high levels of saturated fat has been strongly and consistently associated with coronary disease. It is the major dietary contributor to total blood-cholesterol levels. The consensus today is that blood-cholesterol levels depend less on your intake of cholesterol from foods as on the total amount of saturated fat consumed. Only about 10% to 25% of people find that they lower their blood cholesterol when they consume less cholesterol. Most people experience a minimal effect or no effect. However, almost everyone who lowers saturated-fat intake can lower cholesterol levels by 10% to 20%, especially if he or she is already eating many foods high in saturated fats. One explanation for this is that saturated fats in the diet affect the way the liver handles cholesterol. When saturated fat is low, the liver reacts by clearing cholesterol from the bloodstream.[4]

Dietary sources of fat. According to the National Research Council,[8] animal products, such as red meats, (beef, veal, pork, and lamb), fish and shellfish, separated animal fats (such as tallow and lard), milk and milk products, and eggs contribute more than half of the total fat, three fourths of the saturated fat, and all the cholesterol to the diet of people in the United States. Of these, red meats provide the major source of fat for Americans in all age groups except infants, and ground beef is the single greatest contributor of fat to the American diet. Mayonnaise, salad dressings, and margarine are the chief sources of linoleic acid, an essential fatty acid. Eggs supply the most cholesterol.

Before drawing any conclusions about which foods to eat and which to avoid, it is important to remember that the fat in food is not just saturated or unsaturated, but a mixture. There is considerable variation in the amount of saturated, monounsaturated, and polyunsaturated fat in various foods. It is also a mistake to generalize that all animal fats are more highly saturated than all vegetable fats or that all tropical oils, such as coconut oil, palm kernel oil, and palm oil, are more saturated than animal oils and vegetable oils.

Table 3-3 presents the fat content of common representative foods. Some foods are naturally high in fat calories. For example, dairy products, such as cream cheese, cheddar cheese, and whole milk; beef products, such as hamburger and steak; pork products, such as pork chops, bologna, and frankfurters; and oils, such as butter and margarine, derive from 49% to 100% of their calories from fat. Fish products, vegetables, and fruits are significantly lower in fat. Still, the way food is processed, stored, and prepared can have a dramatic effect on its fat content. For instance, whole milk has more than eight times the fat cal-

TABLE 3-3 Fat content of representative foods

Food	Percentage of total calories from fat*			
	Total	Saturated	Monounsaturated	Polyunsaturated
Egg, whole, raw	64	19	25	8
Butter, pat	100	67	31	4
Margarine, 1 pat, hard	100	20	45	32
Cheese, cream	90	57	25	3
Cheese, cheddar	74	47	20	2
Cheese, cottage	39	25	11	1
Milk, whole	49	30	14	2
Milk, skim	6	4	1	trace†
Frankfurter	82	33	40	3
Bologna, beef	82	34	40	3
Bologna, pork	72	26	36	8
Flounder, baked	9	trace†	tr	trace†
Fish sticks	39	10	18	10
Tuna, canned, oil-packed	38	8	10	17
Tuna, canned, water-packed	7	trace†	tr	trace†
Ground beef	65	25	28	3
Steak, broiled, sirloin	56	24	26	2
Pork chop, broiled	62	23	29	7
Chicken breast, fried, flour-coated	36	10	14	8
Ham, cured, extra-lean	47	15	22	5
Beans, navy	4	tr	trace†	3
Potato, baked	1	tr	trace†	4
Potato chips	61	16	11	31
Ice cream, vanilla, regular	48	28	14	2
Apple	6	1	tr	2
Danish pastry	50	14	29	4

*Rounded off to nearest whole number
†trace = less than 1.9

ories as skim milk, fish sticks fried in oil have four times the fat calories as baked flounder, oil-packed tuna has five times more fat calories than water-packed tuna, and potato chips have 60 times more fat calories than a baked potato.

Just because a food is high in fat does not mean that it is also high in saturated fat. Margarine is a classic example. It is 100% fat, but only 20% of the fat is saturated. Most of the fat calories are monounsaturated or polyunsaturated. Butter is also 100% fat, but 67% of its fat content is saturated. In general, beef and pork products, foods made with butter fat and whole milk, and foods fried in oil are high in saturated fats. To help reduce consumption of total fat, especially saturated fat, choices should emphasize consumption of fruits, vegetables, and whole-grain cereals and other products. They should also emphasize consumption of fish, poultry prepared without the skin, lean cuts of meat, and low-fat dairy products.

Hidden fat. In an effort to reduce the amount of saturated fat in their diet, many people choose foods and snacks whose labels say they are made with "100% pure vegetable oil" or "pure vegetable shortening." The assumption is that because it is a vegetable oil, a pure (100%) oil at that, it is free of saturated fat and better for your health.

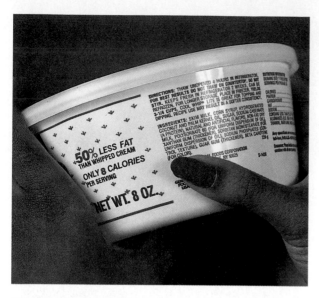

Beware of hidden fat.

Unfortunately this is not necessarily true. Cooking oils are the number 1 source of hidden fat in the American diet.[1]

Several vegetable oils are more highly saturated than lard and beef fat. Coconut oil and palm kernel oil are the two main villains for two reasons: They contain 86% and 81% saturated fat respectively, and they are widely used in making a variety of snack items from crackers and chips to cookies, cake mixes, and granola bars.[9] Figure 3-6 presents a comparison of the type and percentage of fat in various oils and foods. The point is that it is important to look beyond the "vegetable oil" banner displayed prominently on many snack packages and scan the ingredients list for the words "coconut," "palm kernel," and "palm oil." Beware too because many items outside the snack aisle contain palm or coconut oil. For instance, Cool Whip contains both palm kernel and coconut oils, making it more highly saturated than real whipped cream.

Another warning relates to "cholesterol free" claims made on the labels of vegetable oils. Although it is true that vegetable oils do not contain cholesterol, it is also true that they contain varying amounts of saturated fat. And like all saturated fats, they tend to raise cholesterol levels in the blood. So a steady diet of "cholesterol-free" baked goods that are made with, for example, "100% vegetable shortening" can actually raise your cholesterol level if they contain one or more tropical oils.[10]

Tropical oils. With the landslide of publicity against the use of coconut oil and palm kernel oil—also called **tropical oils** because they come from the fruit of the coconut tree or the oil palm tree, which grow easily in the warm, humid climates of Southeast Asia, Africa, Central and South America, and Malaysia—there is a tendency to think that they are all alike.

As it turns out, palm oil is different from palm kernel oil and coconut oil in that it contains significantly less saturated fat and significantly more monounsaturated fat than coconut or palm kernel oils. Because it is stable and resistant to spoilage, it requires little or no hydrogenation. In other words, there is a big difference between palm oil and palm kernel oil, and there may not be as big a difference between palm oil and some of the vegetable oils, especially those that are hydrogenated.

The major point is not to encourage consumption of palm oil but to warn against the tendency to jump to sweeping conclusions about food, even fat. It would be a mistake to think that complete avoidance of tropical oils would significantly lower dietary fat. This would be convenient but not true. Tropical oils make only a minor contribution (less than 3.5%) to total consumption of saturated fat in the United States.[11] The real issue is that Americans consume too many calories from fat of all kinds (Figure 3-7). The healthiest choice is to reduce total oil consumption (See Assessment Activity 3-2).

Dietary guidelines. The American Heart Association has developed a diet (formerly called the Prudent Diet) that achieves a total fat intake of 30% of total calories, with 10% coming from each type of fat (saturated, monounsaturated, and polyunsaturated), and a cholesterol intake below 300 mg per day. The guidelines of the diet are as follows[12]:

- Limit meat, seafood, and poultry to no more than 5 to 7 ounces per day.
- Use chicken or turkey (without the skin) or fish in most main meals.
- Choose lean cuts of meat, trim all the fat that you can see, and throw away the fat that cooks out of the meat.
- Substitute meatless or low-meat main dishes for regular entrees.
- Use no more than 5 to 8 teaspoons of fats and oils per day for cooking, baking, and salads.
- Use low-fat dairy products.

To control cholesterol:

- Use no more than four egg yolks per week, including those used in cooking.
- Limit consumption of shrimp, lobster, sardines, and organ meats.

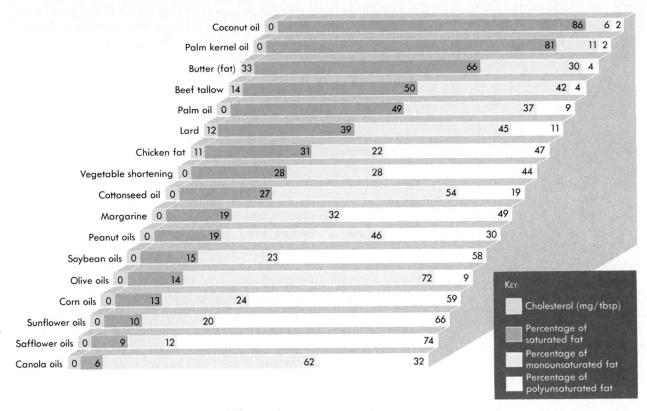

Figure 3-6 Comparison of dietary fats.

Eat Foods With Adequate Starch and Fiber

Starch and fiber belong to the carbohydrate family of nutrients. Carbohydrates are the primary energy source for all body functions and physical activity. They are also the preferred energy source; dietary guidelines recommend that complex carbohydrates make up 48% of the diet.

Carbohydrates supply energy in the form of sugar, or *saccharides.* The simplest form of carbohydrates is the *monosaccharide,* which includes *glucose* and *fructose* (fruit sugar). Fructose is the sweetest of simple sugars. *Disaccharides* are double sugars, meaning that they are pairs of monosaccharides chemically linked together. Included in this group of sugars are *sucrose,* or table sugar, *lactose,* or milk sugar, and *maltose,* or malt sugar. The last group of sugars are the *polysaccharides,* which are composed of many single monosaccharides. Polysaccharides are also called **complex carbohydrates.** They include starch and several forms of fiber.

Starch. Starch is the most significant polysaccharide in human nutrition. A diet high in starch is likely to be lower in fat, especially saturated fat and cholesterol, lower in calories, and higher

Figure 3-7 How much fat is in food?

The amount of fat in food depends on how fat is measured. Measuring fat content by weight will yield a completely different result than measuring fat by calories.

For example, one cup of whole milk weighs 244 g (8.5 oz). Eight of these grams come from fat; thus by *weight*, whole milk is 3.28% fat $(8.5 \div 244 = 3.28\%)$.

Calculating fat weight by calories provides a different picture. Most of the weight of milk (200 g) comes from water, and water has no calories. This leaves 44 g of calorie weight. Because 8 g come from fat and because 1 g of fat yields 9 calories, the fat content of 1 cup of whole milk provides 72 calories. The total percentage $(72 \div 150 = 48\%)$ of the calories is from fat, making it a fattier food than it seems at first glance. (The fat weight by calories for 2%, 1%, and skim milk are 38%, 18%, and 0%, respectively.)

in fiber. These factors together are associated with lower rates of obesity, cardiovascular disease, diabetes, cancer, malnutrition, and tooth decay. An added benefit of starch is that it helps the body maintain a normal blood-sugar level through a slower, more even rate of digestion and glucose absorption. All starch is digested and circulates to the cells as glucose 1 to 4 hours after a meal. This is one reason athletes involved in endurance activities, such as marathons, load up on complex carbohydrates before competition.

All starchy foods are plant foods. Grains, such as rice, wheat, corn, millet, rye, barley, and oats, are the richest food source. The legume family (beans and peas), including peanuts and dried beans (butter beans, kidney beans, black-eyed peas, garbanzo beans, and soybeans), is another good source of starch. It also contains a significant amount of protein. A third source is the tubers, such as potatoes and yams.

Many weight-conscious people mistakenly and unwisely avoid starches, thinking that they are high in calories. What makes starchy foods fattening is how they are served and eaten. For example, a baked potato contains 90 calories, compared with 285 calories in a hamburger of the same weight. It is adding fat in the form of butter, sour cream, margarine, or cheese that adds calories to the potato.

Fiber. One advantage in a diet that is high in starch is that it will almost automatically be high in fiber. Starch and fiber invariably appear together in foods unless the foods are refined or highly processed.

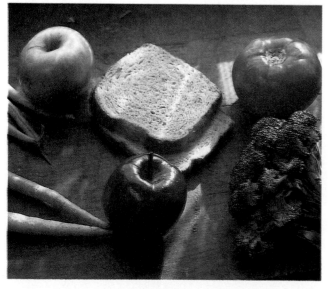

There are many health-related benefits of consuming foods that are higher in fiber.

Fiber (In the past it was called roughage.) is a general term that refers to the substances in food that resist digestion. The amount of fiber in a food is determined by its plant source and the amount of processing to which it is subjected. Generally the more a food is processed, the more the fiber is broken down and the lower the fiber content.

The fiber content shown on food labels is likely to be listed as either dietary fiber or crude fiber. *Dietary fiber* is the actual residue of plant food that resists digestion in the human body. *Crude fiber* is the residue of plant food following a harsh chemical digestive procedure in the laboratory. One gram of crude fiber equals 2 to 3 grams of dietary fiber.

There are two kinds of fiber, *soluble fiber*, which dissolves in hot water, and *insoluble fiber*, which doesn't dissolve in water. Each plant food contains a mixture of fiber types. Some contain mostly soluble fiber; others contain mainly insoluble fiber. But virtually every food is a mixture; almost no food provides a pure form of one type or another.

Soluble fiber. Soluble fiber appears to have several favorable effects. Because it forms gels in water, it adds bulk and thickness to the contents of the stomach and may slow emptying of the stomach, thus prolonging the sense of fullness and possibly helping dieters control their appetites. Studies have shown that soluble fiber lowers blood-cholesterol levels somewhat. It also slows the absorption of sugars from the small intestine, which may be beneficial to diabetics.[13]

Good sources of soluble fiber are fruits, vegetables, and a wide variety of grains. Specific foods include prunes, pears, oranges, apples, dried beans, cauliflower, zucchini, sweet potatoes, and oat and corn bran (see Table 3-4).

Insoluble fiber. Insoluble fiber benefits the body by adding bulk to the contents of the intestine rather than the stomach. This speeds the *transit time,* time of passage, of a meal's remnants through the small and large intestines. This in turn appears to offer several important health benefits:

- It helps prevent constipation because insoluble fiber attracts water into the digestive tract, thus softening the stool.
- Softer stools reduce the pressure in the lower intestine, creating less likelihood that rectal veins will swell and cause *hemorrhoids.*
- It helps prevent compaction of food in the

intestines, which could obstruct the appendix and lead to appendicitis.

■ It stimulates muscle tone in the intestinal wall, which helps to prevent *diverticulosis*, a condition that occurs when the intestine bulges out into pockets, and possibly leading to *diverticulitis*, in which the pockets become infected and sometimes even rupture (see "Common digestive problems" at the end of the chapter).

■ It may reduce the chances of colon cancer. A shorter transit time reduces the exposure of the intestines to cancer-causing agents in the food. Also, insoluble fiber stimulates the secretion of mucus in the colon. Mucus coats the colon wall and may provide a barrier that keeps cancer-causing agents from reaching the colon's cells.

The best source of insoluble fiber is wheat bran. Other good sources include whole grains, dried beans and peas, and most fruit and vegetables, especially those eaten with the skin.

If you are not used to eating fiber-rich foods, gradually add them to your diet over 4 to 6 weeks, using these suggestions[14]:

■ Eat ¼ to ½ cup whole-grain cereal every day. Look for cereals that list wheat bran as their first ingredient and that contain at least 5 grams of dietary fiber per serving.

■ Buy bread that lists "whole wheat" or "stone-ground wheat" as its first ingredient. Breads that don't list these ingredients first are made mostly from refined wheat flour that has been colored brown.

■ To make whole-wheat breads, muffins, or other baked goods, substitute one of the following for 1 cup of white flour: 1 cup minus 2 tablespoons whole-wheat flour, ½ cup white flour and ½ cup whole-wheat flour, or ¾ cup white flour and ¼ cup wheat germ or 100% bran.

■ Add 2 to 3 tablespoons of 100% bran to low-fiber foods, such as breakfast cereal, pudding, or applesauce.

■ Substitute brown rice, millet, or bulgur for white rice and potatoes, add barley to soups and casseroles, and snack on popcorn instead of potato chips or pretzels.

How much fiber?. Most Americans consume between 10 and 13 grams of dietary fiber per day. Some experts recommend that adults raise that level to 20 to 35 grams.[4] Because the high meat content in American diets provides little or no residue, only vegetarians are likely to consume this amount of fiber. Therefore some experts offer

a more reasonable recommendation of about 15 to 20 grams of total dietary fiber per day.[15] This can easily be achieved through consumption of generous amounts of complex carbohydrates.

Like most other nutrients, fiber can be consumed in excess. Too much is no better for you than too little. Indiscriminate consumption of fi-

TABLE 3-4 Fiber content of selected foods

Food	Fiber (grams)
Fruits	
Apple, with peel	4.2
Banana	3.3
Blackberries (1 cup)	9.7
Dates, chopped (1 cup)	15.5
Grapes	1
Orange	2.9
Peach, peeled	2
Pear, with skin	4.9
Prunes, dried, pitted (10)	13.5
Raisins, seedless (1 cup)	9.6
Breads	
Oatmeal bread (1 slice)	0.86
Pumpernickel bread (1 slice)	1.33
Rye bread (1 slice)	1.65
Wheat bread (1 slice)	1.4
Whole-wheat bread (1 slice)	3.17
White bread (1 slice)	0.68
Cereals	
Bran Chex (⅔ cup)	5
Bran flakes (⅔ cup)	5
Cheerios (1¼ cup)	2
Corn flakes (1 cup)	1
Grapenuts (1¼ cup)	2
Raisin Bran (½ cup)	4
Rice Krispies (1 cup)	trace
Shredded Wheat (1 biscuit)	3
Life (⅔ cup)	3
Vegetables	
Lima beans (½ cup)	4.6
Green beans (1 cup)	3.1
Cauliflower (½ cup)	1.3
Corn, canned (½ cup)	6.3
Garbanzo beans (1 cup)	8.6
Greens (1 cup)	2.9
Navy beans (1 cup)	16.5
Baked potato, with skin	4.4
Tomato	2.2
Carrot	2.0

ber may interfere with the body's ability to absorb other essential nutrients. A person who eats bulky foods but has only a small capacity may not be able to take in enough food energy or nutrients. Another point to remember is that a high intake of dietary fiber, for example, 60 grams per day, also requires a high intake of water.[4]

Complex carbohydrates and cancer. Foods associated with decreased cancer risk are commonly found in the complex-carbohydrates group. Consumption of cruciferous vegetables, such as cabbage, broccoli, brussels sprouts, and cauliflower, are thought to help prevent cancer of the gastrointestinal and respiratory tracts. Fruits and vegetables rich in vitamin A have been linked to a reduction in cancer of the ovaries, bladder, larynx, esophagus, and lung. Good sources of vitamin A are carrots, spinach, tomatoes, apricots, peaches, and cantaloupes. Cancer of the stomach and esophagus is less common among people whose diets are rich in ascorbic acid, or vitamin C. Green and yellow vegetables and citrus fruits are excellent sources of vitamin C.

A word of caution is worth noting about the relationship between cancer and diet: It is difficult for scientists to provide firm, solid evidence about the cancer-inhibiting qualities of a particular food. The interaction between food and disease is complex, and it may take 20 to 40 years to determine a relationship between cancer and diet. This is mentioned not so much to give people a reason to disregard dietary guidelines for preventing cancer as to prevent people from mistakenly thinking that if a little bit is good for you, a whole lot is much better. Some of the dietary practices that may help prevent cancer may lead to other toxic conditions if taken to the extreme. Therefore good judgment and moderation are as important here as they are in other nutritional matters.

Avoid Too Much Sugar

The *Dietary Guidelines* recommends that the diet of Americans be limited to 10% sugar. For most people this means cutting sugar consumption in half. The yearly consumption of sugar in 1986 by the average American was 130 pounds, or 20% of total caloric intake.[16] This figure represents an increase of 6 pounds per person per year since 1976, two thirds of which has been hidden in common products by manufacturers. Much of the hidden sugar is not listed as table sugar but as high-fructose corn syrup, the chief sweetening agent used by the food industry today.[8] Consequently, to hide the amount of sugar that is listed on a food label, manufacturers often list the different forms of sugar separately, for example, corn starch, sucrose, and corn syrup. This way, if sugar is the main ingredient, it doesn't appear first on the label.

Diets high in sugar are associated with obesity, malnutrition, heart disease, hypoglycemia, diabetes mellitus, hyperactivity, and tooth decay. Although experts debate the effect of sugar on the first six, there is little doubt that sugar is guilty of contributing to tooth decay.

Dental caries is caused by acid buildup brought about by bacterial growth in the mouth. Bacteria feed on carbohydrates, so it is only natural that sugar be implicated in tooth decay. To negate the effects of sugar on the teeth, brushing is recommended within the first 20 minutes after the mouth bacteria have had access to carbohydrates. If brushing is not practical, rinsing will help wash the sugar off the teeth. An even better action is to floss the teeth. It takes 24 hours for a large enough concentration of bacteria to accumulate on a tooth to produce enough acid to cause dental caries. Therefore flossing once a day can help offset the effect of a high-sugar diet on the teeth.

Nutritive sweeteners. Sweeteners, which provide calories, or food energy, are considered nutritive sweeteners. Each one provides about the same number of calories per gram. Sugars are widespread in nature, occurring in fruits, vegetables, honey, and milk. They are the building blocks of complex carbohydrates, such as starch. All carbohydrates must be broken down into usable energy, blood sugar, also called glucose.

Other common nutritive sweeteners. Included in this group of sweeteners are corn syrup, high-fructose corn syrup, sugar alcohols, and aspartame. *Corn syrup* is often used in foods as a partial or complete replacement for sucrose (table sugar) because it is less sweet and it provides texture. *High-fructose corn syrup* is sweeter than sucrose and is the main nutritive sweetener in soft drinks. Because it is sweeter than sucrose, it can be used in smaller quantities, which in turn allows for a somewhat lower-calorie product. *Sugar alcohols*, such as *sorbitol*, are less sweet than sucrose and are used to add texture to hard candies and gums. *Aspartame*, which is marketed as *Nutrasweet*, has about the same number of calories as sucrose but is 180 to 220 times as sweet. Therefore only a small amount is needed to sweeten products. The taste of aspartame is similar to that of sucrose, and aspartame leaves no aftertaste. Because aspartame is derived partially from an amino acid, phenylalanine, products containing aspartame must be labelled to warn individuals who have the inherited disease *phenylketonuria*. More than 100 studies have analyzed the various effects that aspartame may have on health. Although questions continue to be raised, there is currently no scientific evidence to dispute aspartame's safety.[16]

Non-nutritive   sweeteners. Non-nutritive sweeteners do not contribute any food energy, or calories, to the diet. The most widely used non-nutritive sweetener is *saccharin.* It is approximately 300 times as sweet as sucrose and is colorless, odorless, and water-soluble. Although it has been linked to bladder tumors in second-generation rats fed high doses, studies involving normal consumption of saccharin by humans have not revealed any adverse health effects.[16]

Cyclamate is another non-nutritive sweetener. Cyclamate is 30 times sweeter than sucrose. It has an advantage over saccharin in that it has no aftertaste. The disadvantage of cyclamate is that it was linked with cancer and banned from the marketplace by the Food and Drug Administration (FDA) in the late 1960s. The FDA recently lifted its ban on cyclamate when studies could not prove that it causes cancer. Cyclamate is likely to emerge in the near future as a leading product in the food industry.

Does the use of artificial sweeteners lead to weight reduction? There have never been scientific studies that show that use of artificial sweeteners leads to weight reduction. On the contrary, although sugar substitutes are low in calories, they may actually stimulate the appetite. Unlike sugar, which produces a feeling of *satiety*, or fullness, non-nutritive sweeteners do nothing to ease the appetite and may in fact encourage a craving for sweets by turning on sweet sensors on the tongue without putting sugar into the bloodstream. Even worse, people who use artificial sweeteners may compensate by eating more fats. In a study at Roosevelt Hospital Center in New York City, when aspartame was substituted for sugar, fat intake increased.[17]

Avoid Too Much Salt

Salt contains about 40% sodium by weight and is used widely in the preservation, processing, and preparation of foods. Although sodium is an essential mineral, it is consumed by adults in the United States at levels far beyond the RDA

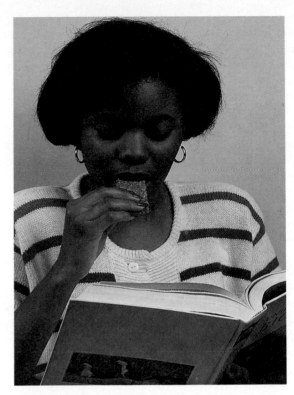

While substituting artificial sweeteners for table sugar helps cut sugar consumption, two thirds of the sugar we consume is "hidden" in other foods.

of 500 milligrams (one tenth of a teaspoon) per day [8] and more than double the 1100 to 3300 milligrams considered safe and adequate.[2] Most people average about 3 to 7 grams of sodium per day, which translates to 7.5 to 18 grams of salt. (A teaspoon of salt contains about 2 grams of sodium; a teaspoon of most dry substances equals approximately 5 grams.) The major health problem associated with consumption of too much sodium is hypertension (see Chapter 5). Approximately 10% of Americans are considered salt sensitive and risk contracting hypertension because of high salt intake.[4]

When trying to cut down on salt consumption, it is important to know that two thirds of the salt consumed is in the form of hidden salt added during the processing of food. Just how much salt is in a processed food can be determined by reading the package label.

Another important point about salt is that the taste buds are not always a good judge of salt content. Some foods that taste salty may be lower in salt content than those that don't taste salty. For example, peanuts taste salty because the salt is on the surface, where the taste buds immediately pick it up. Most people are surprised to learn that cheese contains more salt than peanuts or potato chips and that chocolate pudding contains even more salt.

To cut down on salt consumption:

- Avoid adding salt before tasting food.
- Add little or no salt to food at the table.
- Season food with sodium-free spices, such as pepper, allspice, onion powder, garlic, mustard powder, sage, thyme, and paprika.
- Avoid smoked meats and fish.
- Cut down on canned and instant soups.
- Read labels for sodium content, especially on processed food.

Drink Alcoholic Beverages In Moderation

Excessive use of alcohol is associated with liver disease, some types of cancer, high blood pressure, stroke, and disorders of the heart muscle. It is considered the principal cause of liver *cirrhosis* in the United States. Coupled with cigarette smoking, alcohol consumption increases the risk of developing cancer of the mouth, larynx, and esophagus. Also, alcohol plays a causal role in deaths from accidents, homicide, and suicide and is associated with disrupted family function.

Dietary Guidelines recommends that if an individual drinks alcoholic beverages, he or she should limit them to one or two drinks per day. One drink means 12 ounces of beer, 3 ounces of wine, or 1½ ounces (one jigger) of distilled spirits, each of which contains about 1 ounce of alcohol. A maximum level of alcohol consumption has not been set for women during pregnancy, so pregnant women and women who may become pregnant should refrain from using alcohol.

Nutrient Density

A key strategy for eating well is to select foods that offer significant amounts of nutrients but a small number of calories. If a particular food has a high ratio of nutrients to calories, it is referred to as a nutritionally dense food. This ratio, called **nutrient density,** provides a quantitative basis for judging the nutritional quality of food. The procedure for determining the nutrient density of food consists of adding together the percentage of the RDA for the eight essential nutrients listed on the package label for one serving and dividing by the number of calories per serving (Table 3-5). The higher the score, the higher the nutritional

quality (nutrient density) of the food. If two foods have the same number of calories per serving but one has more nutrients, it is said to be more nutritionally dense. It is possible to compute the nutrient density of any food with a detailed label or any item listed in the food charts in Appendix A.

The concept of nutrient density can help both the health-conscious and weight-conscious person make informed choices. Considering the countless number of foods available and the promises and claims that come with them, there is a need for a way to evaluate foods. Though not perfect, nutrient density is one technique that consumers can use to discriminate in their selection of food.

Food Labels

The FDA oversees the labelling of food products other than meat and poultry. By law the FDA requires that a label identify a product in a language the consumer can understand. It must indicate the manufacturer and the packer or distributor, declare the quantity of contents either in net weight or by volume, and list the common name of each ingredient in descending order of prominence. The definition, scientific names, and uses of some of the more common food ingredients are described in Figure 3-8.

Nutritional labels are required on packages that contain vitamin additives or make specific

▮ TABLE 3-5 Nutrient density

One way to determine the nutritional quality of food is to divide the percentage of the RDA of essential nutrients in one serving by the number of calories. A score of 32 or higher means that a food is nutritionally dense.

Example:	Pizza (cheese)
Calories:	354
Protein	28
Vitamin A	19
Vitamin C	20
Thiamin	25
Riboflavin	29
Niacin	19
Calcium	33
Iron	15
Total:	188
Nutrient density:	53% (188 ÷ 354 = 0.53)

Figure 3-8 Chemical terms on food labels

Preservatives

Chemicals added to food to lengthen their shelf life by inhibiting the growth of microorganisms or by preventing nutrients from breaking down. Sugar, salt, and spices are the most common preservatives. *Chemical names* include butylated hydroxyanisole (BHA), butylated hydroxytoluene (BHT), propyl gallate, calcium propionate, sodium propionate, ethylenediaminetetraaceticacid (EDTA), sodium benzoate, sodium nitrite, sorbic acid, and sulfiting agents. *Purposes and uses:* Retard decomposition of fats and oils, remove metal contamination caused by manufacturing processes, prevent growth of mold and bacteria, prevent food poisoning, and prevent discoloration of food.

Emulsifiers

Substances that enable oil and water to mix, such as those used in salad dressings, chocolates, margarine, ice cream, and baked goods. *Chemical names* include lecithin, monoglycerides, diglycerides, polysorbates 60, 65, and 80. *Purposes and uses:* Prevent various kinds of oils from separating from other ingredients, increase shelf life of some foods, and retard spoilage of some foods.

Thickeners and stabilizers

Agents used to add body to foods and improve their texture and consistency. *Chemical names* include carboxymethylcellulose, carrageenan, locust bean gum, modified starches, and sodium alginate. *Purposes and uses:* Used as a thickener and stabilizer in ice cream, beer, jelly, and cake icing; added to many diet foods because of its water-retention properties; prevent sugar from crystallizing in candy; and improve texture in some brands of baby food.

Flavor enhancers

Chemicals added to foods to improve their natural taste. *Chemical names* include disodium guanylate (GMP) and monosodium glutamate (MSG). *Purpose and use:* Restore flavors lost in food processing.

Other additives

Include such things as sweeteners, dyes, vitamins, and minerals.

What's not on a food label?

It is estimated that there are more than 3000 additives that are not required to be on labels. These include substances used during processing, such as solvents, adhesives, lubricating oils, detergents, and chemicals that seep into food from packaging. Other chemicals not found on labels are those used in early stages of food production, including antibiotics, fertilizers, insecticides, and herbicides.

health claims. Thus if a beverage claims to provide vitamin C or to be sugar-free, it must conform to food-labelling regulations. Food labels must include the following:

- Serving or portion size
- Number of calories and weight in grams of protein, carbohydrates, and fat per serving
- Percentage of the U.S. RDA for protein, five vitamins (vitamins A, C, thiamin, riboflavin, and niacin), and three minerals (calcium, iron, and sodium)

Exceptions to these labelling laws are staples that are made from standard recipes: mayonnaise, ketchup, canned vegetables, milk, ice cream, margarine, some breads, and meat and poultry products.

Although labels now provide some useful information, this is not to say that manufacturers are immune to labelling ploys like those listed below.

Catchy phrasing. One brand of corn chips claims to contain "measurable amounts of important nutrients." The problem is that *measurable* means no less than 2% of the RDA for the nutri-

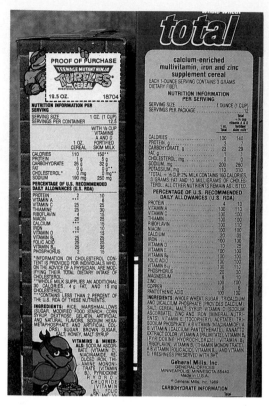

Food labels provide useful information about contents.

ents. Therefore to meet the RDA for a nutrient, it would be necessary to eat 50 bags of corn chips.

"Light," which is mentioned in Chapter 11, is another "catchy" term. For example, *Taco Bell's* Taco Light contains more calories than a taco, Soft Taco Supreme, or Super Combo Taco. According to a company spokesperson, the reason it is called "light" is that its fried, flour-based shell tends to be flakier and easier to chew than corn-based tortilla shells.[18]

Feature missing ingredient. The labels on some packages boast "no cholesterol" but may contain other additives, such as coconut oil, that can be even more objectionable. Rather than to concentrate on what is not in a product, it is just as important to know what is in it.

Invisible nutrients. Fruit, for example, makes more appearances on the outside of a package than on the inside. For instance, a beverage may have a grape taste but have no grapes in the ingredients.

Fortified. Many consumers are eager to buy products that are fortified with vitamins. Although foods fortified with vitamins are healthful, they should not necessarily be preferred over their nonfortified counterparts. It may be more

economical to purchase daily vitamin supplements to go with a nonfortified food. Adding vitamins costs food manufacturers only pennies per package, but the word "fortified" may increase the price significantly.

Manipulation of serving size. Some products claim to have more or fewer nutrients by changing the serving size. One brand of ice cream was labelled "low-fat" after a serving was redefined from 4 ounces to 3½ ounces.

Because American food labels rarely carry complete or accurate nutritional information and because of pressure from consumer groups and public health activists, sweeping changes in food-labelling practices are anticipated by the mid-1990s. Some of these changes include mandatory labelling for nearly all of the U.S. food supply. Future food labels should prove to be easier to read and provide information that makes clear whether a product is high in fat and what health-related terms, such as "low fat," "high fiber," and "light," mean.

Changes In American Eating Patterns

The stereotype of an American family with two parents and several children eating three meals a day appears to be a thing of the past. Changes in the American social picture, including an increase in single-person households, single-parent families, and women in the labor force, have had far-reaching effects on our way of living and subsequently on our eating patterns. Three trends are particularly prominent: snacking, eating at fast-food restaurants, and consuming frozen dinners.

Snacking

Snacks are foods consumed between the three main meals of the day. The majority of Americans have at least one snack per day, and the sale of snack foods is growing at a rate of 10% a year.[15] College students have shown preferences for soft drinks, candies, gum, and fresh fruit as snacks, followed by bakery items, milk, and both corn and potato chips.

Snacking is clearly a trend of the present and the future. But is snacking all bad? Not necessarily. In fact, studies have indicated that adolescents' snacks contribute as much nutrition as do their meals and that their snacking frequency may range upward to as many as seven eating occasions per day. Surveys also show that there is a correlation between snacks and nutritional well-being, meaning that adolescents get more complete nutrition with increases in snacks: those who snack more come closer to meeting the RDA of essential nutrients.[19]

The key issue is not the time or frequency of eating but rather what is eaten. Nutritionally dense foods eaten as snacks are just as good for health as they are when consumed at mealtime. The converse is also true: Foods low in nutrient density eaten at mealtime are just as worthless as they are when eaten as snacks. Although it is true that many Americans consume far too many empty-calorie foods, it is not correct to assume that snack foods are junk foods. Some nutritionists claim that there is no such thing as junk food. The problem occurs when a person's diet is dominated by foods low in nutrient density. With the exception of foods restricted for medical reasons, all foods can contribute to a healthful diet, provided a variety of foods is eaten in the right portions. Rather than to rule out snacking, we need to promote snack foods that enhance wellness.

Fast-Food Eating

Changes in the American family are mirrored in the trend toward eating in fast-food restaurants. Family meals at home are becoming the exception rather than the rule. Breakfasts and lunches are seldom eaten in a family setting by many American families. The evening family dinner also seems to be headed toward extinction. As many as 25% of American households do not have a sit-down dinner as often as five nights a week.[15] Instead, more and more families plan mealtimes at fast-food restaurants. And there are plenty of these restaurants from which to choose. From 1970 to 1980 alone, the number of fast-food restaurants in the United States more than quadrupled—from 30,000 to 140,000. Every day an estimated 46 million Americans eat in fast-food restaurants, ordering, among other things, approximately 200 hamburgers every second.[18]

From a nutritional viewpoint the criticisms of fast-food eating are the same as those of the rest of the American diet: too much protein, fat, calories, and sodium and not enough complex carbohydrates and fiber. In a study[20] of the claims made by popular restaurants, it was found that fast foods are typically high in calories because of their high fat content. The average meal of a cheeseburger, milk shake, and fries supplies about 1,500 calories, 43% of which comes from fat. Chicken and fish are just as fatty as other pro-

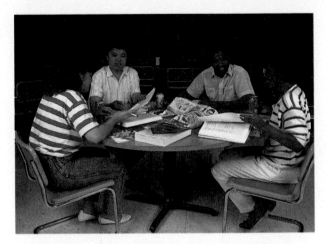

Snacking is clearly a trend of the present as well as the future.

tein sources at fast-food restaurants because they are breaded and fried. Frying has the same effect on potatoes. However, milk shakes get most of their calories from sugars. Table 3-6 gives the percentage of calories from fat, protein, and carbohydrates for selected fast-food items (see the Appendix for the nutritive values of fast-food items). The above study also found that more than half the food items tested contained more than 500 mg of sodium. Some contained more than 1000 mg.

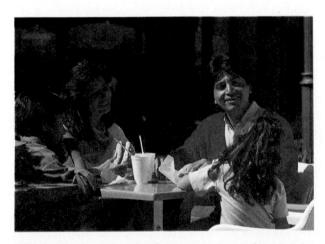

Family meals at fast-food restaurants are becoming the rule rather than the exception.

■ TABLE 3-6 Calorie sources of selected fast-food items

	Calories	Weight (grams)	Percentage of calories from protein	Percentage of calories from carbohydrates	Percentage of calories from fat
Arby's roast beef	350	140	25	36	39
Burger King Whopper	630	261	17	32	51
McDonald's Big Mac	563	204	18	29	53
Wendy's double hamburger	670	285	26	20	54
Church's Fried Chicken (white)	327	100	26	11	63
Church's Fried Chicken (dark)	305	100	29	9	62
Kentucky Fried Chicken Original Recipe (dark)	643	346	22	29	49
Kentucky Fried Chicken extra crispy (dark)	765	376	20	28	52
Long John Silver's fish (2 piece)	366	136	24	23	52
Taco Bell Burrito Supreme	457	225	18	38	43

Eating at fast-food restaurants does not have to be a nutritionally worthless experience. Owners of many restaurants are now aware that Americans are becoming more knowledgeable about the nutrient content of food and are demanding wholesome, safe, and nutritious foods. Consequently, there has been a trend toward more nutritious menus, including salad, pasta, and potato bars. By exercising good judgment in the choice of foods, an occasional meal at a fast-food chain does not have to compromise a well-balanced diet.

Frozen Dinners

Frozen dinners have become part and parcel of the American diet. Consumers spend $4 billion a year on them, and food manufacturers are constantly turning out new lines.[21] The challenge for health-conscious consumers is to determine which ones fit easily into a nutritious diet.

In a study[21] of frozen foods, a panel of judges applied strict criteria to identify entrees that are suitable for people wanting to limit their intake of fat, calories, and sodium while including in their diets essential vitamins and minerals. The results were encouraging. A total of 108 frozen

dishes were judged to be suitable. Thirty-six were "highly recommended" as meeting all of the criteria used in the study. Seventy-two were short in only one of the criteria. While space does not permit these entrees to be listed here (see Annotated Readings for the reference), it is helpful to know how to evaluate these items. By applying the following criteria, you should be able to conduct your own evaluation of frozen dinners:

■ A maximum of 300 calories
■ No more than 30% of calories from fat
■ No more than 800 mg of sodium
■ At least 15 grams of protein

However, it is important to remember that just because a dinner meets the above criteria, it does not necessarily provide every single nutrient. Some meals are likely to be deficient in some nutrients, so they will need to be supplemented. It is necessary to read the labels and add foods that will compensate for missing nutrients.

Planning a Nutrition Strategy for Wellness

Fortunately it isn't necessary to be a nutritionist to form a nutrition strategy that works for you.

A nutrition plan will work only if it is personalized. Several strategies should be helpful in personalizing your nutrition plan.

Assess Your Nutrition

Take an honest look at your eating choices. Analyze your nutrition profile (Assessment Activity 3-3) to determine if you are:

- Eating a variety of foods every day from the basic food groups (remember the 2:2:4:4 guide to eating, p. 39.
- Avoiding high-fat foods (more than the equivalent of 3 teaspoons of fat)
- Including sufficient fiber, including whole grains, dried beans, and fresh fruits and vegetables
- Consuming six to eight servings of water (8 ounces each)
- Limiting high-sugar desserts or sweets to no more than three or four each week
- Restricting your intake of high-salt foods like processed meats
- Consuming no more than one or two drinks a day or letting drinking interfere with your appetite

Make Small Adjustments

Remember the principle of changing health behavior (Chapter 2): the smaller the change, the longer it lasts. For example, rather than vowing to abstain from eating ice cream, make one small change at a time. Reduce the amount or number of servings at first. Try substituting a low-fat brand. If your diet is heavy in salt, gradually substitute sodium-free seasonings. If you have a sweet tooth, try low-sugar snacks. If you eat for fullness, prepare less food or leave food on your plate. Whatever adjustments need to be made, plan an approach that builds on the cumulative effect of many small successes.

Choose Foods For Wellness

Choosing foods for wellness means following the *Dietary Guidelines* for Americans. This means following a diet that

- Is low in highly saturated fat
- Emphasizes complex carbohydrates such as bread, potatoes, and pasta
- Provides six to eight glasses of water throughout the day
- Provides iron and calcium
- Emphasizes fresh fruits and vegetables
- Is low in sugar, salt, alcohol, and caffeine

Common Digestive Problems

Occasionally, people experience some kind of problem with their digestive system. Some of the more common problems include constipation, diarrhea, vomiting, ulcers, hiatal hernia, and diverticulitis. Most of the time these problems run a short course. However, sometimes long-term complications may occur and require medical intervention.

Constipation

Constipation is the condition of having painful or difficult bowel movements. It is important to note that pain and difficulty are the criteria for recognizing constipation, not time. Each person's digestive system responds to food in its own way with its own rhythm. If several days pass between movements but these movements take place without discomfort, the person is not constipated. If the *feces* is hard and is passed with difficulty, discomfort, or pain, the person can be said to be constipated.

Extended constipation is usually the result of stress or changes in routine (such as vacations, prolonged use of laxatives, low-fiber diets, insufficient intake of water or fluids, lack of exercise, and some medicines).

Changes in diet and lifestyle should be sufficient to correct most cases of constipation. Use of laxatives on a regular basis should be avoided because they can create a dependency cycle, in which the intestines become dependent on a laxative to facilitate a bowel movement. Some recommendations for preventing and/or overcoming constipation include:

- Increase physical activity. The muscles in the intestines that push food through the body are improved by any activity that increases the muscle tone of the entire body.
- Increase the fiber content of the diet. Fiber adds bulk to the intestines and absorbs a lot of water, softening the stools.
- Increase fluid intake. Fluids add bulk, which promotes *peristalsis*, or involuntary muscular contraction of the intestines.
- Increase consumption of naturally laxative fruits, such as prunes and figs.
- Rearrange lifestyle to ensure a daily regimen with regular eating and sleeping times.
- Allow time, as the body needs, to have a bowel movement.

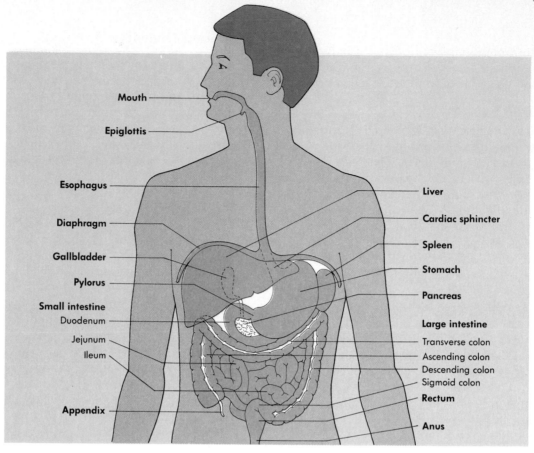

Figure 3-9 Diagram of the digestive system.

Diarrhea

Diarrhea is a condition characterized by frequent loose, watery stools. It indicates that food has moved too quickly through the intestines for fluid absorption to take place or that water has been drawn from the intestinal tract and added to the food residue. Possible causes include food poisoning, such as salmonellosis, food intolerance (lactose or milk intolerance is most common), a spastic or irritable colon, intestinal viruses, stress, and medications.

Diarrhea can become serious if it continues for several days. In an infant it may lead to dehydration in less than a day and require emergency medical treatment.

There are not many effective over-the-counter antidiarrheal medications. It may be necessary to consult a physician to obtain a prescription for a medicine that will allow the intestines to absorb the fluid or depress the contractions of the intestines.

Vomiting

Vomiting is not a disease, but rather it is a symptom of many different diseases. Regardless of the cause the waves of peristalsis reverse direction and expel material from the stomach, through the esophagus, and out the mouth. It is nature's way of getting rid of something irritating.

Simple vomiting is unpleasant, but it is usually no cause for alarm. If it continues long enough or is severe enough, it may be serious and require a doctor's care. In an infant it is especially serious because it can quickly deplete body fluids and cause an imbalance in body *electrolytes,* or body salts, that are essential to the life of cells. When this happens, fluids must be replaced often with intravenous feedings of a salt solution and sugar. This of course requires medical care.

Ulcers

A common digestive problem is ulcers of the stomach (gastric ulcers) or duodenum (duodenal ulcers) (see the diagram of the digestive system, Figure 3-9). A peptic ulcer includes both of these and is the most common type of ulcer. An *ulcer* is a sore of the top layer of cells of the stomach or duodenum. This leaves the underlying layers of cells exposed without protection, and anything that touches the exposed area causes pain. The sore may penetrate the underlying layers, causing bleeding, or may even perforate completely through the stomach or intestinal wall.

Ulcers are thought to be caused by stomach acids. The main portion of the stomach secretes hydrochloric acid and enzymes for the purpose of digesting food. To avoid digesting itself, the lining of the stomach and duodenum produces a protective mucous covering. However, when an excess amount of acid is produced, it overwhelms the mucous covering and erodes through the cells. The result is pain, usually experienced as deep and aching in nature. Sometimes instead of hurting, the ulcer produces only a sharp sense of hunger when the stomach is empty. The pain associated with peptic ulcers typically is present only when the stomach is empty[12] because there is nothing in the stomach to buffer the excess acid. Therefore some foods and antacids can bring soothing, temporary relief.

The most important aspect of treatment for ulcers is controlling or preventing acidity. One common drug therapy is the use of antacids. They are readily available and work best when taken as a liquid 1 to 2 hours after meals and at bedtime.[23] Newer drugs include those that suppress or block acid production, increase the ability of the intestinal wall to resist acid damage, or provide a protective coat for the intestinal wall.

Contrary to popular belief, diet does not seem to be an effective treatment for ulcers although if a particular food causes discomfort, it should be avoided. This is especially true for aspirinlike products, coffee, tea, alcohol, and highly seasoned, spicy foods, as well as cigarette smoking.

For some people stress and tension excite the nerves that control the stomach. This in turn increases acid secretion and may eventually lead to an ulcer. For these people learning how to relax and handle stress may be the best preventive measure for ulcers. If medical treatment is needed, consult a physician. Ulcers are not typically suited for self-treatment.

Hiatal Hernia

"Hiatus" means "opening"; "hernia" means "the protrusion of one body part through another." *Hiatal hernia* occurs when the stomach pushes through the hiatus of the diaphragm (Figure 3-10). This allows food to be trapped in the herniated area of the stomach and, mixed with acid, to be regurgitated back up into the lower portion of the esophagus. This irritates the

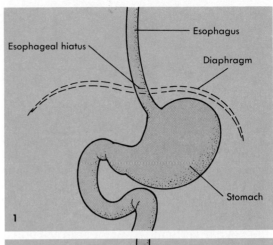
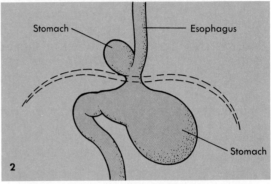
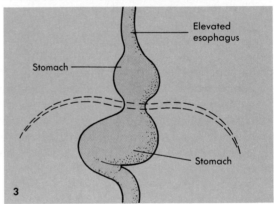

Figure 3-10 Hiatal hernia.

esophagus, causing the burning sensation in the chest typically referred to as *heartburn*. The term "heartburn" is actually a misnomer because the heart is not affected. It would be more accurate to call this condition esophageal burn.

Several guidelines are recommended for persons with hiatal hernia:

▪ Use of antacids may help to relieve the burning sensation. Large hiatal hernias may require surgery.

▪ Avoid eating large meals, which stretch the

stomach. Several small meals are preferable to one large meal.
- In the case of obesity, weight reduction may help.
- Avoid leaning over or lying down immediately after meals.
- Avoid tight-fitting clothes, which compress the intestines against the stomach.

Diverticular Disease

Small, pouch-like swellings known as diverticula sometimes develop in the walls of the intestine (see Figure 3-11). When this happens, a person is said to have *diverticulosis*. Many older people have diverticulosis without ever knowing it because they have no symptoms. Sometimes for no known reason, one or more of the diverticula becomes infected. This condition is called *diverticulitis*.

Symptoms of diverticulosis include cramping and tenderness in the left side of the abdomen, occasional attacks of diarrhea, presence of blood in bowel movements, and bowel movements that are small and hard.

In the case of diverticulitis, severe abdominal pain also may occur in the left side of the abdomen. The pain may start off spasmodically and then become constant. Nausea and fever are also common. Left untreated, diverticulitis can lead to serious complications, cause abscesses, and even rupture, causing a serious medical emergency.

If your bowels behave in an unusual manner for more than a week or two, or if you have persistent pain in the lower part of the abdomen, consult a physician. Diagnostic tests are available to detect diverticular disease. In the case of diverticulosis, ways to minimize pressure within the colon and possibly help prevent more diverticula from forming include the following[24]:
- Eat a diet rich in fiber. Fiber facilitates bowel movements by making the stools soft and easier to pass.
- Drink eight or more cups of liquid every day. Fiber draws water into the stool. Fluids increase the effect of fiber in moving food through the colon.

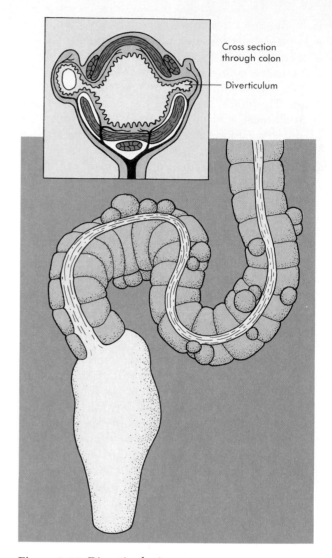

Cross section through colon

Diverticulum

Figure 3-11 Diverticulosis.

- Respond to an urge for a bowel movement. Delaying bowel movements may lead to drier, more compact stools, which can increase the pressure within the colon. This in turn can weaken the wall of the colon and permit a diverticulum to form.
- Avoid laxatives. They can irritate your colon and make you dependent on them for regular bowel movements.

If diverticulitis is present, immediate medical intervention is required.

Summary

- The major nutritional problems of Americans are due primarily to dietary excess and imbalance.
- A good nutritional plan is one that consists of a variety of foods from the basic food groups.
- The recommended diet for Americans calls for an emphasis on complex carbohydrates as the major source of energy.
- The greatest shortcoming of the American diet is the overconsumption of fat, especially saturated fat.
- There is considerable variation in the amount of saturated, monounsaturated, and polyunsaturated fat in various foods. Most foods contain a mixture of these fats.
- A diet high in starch is likely to be lower in fat, especially saturated fat and cholesterol, lower in calories, and higher in fiber.
- Fiber benefits the body by adding bulk to the contents of the intestines, increasing the transit of food

through the body, which reduces the chance of developing colon cancer, and lowering blood-cholesterol levels.
- Consumption of fruits and cruciferous vegetables are associated with a decreased risk of cancer.
- Sugar and salt are consumed in the United States in excessive amounts. Most of the time they are hidden in common products to which they have been added by food manufacturers.
- A food has a high index of nutritional quality when it has a high ratio of nutrients to calories.
- The criticisms of fast-food eating are the same as those of the rest of the American diet: too much protein, fat, calories, sodium, and sugar, not enough complex carbohydrates and fiber.
- Sound nutritional practices may prevent the occurrence of common digestive problems, including constipation, hiatal hernia, and diverticular disease.

 ## Action plan for personal wellness

An important consideration in assuming responsibility for the individual's own quality of life is using information. After reading this chapter, answer the following questions and determine an action plan for enhancing your own lifestyle.

1 Based on the information presented in this chapter and what I know about my family's health history, the issues related to nutrition that I need to be most concerned about are:_____

_____

_____

_____

2 Of the nutrition issues listed in number 1, the one I most need to act on is:_____

3 Possible actions that I can take to improve my ability to form a plan for good nutrition are (try to be as specific as possible):_____

_____

4 Of the actions listed in number 3, the one that I most need to include in an action plan is:_____

_____

5 Factors I need to keep in mind to be successful in my action plan are:_____

_____

_____

Review Questions

1. What is meant by the statement that nutritional diseases of the past have been replaced by diseases of dietary excess and imbalance?
2. What are the importance and implications of variety as it relates to planning a nutritionally bal-

anced diet?
3. What is the difference between a high-quality, complete protein and a low-quality, incomplete protein?
4. What are the similarities and differences between

water-soluble and fat-soluble vitamins?

5. Under what circumstances if any should vitamin and/or mineral supplements be added to a person's daily regimen?

6. What are the rules about water and the functions of it that make water an essential nutrient?

7. What is the difference between saturated and unsaturated fats? What are some food sources for each?

8. What are five dietary practices that will help lower consumption of fat, especially saturated fat?

9. How does a diet high in complex carbohydrates contribute to health and wellness?

10. What are the major benefits of soluble and insoluble fiber in the diet?

11. What is the relationship between cancer and diet?

12. What effects have snacking and fast-food eating had on the nutritional status of Americans?

13. What are six guidelines for planning a diet that satisfies the criteria presented in *Dietary Guidelines for Americans*?

14. What are the similarities and differences among the causes and characteristics of common digestive problems, including constipation, diarrhea, vomiting, ulcers, hiatal hernia, and diverticular disease?

References

1. Office of Disease Prevention and Health Promotion: Disease prevention/health promotion: the facts, Palo Alto, Calif, 1988, Bull Publishing Co.

2. US Department of Health and Human Services: The surgeon general's report on nutrition and health, Washington, DC, 1988, US Government Printing Office.

3. US Department of Health and Human Services: Nutrition and your health: dietary guidelines for Americans, ed 2, Washington, DC, 1985, US Government Printing Office.

4. Wardlaw G and Insel P: Perspectives in nutrition, St Louis, Mo, 1990, Times Mirror/Mosby College Publishing.

5. Council on Scientific Affairs of the American Medical Association: Vitamin preparations as dietary supplements and as therapeutic agents, Contemp Nutrition 13(3,4):2, 1988.

6. Lamb L: Colds, flu and pneumonia, The Health Letter 34(8):3, 1989.

7. Mayer J: Getting the most from the most essential nutrient, Tufts University Diet and Nutrition Letter 4(8):3, 1986.

8. National Research Council: Recommended dietary allowances, ed 10, Washington, DC, 1989, National Academy Press.

9. Beware of snacks made with "pure vegetable oil," Tufts University Diet and Nutrition Letter 5(3):1, 1987.

10. Consumers Union: What's your nutrition IQ? Consumer Report 55(5): 322, 1990.

11. Williams L: Importers' group launches palm oil defense, *Los Angeles Times*, p. IV:5, Feb 2, 1989.

12. The American Heart Association diet: an eating plan for healthy Americans, Dallas, Texas, 1985, The Association.

13. Consumers Union: The fiber furor, Consumer Report 51(10):640, 1986.

14. How to add fiber to your diet, Mayo Clinic Health Letter 8(5):2, 1990.

15. Williams SR: Nutrition and diet therapy, ed 6, St Louis, Mo, 1989, Times Mirror/Mosby College Publishing.

16. The Institute of Food Technologists' Expert Panel on Food Safety and Nutrition: Sweeteners: nutritive and non-nutritive, Contemp Nutrition 12(8):1, 1987.

17. Shell ER: Nutrition sweetness and health, The Atlantic Monthly 256(2):20, 1985.

18. Mayer J: How fast food figures in, Tufts University Diet and Nutrition Letter 8(1):7, 1990.

19. Bigler-Doughton S and Jenkins RM: Adolescent snacks: nutrient density and nutritional contribution to total intake, J Am Diet Assoc 87(12):1678, 1987.

20. Consumers Union: Fast foods, Consumer Report 49:367, July 1984.

21. Mayer J: Special report: more than 100 frozen dinners worth heating, Tufts University Diet and Nutrition Letter 8(2):3, 1990.

22. Duodenal ulcers, Mayo Clinic Health Letter 7(9):1, 1989.

23. Ulcer drugs—old and new, Harvard Medical School Health Letter 11(5):2, 1986.

24. Diverticulosis, Mayo Clinic Health Letter 8(5):2, 1990.

Annotated Readings

1. American Heart Association: The American Heart Association diet: an eating plan for healthy Americans, Dallas, Texas, 1985, National Center of the American Heart Association.
   Practical, concise booklet on ways to plan a diet that reduces the risk of heart diseases. Emphasis is on food choices that are low in saturated fat and cholesterol.

2. Barone J and Barnett R: Eat smart, Am Health 7:64, March 1987.
   The authors explore a unique approach to balanced nutrition that focuses on combining various types of foods and enhancing the body's absorption of vital nutrients.

3. Mayer J: Special report: more than 100 frozen dinners worth heating, Tufts University Diet and Nutrition Letter 8(2):3, 1990.
   Identifies 108 frozen dinners that are suitable for people trying to limit intake of fat, calories, and sodium.

4. National Research Council: Recommended dietary allowances, ed 10, Washington, DC, 1989, National Academy Press.
   Widely regarded as the authoritative source on nutrient allowances for healthy people. Reviews the function of each nutrient in the human body, food sources, usual dietary intake, and effects of deficiencies and excessive intake.

5. Wardlaw G and Insel P: Perspectives in nutrition, St Louis, Mo, 1990, Times Mirror/Mosby College Publishing.
   An extensive, in-depth, comprehensive presentation on all aspects of nutrition.

ASSESSMENT ACTIVITY   3-1

Assessing Your Protein RDA

Directions: Complete the following steps to determine your RDA for protein.

1. How much do you weigh?   _____ pounds
2. Convert weight in pounds to kilograms by   _____ kilograms
   dividing pounds by 2.2.
3. Multiply kilograms by 0.8.   _____ grams
                                                             Your protein RDA

(Example: Someone who weighs 150 pounds needs 54 g of protein. 150 ÷ 2.2 = 68 kg; 68 kg × 0.8 = 54 g of protein.)

ASSESSMENT ACTIVITY   3-2

Assessing Your Maximum Daily Fat Intake

Directions: To figure the maximum number of grams of fat you should consume per day to stay within the dietary guidelines of 30% of total daily calories in fat, complete the following steps:

1. Enter your body weight   _____ pounds
2. Caloric intake   _____ calories
   Multiply your weight by 15. (This gives a rough estimate of
   the number of calories you consume on a daily basis, assuming that you are not in a weight-loss or weight-gain
   program.)
3. Recommended maximum fat calories   _____ calories
   (Multiply caloric intake by 0.3)   _____ grams
4. Recommended maximum fat intake
   Divide maximum fat calories by 9. (This is a necessary step
   because food-composition tables report the fat content of
   foods in terms of grams. Grams can be converted to
   ounces by dividing by 28.)

Example for an individual weighing 185 pounds:

1. Body weight   _____ 185 pounds
2. Caloric intake   _____ 2775 calories
   (185 × 15 = 2775)
3. Recommended maximum fat calories   _____ 822 calories
   (2775 × 0.3 = 822)
4. Recommended maximum intake   _____ 92 grams
   (822 ÷ 9 = 92)

(This amounts to approximately 3 ounces of fat [92 ÷ 28 = 3.3])

ASSESSMENT ACTIVITY

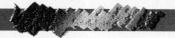

3-3

Nutrition Assessment

Part I: One-day Assessment

One way to determine if you're getting sufficient quantities of the proper nutrients is to keep a record of your diet. Ideally this should cover a time span of at least a week. However, in this exercise you are asked to assess your dietary selections for only *one day*. Therefore it is important to choose a day that is most representative of your overall nutritional practices.

Directions:

1. Use the following form to record your dietary selections. Include all foods and beverages, and specify the amount eaten, how cooked, etc. Don't forget to list condiments and seasonings, such as mustard, ketchup, butter, and dressings, and trimmings, such as lettuce, onions, marshmallows, sugar, etc. The more detailed your record, the more you will learn from this assessment and the more accurate your nutrition assessment will be.

2. Once foods have been listed, refer to the nutritive values of foods (see Appendix) and record appropriate values in the spaces provided. If some foods are not included in the Appendix, refer to package labels if available to determine nutritive values.

3. When you have finished with this assessment, proceed to Part II to determine your nutrition profile.

Part II: Nutrition profile

Food	Calories	Protein (grams)	Vitamin A (iU)	Vitamin C (milligrams)	Thiamin (milligrams)	Riboflavin (milligrams)	Niacin (milli-grams)	Calcium (milligrams)	Iron (milli-grams)
Total*									

*Transfer totals to Part II.

Continued.

Based on the results of your one-day assessment, indicate how you are doing in meeting the RDA for the nutrients listed below.

1. Transfer your totals from Part I to the second column below.

2. Compare these with the RDAs in the third and fourth columns, and indicate how you are doing in the last column.

3. Go to Part III to complete this assessment.

		RDA†		
Nutrients	Total*	Men	Women	How are you doing‡
Protein	_____	56 g	44 g	_____
Vitamin A	_____	1000 (IU)	800 (IU)	_____
Vitamin C	_____	60 mg	60 mg	_____
Thiamin	_____	1.5 mg	1.1 mg	_____
Riboflavin	_____	1.7 mg	1.3 mg	_____
Niacin	_____	19 mg	14 mg	_____
Calcium	_____	800 mg	800 mg	_____
Iron	_____	10 mg	18 mg	_____

*Total values from Part I: One-Day Assessment.

†RDAs for healthy adults.

‡Subtract RDA from your total. A positive value means that you are meeting the RDA for that nutrient; a negative value means that you are deficient in that nutrient.

Part III: nutrition prescription

Directions: Transfer the results from the last column in Part II to the first column below. For the nutrients with a negative value (indicating you are below the RDA), write a prescription of foods that will eliminate the deficiency. Refer to the nutritive values of food (see Appendix A) to identify specific foods and amounts that will provide 100% of the RDA for each nutrient. These foods can be viewed as your nutrition prescription.

Nutrients	How are you doing?	Food prescription
Protein	_____	_____
Vitamin A	_____	_____
Vitamin C	_____	_____
Thiamin	_____	_____
Riboflavin	_____	_____
Niacin	_____	_____
Calcium	_____	_____
Iron	_____	_____

ASSESSMENT ACTIVITY   3-4

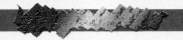

Eating Behaviors to Think About

Directions: Answer the following questions to reveal information about your eating habits, how you developed certain tastes, and your attitude about various foods.

1 When was the last time you tried a new food? What was the food? What were the circumstances?

2 What new foods have you learned to eat during the past year?

3 Name the foods that have been on your "won't try" list (that is, foods that you won't eat under any circumstances).

4 What special events do you celebrate in some way with food?

5 Where is your favorite place to eat?

6 If you were to go on an eating binge, what foods would you be most likely to eat?

7 Describe in detail your favorite meal.

8 Do you consider yourself a slow eater, moderately fast eater, or gulper? What do you think is responsible for your eating pattern?

9 What do you consider to be your good eating habits? Poor eating habits?

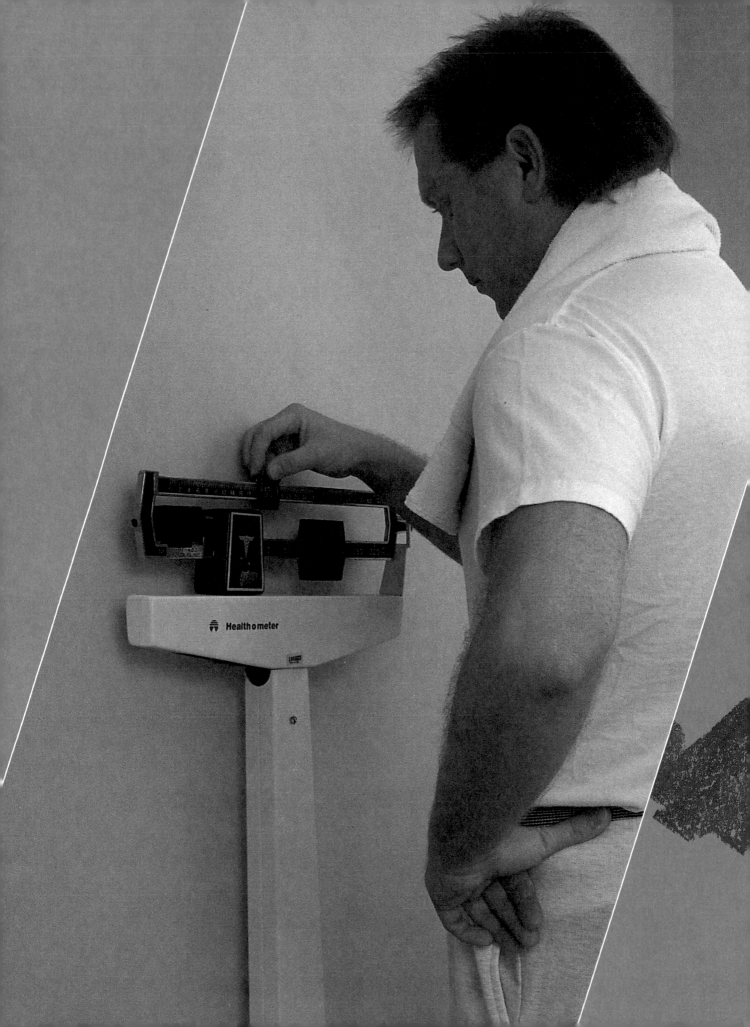

Chapter 4

Overcoming the Diet and Weight Obsession

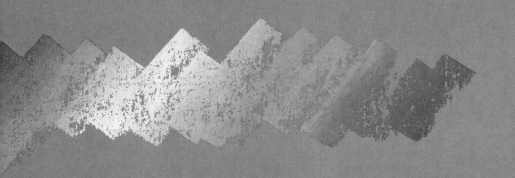

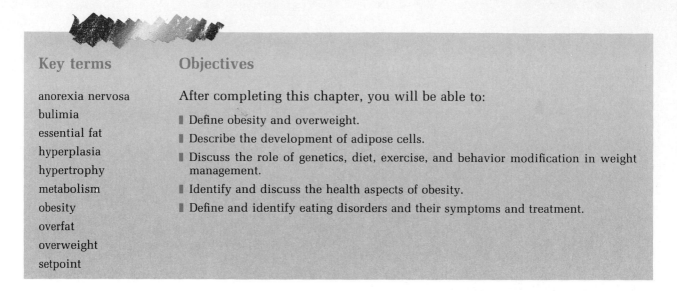

Key terms

anorexia nervosa

bulimia

essential fat

hyperplasia

hypertrophy

metabolism

obesity

overfat

overweight

setpoint

Objectives

After completing this chapter, you will be able to:

▌ Define obesity and overweight.

▌ Describe the development of adipose cells.

▌ Discuss the role of genetics, diet, exercise, and behavior modification in weight management.

▌ Identify and discuss the health aspects of obesity.

▌ Define and identify eating disorders and their symptoms and treatment.

mericans are obsessed with their body weight and the means of losing excess pounds that have accumulated over the years. Why are we so preoccupied, how have we gotten into such a predicament, and what are appropriate solutions to weight management? This chapter attempts to answer these and other important questions.

The Changing Ideal: Thinness on the Wane

American society is dynamic and constantly changing. Trends come and go in a blink of an eye. Just a few years ago the slogan was "thin is in." Today, we are witnessing the inevitable seeds of change. The latest Gallup poll indicates that for both sexes the fit and muscular look is gaining momentum and the thin look is on the way out.[1] From a health and an aesthetic perspective this represents a positive change that was too long in coming. Many dieters starved themselves in an effort to achieve what was for them the impossible dream. Many more women than men superimposed the ultrathin ideal upon themselves even though it was realistically unattainable for most, despite sacrificial efforts. Failure to attain the ultrathin silhouette for many who tried was devastating to both body image and ego.

The thinness mania, pervasive since the 1960s, is finally relenting. Although ultrathinness was unachievable and/or unmaintainable for the majority of aspiring weight watchers, development and maintenance of physical fitness is within the grasp of most if not all people. As opposed to the unhealthy nature of extreme thinness, the pursuit of physical fitness implies development of large energy reserves and confers health benefits that reduce the risks associated with many of today's chronic diseases. Additionally the processes leading to development of physical fitness naturally encourage leanness.

The Gallup pollsters found that only 35% of the women who responded wanted to be thin though 50% claimed that they were satisfied to be average. None of them wanted to be flabby. Forty-eight percent of the men clearly preferred to be muscular, and only 29% preferred the lean look.

This poll uncovered some interesting data regarding how both of the sexes think they are perceived by the other. Sixty-two percent of the women reported having a soft-looking body, and they predicted that this was preferred by men. As it turned out, they were correct because 59% of the men agreed with them. Only 20% of the men were fond of the Fonda-like hard-body look. Interestingly, the women in the study seemed to be unaffected by the men's preference for the soft look because the majority of women aspired to have the hard-body look and wanted to become physically stronger. The emerging ideal of today's woman is one who is muscular, fit, healthy, vibrant, energetic, and feminine. Many contemporary women are living examples of the coalescence of fitness, strength, and femininity.

The desirability of this ideal is affected by a woman's educational level. Sixty-five percent of college-educated women wanted the hard-body look, compared with 27% of women without a college degree. More college-educated men prefer women with muscles than do men who have not earned a college degree.

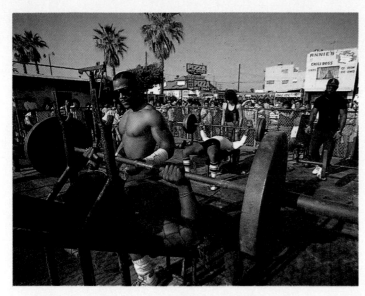

Most men would prefer to look this way.

The Gallup poll also revealed that men were not as preoccupied with body weight as women but that overall muscularity and chest and shoulder size were important and desirable. Women preferred muscular men, but they were not quite as demanding in this preference as men perceived them to be. Females reported that they would be satisfied with an average-sized man: 5 feet, 11 inches tall and weighing 171 pounds.

Obesity: Some Basics

Obesity, or overfatness, refers to an excessive amount of storage fat, which is related to gender; that is, it is defined as body fat that is equal to or greater than 25% of the body weight of males and 30% or greater of the body weight of females. These values are somewhat arbitrary because an optimal health-oriented definition of obesity is unavailable at this time. The point at which fat storage actually increases health risks has not been determined. Methods of assessing the amount of body fat are indirect, and each contains a degree of measurement error. Still, most authorities, as reflected in the guidelines set by the American College of Sports Medicine, agree that obesity begins at 30% of total weight for females, and it occurs between 20% and 25% of total weight for males.[2]

Overweight refers to excessive weight for one's height without regard for *body composition,* which is the ratio of lean versus fat tissue in the body. Because the term *overweight* makes no allowances for body composition, it is a poor criterion to use when making decisions regarding the desirability of weight loss. For example, well-muscled individuals may be overweight and yet

be lean in regard to the amount of body fat. This is not only healthy but, as the Gallup Poll indicates, aesthetic and desirable as well. By the same token, other individuals may be well within the norms for total body weight but **overfat,** that is, they carry a large proportion of their body weight in the form of fat rather than lean tissue. This is unhealthy and unattractive by American social standards.

The evidence that we as a nation are overweight and obsessed with taking corrective measures is reflected in the number of people who are attempting to change their physical appearance. Twenty-four percent of men and 27% of women between the ages of 20 and 74 weigh at least 20% more than what is recommended by nutritionists.[3] These people meet or exceed the definition of clinical obesity as determined by the National Institutes of Health (NIH). Nearly 90% of Americans judge their weight to be excessive. Approximately 35% want to lose at least 15 pounds; 30% of the women and 16% of the men are dieting at any given time; 31% of women age 19 to 39 diet at least once per month; and 16% consider themselves to be perpetual dieters.

The obsession with weight control does not stop with adults; it permeates all age groups. Eighty percent of fourth-grade girls have had at least one experience with dieting. Approximately 20% of this nation's children and adolescents between the ages of 5 and 17 are obese. This figure is 40% higher than 20 years ago.[4] This trend was also observed in the National Children and Youth Fitness Study (NCYFS).[5] *Skinfold measures* (a method of determining the amount of body fat and expressing it as a percentage of total weight) on elementary-school children were sig-

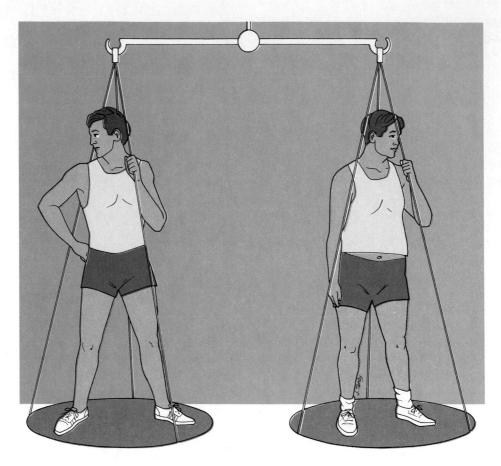

Many people who are the same age, height, and sex may weigh the same, but one can be overfat while the other is not.

nificantly higher in 1986 than they were two decades ago. Weight management is difficult for obese children, and it may be worsened by the tendency for them to develop more fat cells than children of normal weight. Obese children, who are often the progeny of obese parents, have a much higher probability of becoming obese adults than children of normal-weight parents. Americans of all ages are attempting to slim down to achieve their perceived optimal or ideal size. But many of them are, no doubt, using approaches that are guaranteed to fail.

Factors That Affect Body Weight

Diet, exercise, and heredity are the major factors currently associated with the loss or gain of body weight. Until recently, advice to overfat persons has been simplistic and imprecise. For example, the suggestion that a person simply "cut back on calories" ignores many essential elements of healthy eating. It does not provide information on the nutritional changes that are appropriate for successful weight management. Sec-

ond, the term *weight loss* is too generic and implies that indiscriminate weight loss—liquid, fat, and protein—represents a successful program. Advice to aspiring weight watchers can be enhanced by including the following points:

- The success of a weight-management program should be measured by the amount of fat lost rather than by muscle or fluid loss.
- The term *weight loss* should be replaced by the more specific term *"fat-weight loss."*
- It is important to reduce calories from fatty foods and calorically dense and nutritionally poor foods, such as alcohol and sugar-laden snacks, and to increase the proportion of calories derived from foods high in complex carbohydrates, such as potatoes and pasta.
- Exercise that meets the prescribed specifications for fat loss through appropriate manipulation of intensity, frequency, duration, and type should be an integral component of the program.
- Behavior-modification strategies can positively supplement a successful program.
- Successful, permanent weight loss is rarely

the result of following a diet for "X" number of weeks; rather it is the result of healthy lifestyle changes that can be pursued throughout a lifetime.

Development of Obesity

Adipose cells (fat cells) grow by **hypertrophy** (an increase in size) and **hyperplasia** (an increase in number). Obesity occurs when fat cells increase excessively in size and/or number. Obesity that results from an increase in the size of fat cells is hypertrophic, obesity that results from an increase in the number of fat cells is hyperplastic, and obesity that results from an increase in both the size and number of fat cells is hypertrophic/hyperplastic.

Adipose cells follow a normal pattern of growth and development. They increase significantly in size during the first 6 months of *postnatal* (after birth) life, and by 1 year of age they are similar in size to those of adolescents.[6] From 1 year of age to puberty, the size of fat cells remains essentially stable, but the cells proliferate in number, so growth is hyperplastic during this period. During puberty both size and number of fat cells increase substantially.

Childhood obesity and juvenile-onset obesity are usually due to the combined effects of hypertrophy and hyperplasia of fat cells. Of adult-onset obesity, 80% to 90% tends to be primarily hypertrophic, but extreme obesity in adulthood may be hyperplastic as well.[7]

Adipose cells have a long lifespan. If adult obesity is both hypertrophic and hyperplastic, is it more difficult to lose weight than if adult obesity is due to hypertrophy alone? There is some evidence that an increased *number* of fat cells increases the body's reluctance to reduce fat stores. It is indeed possible that the needs of adipose cells require that they store at least nominal amounts of fat.[8] If this intriguing proposition is correct, more fat cells would result in more fat storage, and this would certainly complicate efforts to lose weight. This is speculative, but it is known that the longer a person remains obese, the more intractable the condition becomes. (See Figure 4-1.)

Gender differences in depositing subcutaneous fat become noticeable during and after puberty. Males distribute fat primarily in the upper half of the body, but females tend to deposit it in the lower half (Figure 4-2). The percentage of fat in the body reaches peak values during early adolescence for males and then declines during the

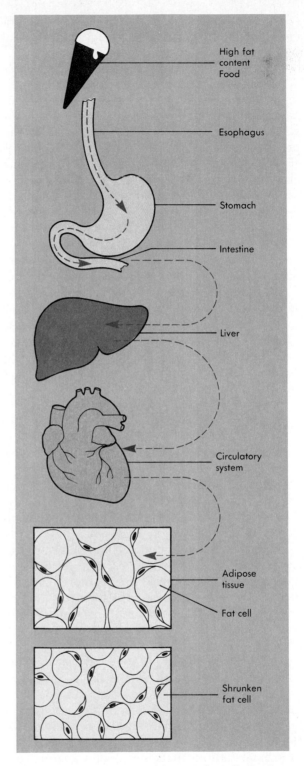

Figure 4-1 Fat can be manufactured in the body from any food and stored when calorie intake exceeds expenditure. Fat droplets travel to the liver from the stomach and intestines, and then enter the circulatory system where they are delivered to the cells and organs. Excess fats are stored in adipose tissue. When more energy is needed, fats are released from adipose cells. If the energy needs continue, the cells will shrink.

remainder of adolescent growth. Females experience a continuous increase in the percentage of fat from the onset of puberty to age 18.

From approximately 2 years of age, obese children develop a greater number of fat cells than children of normal weight. Some evidence has suggested that overfeeding during infancy stimulates development of excess fat cells and predisposes affected children to later obesity. However, more recent evidence indicates that obesity later in life is unaffected by overfeeding early in life, though underfeeding in early life does not guarantee that obesity will be prevented in later life.[3] Neonatal adiposity is not a good predictor of adult obesity. Studies have shown that most infants who are obese tend to slim down to normal weight by age 9. Although several longitudinal studies (research methods in which the same subjects are studied over a long period) have shown that obese infants do not become obese adults, approximately 80% of obese children remain obese during adulthood. Obviously certain forces become operative between infancy and childhood that contribute to adult obesity.[8]

Causes of Obesity

Obesity is a complex eating disorder with multiple causes, including heredity, diet, lack of exercise, and behavioral considerations. It was formally declared a disease a few years ago by the National Institutes of Health Development Conference.[9]

The laws of thermodynamics indicate that energy cannot be destroyed; it is used for work or converted into another form. Accordingly the progressive accumulation of stored fat in the body is the result of consumption of more calories (energy) than are expended. Following the principles of thermodynamics, food energy in excess of the body's need is converted to fat and becomes stored energy in adipose cells. Although this relationship has been demonstrated many times in population studies, it appears that it may not apply to a small number of individuals. However, for the majority of people excessive caloric intake and/or deficient energy expenditure are responsible for their obesity. For the few exceptions one or several of the following may apply[7]:

- It is possible that obesity develops and is maintained because the mechanisms that regulate food intake are impaired.
- Obesity is often a genetic or familial disorder.

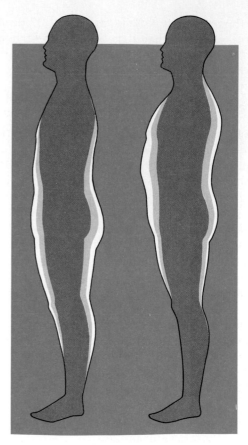

Figure 4-2 Feminine versus masculine deposition of fat.

- Obesity is more prevalent among women than men. This relationship is sustained at all age levels; it increases with age for both sexes but decreases in people who are involved in consistent, vigorous physical activity and in people of higher socioeconomic status.

The Effects of Genetics

Studies of adoptees. The genetic influence on weight control is becoming more clearly established. Researchers at the University of Pennsylvania examined the relative obesity and the body type of adults who had been adopted during childhood.[10] They classified 540 adoptees in the following categories: thin, median weight, overweight, and obese. They found that the subjects resembled their biological parents rather than their adoptive parents even though for many years, including the early, formative ones, they learned and practiced the lifestyle of the latter.

Studies of identical twins. The same research team from the University of Pennsylvania studied identical and fraternal male twins for more than 25 years.[11] Height, weight, and *body mass index (BMI)*, a measure of relative obesity, were measured initially when the subjects entered the military and again 25 years later. *Identical twins* are excellent subjects for these studies because, having emanated from the same egg, they have an identical genetic make-up. Any physical differences that occur in one of a pair of identical twins can be attributed to environmental and/or lifestyle factors. The identical twins in this study were very similar in height, weight, and BMI when they entered the military and again 25 years later. Each member of the pair gained the same amount of weight at approximately the same time in life. The similarity in the identical twins was twice that observed in *fraternal twins* (twins who emanate from separate eggs and do not have identical genes). This supports the notion that obesity and fat deposition are under substantial genetic control. Another group of researchers fed identical twins 1000 calories per day more than they needed for 22 days.[12] Each member of the set gained about the same amount of weight, and their weight was distributed in the same places. Once again the amount and distribution of weight gain seemed to be controlled by genetic factors.

The setpoint theory. The *setpoint theory* of weight control also reflects the role of genetics. Proponents of this theory suggest that the body prefers to maintain a certain weight and it defends this weight quite vigorously. More specifically, each person has an internal **setpoint** for fatness that the body seems to regulate by adjusting hunger, appetite, food intake, and energy expenditure. Researchers have demonstrated that human and animal subjects who have been put on low-calorie and/or high-calorie diets lose and gain only to a certain level. When the diet ends, they spontaneously return to their approximate original weight.

Dieting denies the body, so it takes a conscious effort to ignore natural signals to eat. Interestingly, dieting does not seem to lower the setpoint. If the setpoint were lowered with dieting, all dieters would stabilize at lower weights and would not return to prediet weight. Americans are consuming about 10% fewer calories today than 20 years ago, yet they weigh about 4 to 5 pounds more.

Proponents of the setpoint theory argue that vigorous exercise pursued regularly lowers the setpoint and thereby lowers the level of fat that the body will accept and defend. Exercise induces the body to stabilize at a lower body weight, which is precisely what dieters are trying to do. This is a classic case of a genetic inclination being modified through appropriate lifestyle behavior. It supports the idea that heredity is not destiny. Living a healthy life—through regular exercise, sound nutritional habits, and maintenance of normal weight—cannot negate heredity, but it can modify it, allowing people to have longevity and high quality of life and to fulfill their aesthetic potential.

The Effects of Diet

Statistics gathered in the last few years clearly show that dieting is the method of choice for the majority of Americans who are attempting to lose weight. It is noteworthy that dieting has not worked except temporarily for most people, and it probably never will. What is even more intriguing is that the majority of those who have failed are willing to repeat the same approach in a modified form again and again as they seek that magic bullet—the miraculous diet that will transform them from fat to thin people, preferably with minimal effort and in the shortest time possible.

The success rate of diet-only strategies is dismal. Only 5% of all dieters are successful in reducing to a target weight and maintaining that weight for more than 1 year.[13] Maintaining postdiet weight is one of the major failures of weight loss through dieting because dieters do not learn the habits and behaviors needed to remain at the new weight. As a result they lose and regain weight many times in their lives. This pattern of repeated weight loss and gain, known as *weight cycling* (also known as "yo-yo" or "seesaw" approaches to weight loss), is potentially harmful as well as counterproductive. Cycle dieters lose significant amounts of muscle tissue and gain fat in its place. This lowers the *basal metabolic rate (BMR)*, which represents the number of calories needed to sustain life, because muscle is metabolically more active and uses more calories than fat under all circumstances of life. Replacing muscle with fat lowers the body's caloric needs, which increases the effort required to continue to lose weight. It also significantly changes one's physical appearance.

The BMR is measured while the individual is in a thermally neutral environment in a resting and fasted state. BMR is the number of calories needed to keep the heart beating, the lungs moving air in and out, and the liver, kidneys, and all other organs functioning. Maintenance of BMR is the body's primary consumer of calories. Ap-

TABLE 4-1 Average weight lost by groups

Weight-loss strategy	Fat tissue loss (pounds)	Lean tissue change (pounds)	Total weight loss (pounds)
Diet only	−9.3	−2.4	−11.7
Exercise only	−12.6	+2.0	−10.6
Diet and exercise	−13.0	+1.0	−12.0

+ = Lean tissue gain
− = Total weight or lean tissue loss

proximately 65% to 70% of the energy liberated from food is expended to support BMR.[14] See Assessment Activity 6-1 at the end of the chapter to learn how to estimate your BMR.

The goals of a weight-loss program are to lose fat weight and to retain or gain muscle weight so that BMR will not be affected negatively. This cannot be accomplished by diet-only approaches to weight loss. This concept was exemplified in a study of young and middle-age overweight women who were grouped into three weight-loss strategies, each configured to produce a conservative 1-pound loss per week.[15] Table 4-1 presents the results of this study.

All three groups lost essentially the same amount of body weight. The important outcome was that 2.4 pounds, or 21% of the total amount of weight lost by the "diet-only" group, was in the form of lean tissue. This occurred despite a nutritionally sound diet of modest caloric restriction. The other two groups lost fat and gained, rather than lost, lean tissue. Maintaining the strength of the muscular system and/or enhancing it while losing weight is crucial to success.

One of the major deficiencies of diet-only strategies was demonstrated in animal studies. Rats who were cycled required 21 days to lose a specified amount of weight and 46 days to regain it during the first cycle.[16] On the second cycle on the same diet, it took the rats twice as long (40 days) to lose the same amount of weight, but it was regained 3 times as fast (14 days). With each succeeding cycle, more muscle was lost, and more fat was regained. Evidence emerging from human studies demonstrates that people may react in a similar fashion to weight cycling.

Cycle dieting increases the efficiency with which the body converts food to fuel. As a result,

fewer calories supply more of the energy, and the calories saved are converted to fat. Cycling may enhance the activity of *lipoprotein lipase*, an enzyme that increases the body's ability to store fat. Repeated cycling may alter the number and/or size of the fat cells, predisposing the individual to the gaining and storage of fat. Finally, cycle dieting promotes a masculine pattern of fat deposition, which is positively related to a number of chronic diseases. This will be discussed later in this chapter under the heading "The Health Aspects of Obesity."

Most dieters fall into the cycle pattern of dieting and, without including exercise, they are plagued by rebound weight gain and failure. The message from this is quite clear: Do it right the first time and keep the weight off because each failed attempt contributes to the body's reluctance to part with its pounds.

In addition to the adverse effects on BMR, diets very low in calories (800 calories per day or fewer), including those that have been promoted as having a "protein-sparing effect" (conserving lean tissue), have often been associated with medical complications, including *cardiac arrhythmias* (irregular heart rate that is sometimes intractable) and sudden death.[17] Diets very low in calories produce distinctive and abnormal *electrocardiographic (EKG)* rhythm patterns that are most likely caused by protein loss from the *myocardium* (heart muscle) and/or cell-membrane instability from rapid weight loss.[18]

Low-calorie diets (800 to 1000 calories per day) result in atrophy of the heart muscle. When low-calorie diets are accompanied by regular exercise, the muscle loss is minimized, but it still occurs.[19] However, regular exercise combined with a *moderate-calorie diet* (1300 to 1600 calories per day) results in loss of body weight and gain of cardiac muscle. Exercise-induced cardiac hypertrophy results in a stronger, more efficient heart. Health professionals have been warning against the use of diets low or very low in calories as weight-loss strategies for a number of reasons. The loss of cardiac muscle is surely one of the major drawbacks.

A widely held assumption is that obese people eat more than people of normal weight. However, evidence indicates that they usually eat no more and they sometimes eat less than normal people.[20] Studies of obese people have shown that the beginning of their weight gain could be traced back to a time in their lives when a decrease in physical activity, not an increase in food consumption, occurred. This pattern is frequently observed in people who are in the process of establishing a career. Although appetite and food consumption are not increased, the time and attention once devoted to physical activity decreases, resulting in an imperceptible yet relentless weight gain.

Our position regarding dieting in the conventional sense is that it is an ineffective weight-management method. The expectation that temporary changes in eating habits will lead to permanent weight loss is unrealistic and naive. Diets don't work. Sensible and permanent dietary changes that depend on wise food choices are not only an excellent way to cut calories but also a healthy way to eat. For example, Table 4-2 dem-

onstrates how to trim calories that come from fat and cholesterol by making appropriate substitutions. This table provides healthy substitutions for selected foods. To use this table, simply refer to the left column, which contains popular but calorically dense and fat-laden foods, and then refer to the middle column for an appropriate substitute. Observe the savings in calories, fat, and cholesterol in the right column as a result of the substitution.

There are many diets on the market, some of which are nutritionally sound and many of which are not. Some are potentially hazardous, and many are based on faulty nutritional and physiological concepts. Some require that food

▌ TABLE 4-2 Food substitutions that reduce fat, cholesterol, and calories

Instead of eating	Substitute	To save*
1 croissant	1 plain bagel	35 calories, 10 g fat, 13 mg cholesterol
1 cup cooked egg noodles	1 cup cooked macaroni	50 mg cholesterol
1 whole egg	1 egg white	65 calories, 6 g fat, 220 mg cholesterol
1 oz cheddar cheese	1 oz part-skim mozzarella	35 calories, 4 g fat, 15 mg cholesterol
1 oz cream cheese	1 oz cottage cheese (1% fat)	74 calories, 9 g fat, 29 mg cholesterol
1 teaspoon whipping cream	1 tablespoon evaporated skim milk, whipped	32 calories, 5 g fat
3.5 oz skinless roast duck	3.5 oz skinless roast chicken	46 calories, 7 g fat
3.5 oz beef tenderloin, choice, untrimmed, broiled	3.5 oz beef tenderloin, select, trimmed, broiled	75 calories, 10 g fat
3.5 oz lamb chop, untrimmed, broiled	3.5 oz lean leg of lamb, trimmed, broiled	219 calories, 28 g fat
3.5 oz pork spare ribs cooked	3.5 oz lean pork loin, trimmed, broiled	157 calories, 17 g fat
1 oz regular bacon, cooked	1 oz Canadian bacon, cooked	111 calories, 12 g fat
1 oz hard salami	1 oz extra-lean roasted ham	75 calories, 8 g fat
1 beef frankfurter	1 chicken frankfurter	67 calories, 8 g fat
3 oz oil-packed tuna, light	3 oz water-packed tuna, light	60 calories, 6 g fat
1 regular-size serving french fries	1 medium-size baked potato	125 calories, 11 g fat
1 oz oil-roasted peanuts	1 oz roasted chestnuts	96 calories, 13 g fat
1 oz potato chips	1 oz thin pretzels	40 calories, 9 g fat
1 oz corn chips	1 oz plain air-popped popcorn	125 calories, 9 g fat
1 tablespoon sour-cream dip	1 tablespoon bottled salsa	20 calories, 3 g fat
1 glazed doughnut	1 slice angel-food cake	110 calories, 13 g fat, 21 mg cholesterol
3 chocolate sandwich cookies	3 fig-bar cookies	4 g fat
1 oz unsweetened chocolate	3 tablespoons cocoa powder	73 calories, 13 g fat
1 cup ice cream (premium)	1 cup sorbet	320 calories, 34 g fat, 100 mg cholesterol

*The values listed are the most significant savings; smaller differences are not shown. Weight given for meats are edible portions.

■ **TABLE 4-3** *The Walking Magazine's guide to 1989's most popular diets*

Type	Description	Weight loss	Health drawbacks	Pros/cons
Balanced (available in book stores) Weight Watchers Quick Success Program (Weight Watchers International) Jane Fonda's New Workout & Weight Loss Program I Don't Eat (But I Can't Lose Weight) Complete University Medical Diet Jane Brody's Nutrition Book Fit or Fat Target Diet Popcorn Plus Diet Getting Thin Setpoint Diet Nautilus Diet	Recommends 1000 or more calories/day. At least 50% carbohydrate, less than 30% fat, 15% to 20% protein. Variety of foods from four basic food groups. (Regular exercise and lifestyle changes.)	1 to 2 lb./week. Promotes permanent loss of fat, especially if combined with regular exercise.	None (no side effects in healthy people). Diet includes an adequate amount of food in all the major food groups. No specialized medical supervision necessary in healthy people.	Provides variety and good nutrition. Combined with exercise, diet can be used as a basis of lifelong weight control. No vitamin supplementation necessary. Weight lost is fat, not muscle.
High Carbohydrate Bloomingdale's Eat Healthy Diet Pritikin Permanent Weight Loss Manual	Calorie level varies. Encourages increasing carbohydrate intake to more than 60% of diet. Can severely restrict protein and fat intake. Some advocate exercise and positive lifestyle changes.	Gradual or rapid, depending on calorie intake.	May be too low in protein and require vitamin and mineral supplements.	If protein level and calorie intake are adequate, high-carbohydrate diets are safe and effective. However, they may be so restrictive that they can be hard to stick to.
Formula/Rx (available through a physician or hospital-run program) HMR (Health Management Resources) Medifast Optifast	Suggests only 800 calories or less/day. Requires dieters to forgo food for about 12 weeks and eat only a protein supplement. After initial fast, food is gradually reintroduced. May encourage exercise and lifestyle changes.	Very rapid, 3 to 4 lb./week. Protein supplements claimed to reduce loss of muscle tissue. Unknown: whether dieters keep weight off.	Can produce severe metabolic disturbances, heart beat irregularities, hair loss, dehydration, kidney problems and sense of feeling cold. Vitamins and mineral supplements required.	Expensive. Cost can run as high as $500 per month. Only for obese people (20% or more overweight), to off-set a weight-related health problem, or who have failed on other diets. Requires close medical supervision.

Type / Examples	Description	Weight Loss	Nutrition	Eating Habits
Formula/OTC (over the counter) Nutrament Slender Slim Fast	May advocate less than 1000 calories/day. Replaces one or more meals with a low-calorie shake or food bar that contains some combination of protein, carbohydrates, fats, vitamins, minerals.	Can be rapid, 3 or more lb./week if daily calorie level falls below 1000. May promote water and muscle loss. Weight often regained.	May be low in protein, carbohydrates, vitamins or minerals. Can be dangerous if used for sole source of nutrition.	Teaches reliance on patented products, not on sound, lifelong eating habits.
Low Carbohydrate/High Protein Dr. Atkins' Diet Revolution Complete Scarsdale Medical Diet Doctor's Quick Weight Loss Diet (Stillman, "water diet") 35-Plus Diet for Women	Calorie level varies. Severely restricts carbohydrates, such as bread, cereals, grains, starchy vegetables.	Rapid, 3 or more lb./week. Promotes loss of water and muscle tissue. Weight usually regained.	Usually unbalanced. May be very high in saturated fat and cholesterol. Can cause fatigue, headaches, nausea, dehydration and dizziness.	Does not promote good eating habits. Nutritional claims are unsound.
Very Low Calorie Diet Principal Rotation Diet	Suggests less than 1000 calories/day for part of diet or for its entirety. Based on low-fat, high-carbohydrate foods.	Rapid, 3 or more lb./week. Initial loss is water and muscle, not fat. Weight usually regained.	May be unbalanced and require vitamin and mineral supplements.	Usually does not teach long-term good eating habits.
Food Combination Beverly Hills Diet Fit for Life Rice Diet Report	Usually less than 1000 calories/day. Often makes false claims that specific foods or combinations burn fat; suggests eating one type of food, to exclusion of others.	Can be rapid, depending on calorie intake. Weight generally regained.	Unbalanced. May be dangerously low in protein; often deficient in vitamins and minerals. Can result in dizziness, diarrhea, gas, hair loss, brittle nails and loss of vital muscle tissue.	Based on unsound nutritional guidelines. Weight is lost because of reduction in calories, not magic food formula; can be dangerous. May be extremely restrictive and monotonous.

be eaten in a certain order and severely restrict allowable foods. Some require medical supervision. Seem confusing? Refer to Table 4-3 for a comparative summary of some of today's most popular weight-loss methods.

The Effects of Exercise

Exercise has been one of the most neglected aspects of weight management. Not many years ago it was a common practice to discourage exercise for dieters in the mistaken belief that it would stimulate the appetite at a time when calorie restriction was in order. A second unfounded notion was centered on the belief that the calories used during physical activity were too few to have a substantial effect on weight loss. The consensus was that the results were not worth the effort. Fortunately the public is slowly coming to realize that these assertions were erroneous. Today, the research evidence regarding the effectiveness of exercise in weight management is so compelling that most authorities agree that the prevalence of obesity in the United States is primarily due to physical inactivity—not overeating.

History indicates that life today is considerably different from life in the first 2 to 3 decades

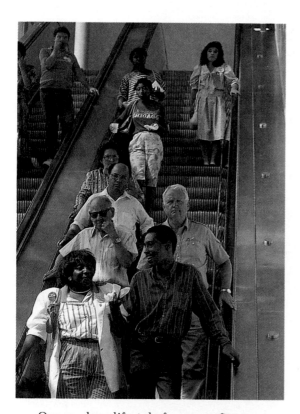

Our modern lifestyle fosters unfitness.

of this century. Scientific and technological advances have made us functionally mechanized. Labor-saving devices permeate all phases of life—our occupations, home life, and leisure-time pursuits—always with the promise of more and better to come. Each new invention helps to foster a receptive attitude toward a life of ease, and we have become enamored with the easy way of doing things. The mechanized way is generally the most expedient way, and in our time-oriented society, this has become another stimulus for us to indulge in a sedentary life.

Today, exercise for fitness is contrived; it is programmed into our lives as an entity separate from our other functions. On the other hand, the energy expenditures of our forefathers were integrated into their work, play, and home life. Physical fitness was a necessary commodity, and fit people were the rule rather than the exception. Tilling the soil, digging ditches, and working in factories were physically demanding jobs. Lumberjack contests and square dances were vigorous leisure pursuits. Being a wife and taking care of home and family required long hours at strenuous tasks. In the early years of this century, one third of the energy for operating the factories came from muscle power. By 1970 this figure had dropped to less than 1%. This decrease reflects the declining energy demand of our jobs.

The turn of the century found 70% of the population working long, hard hours in the production of food. Children of this era walked several miles to school and did chores when they returned home. Today, less than 3% of the population—using highly mechanized equipment—is involved in the production of food, and their children ride to school. Adults drive to the store, circle the parking lot to get as close as possible to the entrance to buildings, and ride elevators and escalators while there. We mow the lawn with a riding mower, play golf with a cart, wash dishes and clothes in electric appliances, and change television channels and open garage doors with a remote control.

These are simply observations of life in America and are intended not to imply that the fruits of science and technology be devalued but rather that their results and their effects on us be viewed in perspective and acted on accordingly. Mechanization has invaded our leisure time. It is in this area that we must willfully commit some time to vigorous activity because it has been effectively removed from other areas of life.

People have inhabited the Earth for many cen-

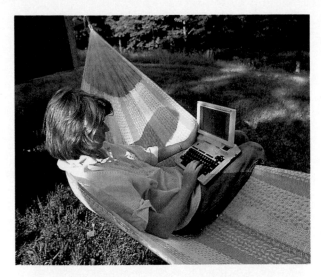

Technological advances have contributed to a sedentary lifestyle.

TABLE 4-4 Estimated caloric cost of selected activities

Activity	Calories/min/lb*
Aerobic dance (vigorous)	0.062
Basketball (vigorous, full-court)	0.097
Bathing, dressing, undressing	0.021
Bed-making (and stripping)	0.031
Bicycling (13 mph)	0.071
Canoeing (flat water, 4 mph)	0.045
Chopping wood	0.049
Cleaning windows	0.024
Cross-country skiing (8 mph)	0.104
Gardening: digging	0.062
Hedging	0.034
Raking	0.024
Weeding	0.038
Golf (twosome carrying clubs)	0.045
Handball (skilled, singles)	0.078
Horseback riding (trot)	0.052
Ironing	0.029
Jogging (5 mph)	0.060
Laundry (taking out and hanging)	0.027
Mopping floors	0.024
Peeling potatoes	0.019
Piano playing	0.018
Rowing (vigorous)	0.097
Running (8 mph)	0.104
Sawing Wood (crosscut saw)	0.058
Shining shoes	0.017
Shoveling snow	0.052
Snowshoeing (2.5 mph)	0.060
Soccer (vigorous)	0.097
Swimming (55 yd/min)	0.088
Table tennis (skilled)	0.045
Tennis (beginner)	0.032
Walking (4.5 mph)	0.048
Writing while seated	0.013

*Multiply calories/min/lb by your body weight in pounds and then multiply that product by the number of minutes spent in the activity.

turies, but only the last 75 years have generated such drastic changes in lifestyle. Our basic need for physical activity has not changed. Our bodies were constructed for and thrive on physical work, but we find ourselves thrust into the automobile, television, and sofa age. We simply have not had enough time to adapt to this new sedentary way of living. Perhaps 100,000 years from now the sedentary life will be the healthy life. But at this stage of our development, the law of use and disuse continues to work. That which is used becomes stronger and that which is not used becomes weaker. For simple verification of this physiological principle, just observe the results of having a leg in a cast for 8 weeks and note the atrophy that occurs to the limb during that time.

Exercise uses calories. One of the obvious benefits of exercise is that it burns calories. They are consumed according to body weight, so heavier people burn more calories per minute than lighter people for the same activity. Table 4-4 includes selected physical fitness activities and a few common physical activities. To use it, simply multiply your body weight by the coefficient in the calories/min/lb column and then multiply this value by the number of minutes spent participating in the activity. For example, a 170-pound person who walks at 4.5 mph for 30 minutes will expend 245 calories. This was determined by finding the coefficient for walking 4.5 miles per hour and proceeding as follows:

1. Multiply body weight by calories/min/lb (170 pounds × 0.048 = 8.16 calories/min/lb)
2. Multiply calories/min/lb by the exercise time in minutes.

(8.16 calories/min/lb × 30 min = 244.8 calories/30 min)

There are 3500 calories in one pound of fat. If this person performs this exercise daily, he or she will lose 1 pound in approximately 14 days or 25.5 pounds in 1 year, provided caloric intake is unchanged. The annual weight loss for this person is calculated as follows:

1. $\dfrac{3500 \text{ calories/lb/fat}}{245 \text{ calories/day}} = 14.3 \text{ days}$

2. $\dfrac{365 \text{ days/year}}{14.3 \text{ days}} = 25.5 \text{ lbs}$

Follow the example in Assessment Activity 4-2 and apply the directions to your situation or to a hypothetical situation of your choosing.

Aerobic exercises, such as walking, jogging, cycling, swimming, and rowing, contribute significantly to weight loss. According to the American College of Sports Medicine (ACSM), optimal benefits are derived from activities that burn 300 to 500 calories per exercise session. Use Table 4-4 to determine the number of minutes that you should participate in your favorite activities to burn a minimum of 300 calories.

Deconditioned people should start slowly and gradually progress through time to using 300 to 500 calories per exercise session. Second, for the purpose of weight loss, all of the calories do not have to be expended in one exercise session. Three 15-minute walks in a day would total 45 minutes and a substantial expenditure of energy. Actually any physical activity above the amount normally done in a day is a bonus for weight control. The cumulative effect of activities such as walking up stairs, mowing the lawn, and mopping floors can be combined with a structured exercise program to produce steady, safe weight loss. No physical activity is insignificant when viewed in the context of its contribution to weight management.

Exercise and appetite: eat more, weigh less. To the uninitiated, the title of this section must seem paradoxical if not impossible. How can a person eat more and weigh less? It sounds like a bit of sorcery or hocus-pocus from a carnival pitchman or like trying to catch smoke with a net. Wouldn't it be nice to have your cake and eat it too, literally—without gaining weight? Many people are doing it. Exercise either stabilizes or increases the appetite, depending to some extent on the individual's body weight at the start of the program. This was exemplified by the results of studies at St. Luke's Hospital in New York.[21] Obese women lost 15 pounds after 57 days of moderate-intensity exercise on a treadmill. Their

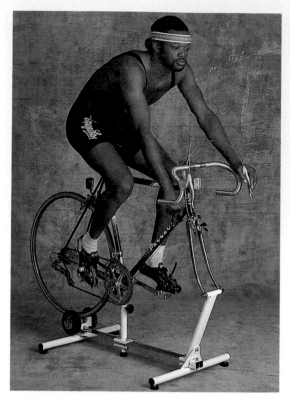

Physical activity, which develops muscle tissue, can also increase metabolism.

voluntary food intake during the 2 months of exercise was essentially the same as before the start of the exercise program. On the other hand, women of normal weight for their height had an immediate surge in appetite. Their food consumption increased when they began exercising, but they neither gained nor lost weight during the 2-month period.

Wood[22] investigated the effect of a year of jogging on previously sedentary middle-age men. The men were encouraged to not reduce their food intake or to lose weight during the time of the study. At the end of 1 year, the men who ran the most miles lost the most fat, but conversely they also had the greatest increase in food intake. Also, the more fat the men lost, the more they increased their food intake. It has been repeatedly demonstrated that men and women joggers consume more calories and yet are slimmer than sedentary people of the same age and sex. Exercise is the only viable method for losing weight while eating more calories.

Exercise stimulates metabolism. Metabolism, the total of all of the chemical reactions that occur within the cells of the body, is measured in calories. Metabolism is affected by age, gender, secretions from endocrine glands, nutritional status, sleep, fever, climate, body surface area, and amount of muscle tissue. The majority of the calories expended during a 24-hour period go to support basal metabolism. Because men have more muscle tissue than women, their BMRs average 5% to 10% higher.

BMR declines with age, but age itself has relatively little effect on this change. It seems that the acquired changes that accompany aging—primarily physical inactivity and muscle loss—are essentially responsible for the decline in BMR. The annual decrease in BMR beginning at 25 or 30 years of age, though imperceptible, has serious ramifications for weight management and accounts for a significant amount of the weight gained with age. Authorities estimate that the loss of active protoplasm (mostly muscle tissue) is equal to 3% to 5% every decade after age 25-30. The loss of muscle tissue and subsequent decline in BMR produce changes in body composition. This is evident when the data in Table 4-5 are examined.

The examples in Table 4-5 are hypothetical, but they are based on fact. The lean-tissue values in the table apply to men. The process applies to women as well but to a lesser degree, simply because they have less muscle tissue to lose.

Subject 1 is most representative of the typical American man who loses muscle, replaces it with fat, and then gains additional fat. Fat is less dense than muscle, so a pound of it takes up 18% more room in the body than a pound of muscle. Subject 2 is inactive but manages to maintain his body weight while aging. However, his inactive lifestyle has resulted in muscle loss, and the accompanying reduction in BMR demands that he keep a tight reign on his appetite to prevent weight gain. He weighs the same at the age of 60 as he did at age 20, but his body composition has changed significantly, as evidenced by his reflection in the mirror and the fit of his clothes. It

should now be clear that body dimensions change when we exchange fat for muscle even without gaining weight. Subject 3 is inactive, but he compensates for the expected muscle loss by controlling food consumption so that he weighs 15 pounds less at age 60 than he did at age 20. His body composition has changed because the loss of muscle tissue means that he is smaller all over. This subject is perpetually dieting—a strategy that is virtually impossible for most people to follow. Subject 4 has been physically active throughout life. There is little muscle loss and no fat gain. Many examples of this modern phenomenon can be seen jogging, cycling, swimming, etc. Exercises and physical activities that develop and maintain muscle tissue will preserve and/or enhance BMR, resulting in improved quality of life and a youthful and healthy appearance for many decades.

Combining Dietary Modification and Exercise

In its simplest terms, weight management involves control of caloric intake versus caloric expenditure. Weight gain results when calories consumed are greater than calories expended, weight loss occurs when the amount of calories consumed is less than the amount of calories expended, and weight maintenance occurs when the amount of calories consumed equals the amount of calories expended. Because caloric consumption and caloric expenditure are involved in weight management, it makes sense to manipulate both to be effective. Combining sensible exercise and sensible changes in eating habits that can be maintained for life is the most effective approach to permanent weight management. Table 4-1, which summarizes the results of the Zuti and Golding study, shows the effectiveness of combining exercise and changed eating habits on total weight loss, fat loss, and lean-tissue gains of young and middle-aged women. Leon and others[23] observed a similar effect in men.

TABLE 4-5 Effects of physical inactivity on body composition

Subject	Body weight at age 20	Body weight at age 60	Activity level	Lean tissue	Fat	Body composition
1	150 lbs	165	Inactive	Lost 12%-20%	Gain	Changed
2	150 lbs	150	Inactive	Lost 12%-20%	Gain	Changed
3	150 lbs	135	Inactive	Lost 12%-20%	Gain	Changed
4	150 lbs	150	Active	No Loss	No Gain	Unchanged

Subjects in this study walked for 90 minutes per day 5 days per week, progressively increasing their speed and consequently their energy expenditure over 16 weeks. The average total loss was 12.5 pounds, fat loss was 13 pounds, and lean-tissue gain was 0.5 pounds. Combining nutritional changes with regular exercise meets the goals of weight management most effectively—it promotes weight loss, fat loss, and lean-tissue gain.

Behavioral Effects

There is some evidence that obese people are more likely than normal-weight people to eat in response to external cues. A clock that says it is suppertime, media messages advertising food and beverages, the sight, sounds, and aroma of food, and so on are more apt to elicit eating behavior in the obese. This is the basis of the "externality" hypothesis, that if people can learn to eat in response to external cues, they can also learn to recognize cues that stimulate eating behavior, substitute other behaviors for eating, and use techniques that decrease the amount of food eaten. As a result of this training, the response to external cues should be reduced and replaced by attention to internal hunger signals. Many techniques have been developed over the past 2 decades that may assist people in resisting the tendency to eat indiscriminately or to overeat. Refer to Figure 2-7 in Chapter 2 for a brief list of some of the techniques that have been successful for some but not all people. Rarely have these techniques produced large weight losses (as much as 40 pounds), and rarely has the loss been maintained. However, these techniques may be useful

as a supplement to sensible food choices and sensible exercise.

Behavioral and psychological hypotheses have been developed to explain the development and perpetuation of obesity in population groups. These hypotheses have attempted to account for differences between normal-weight and obese persons. Although each of the hypotheses is supported by some research, none has been able to account consistently for group differences, and the behavioral and psychological determinants might be the result of obesity rather than the cause.[24] Table 4-6 presents the hypotheses that have been studied.

Health Aspects of Obesity

Obesity was formally declared a disease by a medical panel that was convened by the National Institutes of Health (NIH).[9] The panel simply confirmed what had been known for years: morbidity occurs more frequently and with greater severity, and mortality occurs at an earlier age among obese people compared with those of normal weight. High-level wellness cannot be achieved by obese people because the quality of their lives is diminished by the hazards that are associated with obesity. Obesity coexists with and/or is a precursor of the chronic diseases that kill Americans. It is highly correlated with coronary heart disease, stroke, atherosclerosis, and diabetes—four of the top ten killers of Americans.[25] Obesity contributes to the formation of gallstones, respiratory disorders, and degenerative changes in the joints, particularly those of the knees and hips. It predisposes men to cancer of the colon, rectum, and prostate and women to cancer of the ovaries, uterus, and breasts. Researchers at Harvard's School of Public Health reviewed 25 studies regarding the relationship between body weight and health.[26] They concluded that excess weight caused premature death and that each extra pound increased the death rate by 1% in men 30 to 49 years of age and 2% for men age 50 to 62. Every excess pound counts.

The link between obesity and chronic diseases is well established, but evidence has emerged indicating that the distribution of fat is a risk equally as important as the amount of fat (see Assessment Activity 4-3).

In addition to the medical hazards, obese people suffer from economic and social discrimination, poor body image, and poor self-concept. Obese people pay higher premiums for health in-

---

TABLE 4-6 Selected behavioral and psychological hypotheses to account for obesity

- Abnormal eating styles
- External eating cues
- Response to appetizing food
- Taste perception
- Restrained eating—response to calorie restriction
- External locus of control
- Preference of immediate gratification
- Neurotic personality traits
- Response to anxiety or depression

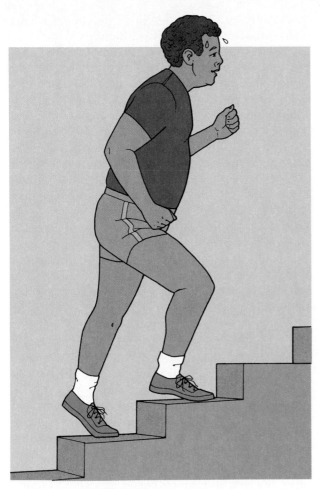

Physical activities are more difficult for the obese but, due to their size, they burn more calories per unit of exercise.

surance or are denied coverage, obese children are often ridiculed by their slim peers, and armed forces personnel are forced out of the military if they gain weight beyond an acceptable level.

Fortunately obesity is reversible, and so too are many of the risks with which it is associated. The preferred course of action would be to prevent obesity from occurring rather than to try to deal with it after the fact. Preventing obesity requires knowledgeable management of dietary and exercise habits, the essentials of which should be taught and practiced in the home. Parents can be effective models for their children.

Eating Disorders

Anorexia nervosa (anorexia), bulimarexia nervosa (bulimia), and pica are eating disorders. Anorexia and bulimia are familiar to most Americans although pica is not.

Although they share some characteristics, anorexia and bulimia are different eating disorders. The common factor between the two is an intense fear of becoming overweight. However, the methods used by persons with the disorders to attain this goal differ. Starvation is the primary strategy of the anorectic, but the bulimic gorges and then purges by vomiting or by using diuretics and laxatives. Bulimics seldom starve to the point of emaciation; instead they are often moderately overweight.[27] Most bulimics do not become anorectic, but many anorectics practice bulimic behavior. On the other hand, pical behavior has nothing to do with weight loss. It is a morbid appetite for unusual or unfit food.

Victims of both of these disorders are predominantly young females who come from middle or upper-class families, are well educated, high achievers, and perfectionists who have low self-esteem regardless of their successes.[27] Only 6% to 10% of all anorectics are male. Anorexia and bulimia usually occur during or immediately after puberty, a stage of accelerated growth characterized by confusion for the majority of adolescents.

Anorexia Nervosa

Anorexia nervosa is defined as a "serious illness of deliberate self-starvation with profound psychiatric and physical components."[28] Although specific causes of anorexia have not been identified, a combination of interacting factors, including organic, psychodynamic, familial, and sociocultural factors, presumably contribute to the disorder.[28] Support for an organic influence has centered on the hypothalamus (the portion of the brain reputed to house the appetite center) and the pituitary gland (the master gland of the body). Evidence supporting a genetic influence is weak, but the fact remains that the disease occurs more frequently among sisters, particularly those who come from families with a higher than normal incidence of various psychopathologies.[24] Psychodynamic causes take various forms, the most popular of which centers on the trauma experienced by young girls whose mothers are excessively domineering and unempathetic. This proposition is more theory than fact at this time. Sociocultural theories focus on the compulsion of adolescent girls to become and remain lean. This exaggerated goal manifests itself at a time when girls are naturally depositing fat, when exercise is not "cool," and when high-calorie fast foods are readily available.

Figure 4-3 Criteria for diagnosing anorexia nervosa

1. Weight change
   a. Unwilling to maintain minimal normal body weight for the person's age and height
   b. Weight loss that leads to the maintenance of a body weight that is 15% below normal
   c. Failure to gain the amount of weight expected during a period of growth, resulting in a body weight that is 15% below normal
2. Inordinate fear of gaining weight and/or becoming fat despite being significantly underweight
3. Disturbed and unrealistic perceptions of body weight, size, or shape. The person "feels fat" although he or she is emaciated and may perceive that one specific part of the body is "too fat."
4. Absence of at least three menstrual cycles for women when they would normally be expected to occur. Amenorrheic women are those whose menstrual cycle normalized only during administration of hormone therapy.

Anorexia is characterized by extreme weight loss, amenorrhea (absence of a menstrual period), and a variety of psychological disorders culminating in an obsessive preoccupation with the attainment of thinness. Fortunately most anorectics recover fully after one experience with the disease. But for 10% to 15% of its victims the disease becomes episodic and relentless, resulting in death from the consequences of starvation.[29] Figure 4-3 gives the criteria that have been developed by the American Psychiatric Association for diagnosing anorexia.

When confronted, anorectics typically deny the existence of a problem and the weight-loss behaviors that have resulted in their emaciated physical appearance. They also avoid medical treatment, refuse the well-intended advice of family and friends regarding professional assistance, and/or submit to treatment under protest. Anorexia is a subtle disease, and anorectics become secretive in their behaviors. They become evasive, and many hide their disease in deep de-

nial even while undergoing treatment. This makes diagnosis especially difficult.

The course of treatment for anorexia is complex, involving a coordinated effort by several health care specialists. Hospitalization is often required because anorectics may have to be fed intravenously or by some other method if they cannot or will not eat. Medications that stimulate the appetite and medications that calm the patient are usually necessary. Nutritional counseling and psychological counseling—individual, group, and family—are integral components of treatment. Finally, behavior-modification techniques are employed to complete a well-rounded treatment effort designed to change the perceptions and lifestyle of the anorectic. At this point, there is no single treatment that has proven to be unusually successful in the treatment of anorectic patients.

Bulimia (Bulimarexia Nervosa)

Bulimia is characterized by alternate cycles of binge eating and restrictive eating. Binges are usually followed by purging, primarily by self-induced vomiting supplemented with the use of laxatives and diuretics. The physical and psychological ramifications of such a struggle include esophageal inflammation, erosion of tooth enamel caused by repeated vomiting, the possibility of electrolyte imbalances, and altered mood states, particularly anxiety and depression.

The diagnostic criteria for bulimia are given in Figure 4-4.

Bulimia is treated in a manner similar to that used for anorexia except that it usually does not require hospitalization. In addition to nutritional and psychological counseling, treatment often includes antidepressive medication because bulimia is associated with clinical depression.

Pica

Pica is a lesser known, poorly understood eating disorder. "Pica is the intentional and compulsive consumption of substances not commonly regarded as food."[24] It is an "international" practice affecting all races and both sexes. This disorder is classified into four categories: (1) geophagia: consumption of earth and clay, (2) amylophagia: consumption of starch or paste, (3) pagophagia: consumption of ice, and (4) miscellaneous: consumption of ash, chalk, plaster, wax, antacids, paint chips, and other substances.

Several theories have emerged to explain these eating behaviors, but none is valid. One

Figure 4-4 Criteria for diagnosing bulimia

▮ Episodic binge eating characterized by rapid consumption of large quantities of food in a short time.
▮ At least two eating binges per week for at least 3 months.
▮ Loss of control over eating behavior while eating binges are in progress.
▮ Frequent purging after eating, using techniques such as self-induced vomiting, laxatives, or diuretics, engaging in fasting or strict dieting, or engaging in vigorous exercise.
▮ Constant and continual concern with body shape, size, and weight.

theory indicates that pical behaviors are the result of nutritional deficiencies, but these behaviors are exhibited by some people who are not nutritionally deficient. Other hypotheses include alleviation of stress, prevention of nausea during pregnancy, and obtaining nutrients, such as iron or calcium. None of these hypotheses has been substantiated by research. Obviously some of these behaviors are hazardous. For example, some of them can cause lead poisoning and iron-deficiency anemia.

Underweight

A small number of people who are not anorectic or bulimic happen to be naturally thin, and some of them are dissatisfied with their appearance. Being underweight presents as much of a cosmetic problem for the affected individual as obesity does for the obese person. Many underweight people find it more difficult to gain a pound than obese people find losing one.

In their attempts to gain weight, many very lean people have consumed large quantities of food, particularly those that are rich in calories. Unfortunately these are foods that are high in fat and sugar. This is an unhealthy eating pattern for anyone, regardless of body weight. The preferred approach is to combine muscle-building exercises with three well-balanced nutritious meals supplemented by two nutritious snacks. The amount and type of weight gain should be closely monitored. Fat stores should not be increased unless the individual is extremely thin and on the verge of dipping into his or her stores of essential fat. **Essential fat,** found in organs, muscles, bone marrow, intestines, and the central nervous system, is necessary for individuals to function biologically as human beings, and it is necessary to support life processes. Essential fat in men constitutes about 3% of the total body weight, whereas in women it constitutes 10% to 12% of total weight. The difference between men and women is due to sex-specific essential fat that is vital for maintenance of fertility. Values for essential fat plus storage fat that are consis-

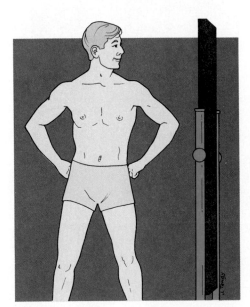
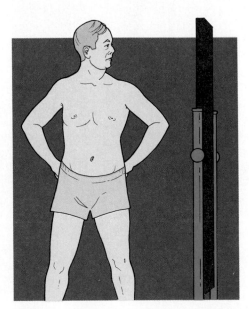

Joe at age 25. Joe at age 55.

tent with healthy leanness would be 8% to 12% for men and 16% to 20% for women.

Measuring Body Composition

Optimal body weight is not necessarily reflective of optimal body composition. This was illustrated by a comparison of young and middle-aged men who were within 5% of their ideal weight as determined by height, weight, and frame-size charts. Although both groups were within the ideal range, the middle-aged subjects had twice the amount of fat as the young subjects, This amount was reflected in their somewhat flabby body composition. Height and weight charts and bathroom scales are not indicators of body composition, nor are they reliable reference points to use for weight management.

Body composition can be determined by techniques that separate body fat from lean body mass. All of these techniques are indirect, so all of them contain some degree error in measurement.

Hydrostatic Weighing

Hydrostatic weighing, one of the most accurate of the measurement techniques, involves weighing subjects while they are completely submerged in water (Figure 4-5). Subjects may contribute to optimal accuracy if they can exhale the maximal amount of air possible from the lungs and can sit still for 6 to 10 seconds while completely submerged. Accuracy is further enhanced if the technician has the equipment to measure residual air (the amount of air remaining in the lungs following a maximal exhalation).

The equipment required for hydrostatic weighing includes an autopsy scale with a capacity of approximately 8 kg. The scale is suspended over a tank of water that is at least 3-feet deep. The subject sits suspended chin-deep, exhales completely, and bends forward from the waist

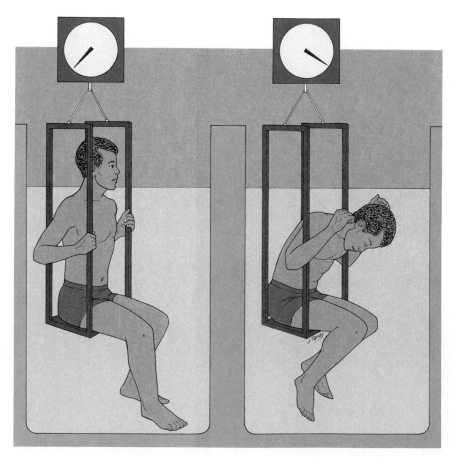

Figure 4-5 Underwater weighing apparatus: **A,** Subject in the ready position for underwater weighing. **B,** Subject in the process of being weighed.

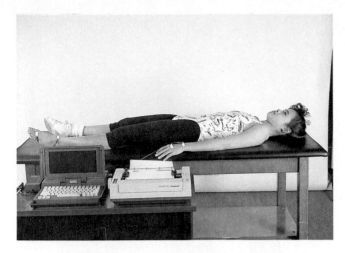

Figure 4-6 Bioelectrical impedance.

until entirely submerged. This position is maintained for 6 to 10 seconds to allow the scale to stabilize. Five to 10 trials are required, and the underwater weight is attained by averaging the three heaviest readings. The subject's net underwater weight is calculated by subtracting the weight of the seat and its supporting structure, plus a weight belt if needed, from the gross underwater weight.

Bioelectrical Impedance

Bioelectrical impedance is a relatively new and simple method of determining body composition. The equipment is portable, computerized, and expensive, but it is safe, noninvasive, quick, and convenient to use (Figure 4-6). A harmless electrical current is sent through the supine body via electrodes attached to the right hand and foot. Water is an excellent conductor of electricity, but fat, which is essentially anhydrous (lacking water), is a nonconductor. Lean body mass includes all tissues of the body except fat so that the two components can be separated. The measurement of electrical conductance or impedance is the tissue resistance to the transmission of an electrical current. The determination of total body water is used to calculate lean weight, fat weight, and percentage of body fat. This measurement correlates positively and highly with hydrostatic weighing.

Skinfold Measurements

Skinfold measurements are one of the least expensive and most economical methods of measuring body composition in terms of the cost of equipment and the time required to determine the fat content of the body. Skinfold calipers may

cost as little as $10 and as much as $450 for computerized models. The most accurate calipers maintain a constant jaw pressure of 10 g/mm^2 of jaw surface area.

The thumb and index finger are used to pinch and lift the skin and the fat beneath it. The caliper is placed beneath the pinch as described and illustrated in Figures 4-7 through 4-11. Use Tables 4-7 and 4-8 to convert the sum of millimeters of skinfold thickness to percentage of body fat. (Note that Table 4-7 is for men and 4-8 is for women.)

College-age women in the United States average 22% to 27% of their total weight as fat while men of the same age carry 15% to 18% of their total weight as fat. The optimal or desirable percentage body fat for women is 16% to 18%; the optimal percentage for men is 10% to 12%. Calculating desirable body weight is a simple procedure when the percentage of body fat is known. The following example is for a 148-pound female whose body fat is equal to 30% of total weight. She wishes to reduce to 17% body fat. The calculations are shown on p. 99.

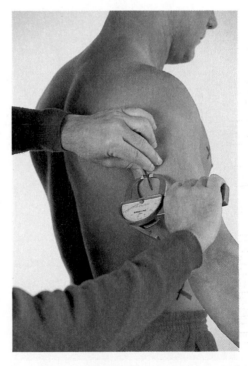

Figure 4-7 Triceps skinfold measurement. Take a vertical fold on the midline of the upper arm over the triceps, halfway between the acromion and olecranon processes (tip of the shoulder to the tip of the elbow). The arm should be extended and relaxed when the measurement is taken. All skinfold measurements should be taken on the right side.

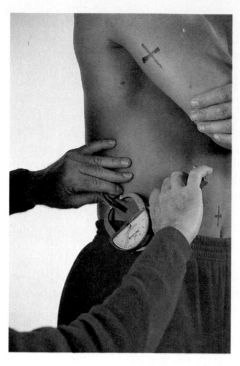

Figure 4-8 Suprailium skinfold measurement. Take a diagonal fold above the crest of the ilium directly below the midaxilla (armpit).

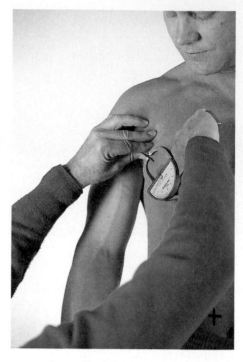

Figure 4-10 Chest skinfold measurement. Take a diagonal fold one-half of the distance between the anterior axillary line and the nipple.

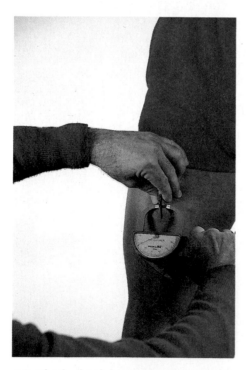

Figure 4-9 Thigh skinfold measurement. Take a vertical fold on the front of the thigh midway between the hip and the knee joint. The midpoint should be marked while the subject is seated.

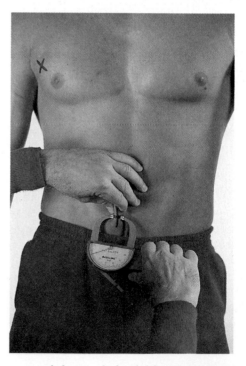

Figure 4-11 Abdominal skinfold measurement. Take a vertical fold about one inch from the navel.

TABLE 4-7 Percentage of fat estimated for men (sum of chest, abdomen, and thigh skinfolds)

Sum of skinfolds (mm)	Age to last year								
	Under 22	23-27	28-32	33-37	38-42	43-47	48-52	53-57	Over 57
8-10	1.3	1.8	2.3	2.9	3.4	3.9	4.5	5.0	5.5
11-13	2.2	2.8	3.3	3.9	4.4	4.9	5.5	6.0	6.5
14-16	3.2	3.8	4.3	4.8	5.4	5.9	6.4	7.0	7.5
17-19	4.2	4.7	5.3	5.8	6.3	6.9	7.4	8.0	8.5
20-22	5.1	5.7	6.2	6.8	7.3	7.9	8.4	8.9	9.5
23-25	6.1	6.6	7.2	7.7	8.3	8.8	9.4	9.9	10.5
26-28	7.0	7.6	8.1	8.7	9.2	9.8	10.3	10.9	11.4
29-31	8.0	8.5	9.1	9.6	10.2	10.7	11.3	11.8	12.4
32-34	8.9	9.4	10.0	10.5	11.1	11.6	12.2	12.8	13.3
35-37	9.8	10.4	10.9	11.5	12.0	12.6	13.1	13.7	14.3
38-40	10.7	11.3	11.8	12.4	12.9	13.5	14.1	14.6	15.2
41-43	11.6	12.2	12.7	13.3	13.8	14.4	15.0	15.5	16.1
44-46	12.5	13.1	13.6	14.2	14.7	15.3	15.9	16.4	17.0
47-49	13.4	13.9	14.5	15.1	15.6	16.2	16.8	17.3	17.9
50-52	14.3	14.8	15.4	15.9	16.5	17.1	17.6	18.2	18.8
53-55	15.1	15.7	16.2	16.8	17.4	17.9	18.5	19.1	19.7
56-58	16.0	16.5	17.1	17.7	18.2	18.8	19.4	20.0	20.5
59-61	16.9	17.4	17.9	18.5	19.1	19.7	20.2	20.8	21.4
62-64	17.6	18.2	18.8	19.4	19.9	20.5	21.1	21.7	22.2
65-67	18.5	19.0	19.6	20.2	20.8	21.3	21.9	22.5	23.1
68-70	19.3	19.9	20.4	21.0	21.6	22.2	22.7	23.3	23.9
71-73	20.1	20.7	21.2	21.8	22.4	23.0	23.6	24.1	24.7
74-76	20.9	21.5	22.0	22.6	23.2	23.8	24.4	25.0	25.5
77-79	21.7	22.2	22.8	23.4	24.0	24.6	25.2	25.8	26.3
80-82	22.4	23.0	23.6	24.2	24.8	25.4	25.9	26.5	27.1
83-85	23.2	23.8	24.4	25.0	25.5	26.1	26.7	27.3	27.9
86-88	24.0	24.5	25.1	25.7	26.3	26.9	27.5	28.1	28.7
89-91	24.7	25.3	25.9	26.5	27.1	27.6	28.2	28.8	29.4
92-94	25.4	26.0	26.6	27.2	27.8	28.4	29.0	29.6	30.2
95-97	26.1	26.7	27.3	27.9	28.5	29.1	29.7	30.3	30.9
98-100	26.9	27.4	28.0	28.6	29.2	29.8	30.4	31.0	31.6
101-103	27.5	28.1	28.7	29.3	29.9	30.5	31.1	31.7	32.3
104-106	28.2	28.8	29.4	30.0	30.6	31.2	31.8	32.4	33.0
107-109	28.9	29.5	30.1	30.7	31.3	31.9	32.5	33.1	33.7
110-112	29.6	30.2	30.8	31.4	32.0	32.6	33.2	33.8	34.4
113-115	30.2	30.8	31.4	32.0	32.6	33.2	33.8	34.5	35.1
116-118	30.9	31.5	32.1	32.7	33.3	33.9	34.5	35.1	35.7
119-121	31.5	32.1	32.7	33.3	33.9	34.5	35.1	35.7	36.4
122-124	32.1	32.7	33.3	33.9	34.5	35.1	35.8	36.4	37.0
125-127	32.7	33.3	33.9	34.5	35.1	35.8	36.4	37.0	37.6

TABLE 4-8 Percentage of fat estimated for women (sum of triceps, suprailium, and thigh skinfolds)								

Sum of skinfolds (mm)	Age to last year							
	Under 22	23-27	28-32	33-37	38-42	43-47	48-52	53-57	Over 57
23-25	9.7	9.9	10.2	10.4	10.7	10.9	11.2	11.4	11.7
26-28	11.0	11.2	11.5	11.7	12.0	12.3	12.5	12.7	13.0
29-31	12.3	12.5	12.8	13.0	13.3	13.5	13.8	14.0	14.3
32-34	13.6	13.8	14.0	14.3	14.5	14.8	15.0	15.3	15.5
35-37	14.8	15.0	15.3	15.5	15.8	16.0	16.3	16.5	16.8
38-40	16.0	16.3	16.5	16.7	17.0	17.2	17.5	17.7	18.0
41-43	17.2	17.4	17.7	17.9	18.2	18.4	18.7	18.9	19.2
44-46	18.3	18.6	18.8	19.1	19.3	19.6	19.8	20.1	20.3
47-49	19.5	19.7	20.0	20.2	20.5	20.7	21.0	21.2	21.5
50-52	20.6	20.8	21.1	21.3	21.6	21.8	22.1	22.3	22.6
53-55	21.7	21.9	22.1	22.4	22.6	22.9	23.1	23.4	23.6
56-58	22.7	23.0	23.2	23.4	23.7	23.9	24.2	24.4	24.7
59-61	23.7	24.0	24.2	24.5	24.7	25.0	25.2	25.5	25.7
62-64	24.7	25.0	25.2	25.5	25.7	26.0	26.7	26.4	26.7
65-67	25.7	25.9	26.2	26.4	26.7	26.9	27.2	27.4	27.7
68-70	26.6	26.9	27.1	27.4	27.6	27.9	28.1	28.4	28.6
71-73	27.5	27.8	28.0	28.3	28.5	28.8	29.0	29.3	29.5
74-76	28.4	28.7	28.9	29.2	29.4	29.7	29.9	30.2	30.4
77-79	29.3	29.5	29.8	30.0	30.3	30.5	30.8	31.0	31.3
80-82	30.1	30.4	30.6	30.9	31.1	31.4	31.6	31.9	32.1
83-85	30.9	31.2	31.4	31.7	31.9	32.2	32.4	32.7	32.9
86-88	31.7	32.0	32.2	32.5	32.7	32.9	33.2	33.4	33.7
89-91	32.5	32.7	33.0	33.2	33.5	33.7	33.9	34.2	34.4
92-94	33.2	33.4	33.7	33.9	34.2	34.4	34.7	34.9	35.2
95-97	33.9	34.1	34.4	34.6	34.9	35.1	35.4	35.6	35.9
98-100	34.6	34.8	35.1	35.3	35.5	35.8	36.0	36.3	36.5
101-103	35.3	35.4	35.7	35.9	36.2	36.4	36.7	36.9	37.2
104-106	35.8	36.1	36.3	36.6	36.8	37.1	37.3	37.5	37.8
107-109	36.4	36.7	36.9	37.1	37.4	37.6	37.9	38.1	38.4
110-112	37.0	37.2	37.5	37.7	38.0	38.2	38.5	38.7	38.9
113-115	37.5	37.8	38.0	38.2	38.5	38.7	39.0	39.2	39.5
116-118	38.0	38.3	38.5	38.8	39.0	39.3	39.5	39.7	40.0
119-121	38.5	38.7	39.0	39.2	39.5	39.7	40.0	40.2	40.5
122-124	39.0	39.2	39.4	39.7	39.9	40.2	40.4	40.7	40.9
125-127	39.4	39.6	39.9	40.1	40.4	40.6	40.9	41.1	41.4
128-130	39.8	40.0	40.3	40.5	40.8	41.0	41.3	41.5	41.8

1. Find fat weight (FW) in pounds.

FW (lbs.) =

$$\frac{\text{body weight (BW)} \times \text{percentage of fat}}{100}$$

$$= \frac{148 \times 30}{100}$$

$$= \frac{4440}{100}$$

$$= 44.4 \text{ lbs.}$$

2. Find lean weight (LW) in pounds.

$$\begin{aligned} \text{LW (lbs.)} &= \text{BW} - \text{FW} \\ &= 148 - 44.4 \\ &= 103.6 \text{ lbs.} \end{aligned}$$

3. Find desirable body weight (DBW) in pounds.

$$\text{DBW (lbs)} = \frac{\text{LW}}{1.0 - \text{percentage of fat desired}}$$

Convert the percentage of fat desired (17%) to a decimal (0.17)

$$= \frac{103.6}{1.0 - 0.17}$$

$$= \frac{103.6}{0.83}$$

$$= 124.8 \text{ lbs.}$$

This subject needs to lose 23.2 lbs. (148 − 124.8) to achieve her goal of 17% body fat. To compute your desirable body weight, turn to Assessment Activity 4-4 at the end of this chapter. Those who are concerned with weight loss will be interested to know that there is evidence supporting a best time for exercise for the achievement of this objective. Figure 4-12 provides the times and the rationale.

Physical activity is one of the major components of weight management because it uses calories and accelerates metabolism. Metabolism increases substantially during physical activity, and it remains elevated for a period after exercise. The intensity and duration of an exercise session and the individual's level of fitness determine the length of the recovery period. The calories used during recovery, until metabolism returns to preexercise levels, contribute to weight loss.

Figure 4-12 Exercise for weight loss: is there a best time?

There may be times during the day when exercise exerts a greater effect on weight loss. The two times most often suggested are before breakfast and before the evening meal.

Runners participated in two 30-minute runs: one after an overnight 12-hour fast (before breakfast) and another after a 3- to 4-hour fast (after lunch). The same number of calories were used for each run, but two thirds of the calories used before breakfast came from fat, compared to one-half of the calories from fat after lunch. Low circulating levels of insulin in the morning were probably responsible for the difference in the percentage of fuels used. Insulin is a hormone secreted by the pancreas that increases the utilization of glucose by the tissues of the body. Low insulin levels inhibit the use of glucose, so the body shifts to fat as a source of fuel—and isn't fat loss the goal of weight reduction?

Exercise before the evening meal may accomplish two goals simultaneously. First, it may alleviate the stress that has accumulated during the day. Second, exercise that is intense enough to raise body temperature will suppress the appetite temporarily so that meals taken during this time will result in fewer calories consumed.

Putting It All Together

This chapter began by asking these questions: (1) Why are Americans preoccupied with their body weight? (2) How do we find ourselves in such a predicament? (3) What can we do about it?

We are preoccupied with our body weight for several reasons. First, our culture emphasizes and deifies the youthful, lean body. This attitude permeates our daily lives. We cannot escape the message of advertisers, clothing designers, models, and media that reinforce the desirability of the slim silhouette. Fatness is not synonymous with aesthetics. Second, obese people have been the victims of social and economic discrimination. Third, most obese people suffer from poor self-esteem, poor body image, and social disapproval. Fourth, obesity is a health hazard; it is a disease that is also associated with other catastrophic diseases. Fifth, obese people are often perceived as weak-willed, lazy people who eat too much.

We find ourselves in the predicament of having to make an effort to achieve and maintain a desirable appearance because our lifestyles have changed significantly in the last 5 or 6 decades. Muscle power has been replaced by machine power, and labor-saving devices pervade all segments of our lives. Refrigeration, freezing, dehydration, and other methods of preserving foods have provided Americans with the opportunity to have access to foods all year that were previously available only seasonally. Fast foods and processed foods are convenient, affordable, and time-saving, but they are also high in calories, fat, and preservatives.

What is the solution to weight management, considering the changes that have occurred? This chapter has attempted to answer this question, but the following represent some important concepts: First, a Gallup Poll has shown that a change in attitude from the thin look to the fit and muscular look is emerging. Second, diet strategies by themselves have proved to be ineffective in producing long-term weight loss. In fact, repeated dieting facilitates weight gain. Third, obesity is a health hazard, but muscular development is not. Fourth, the solution to weight management involves a combination of sensible eating and sensible, consistent exercise. Become and remain physically active, and eat wisely. Although this approach requires some effort—but not an extraordinary amount—the results are not only predictable but also eminently worthwhile.

Summary

- The thin look is becoming passé and is being replaced by the fit and muscular look.
- Obesity is defined as body fat that is equal to or greater than 25% of the body weight of men and 30% or greater of the body weight of women.
- There are more overweight children today than there were 20 years ago.
- Obese children who are the progeny of obese parents have a greater chance of becoming obese adults than children of normal-weight parents.
- Diet, exercise, and heredity are the major factors associated with the loss or gain of body weight.
- Obesity has been declared a disease by the National Institutes of Health.
- The development and distribution of body fat is under substantial genetic control.
- Only 5% of all dieters are able to reach a target weight and maintain that weight for more than 1 year.
- Cycle dieting is ineffective as a weight-management strategy.
- Approximately 65% to 70% of the energy liberated from food is expended to support the BMR.
- Diet-only strategies result in the loss of lean body weight.
- Weight gain is more due to physical inactivity than to overeating.
- Exercise burns calories, stimulates metabolism, and brings appetite in line with energy expenditure.
- BMR declines because of muscle loss as people age and become inactive.
- Behavioral techniques may be a good supplement to exercise and dietary modification for the purpose of weight management.
- Obesity is positively related to the chronic diseases that are the major killers and disablers of Americans.
- Anorexia and bulimia are two potentially destructive eating disorders with complex causes.

Action plan for personal wellness

An important consideration in assuming responsibility for one's own quality of life is using information. After reading this chapter, answer the following questions and determine an action plan for enhancing your own lifestyle.

1 Based on the information presented in this chapter and what I know about my family's health history, the health problems and issues that I need to be most concerned about are:_____

_____

_____

2 Of the health concerns listed in number 1, the one I most need to act on is:_____

_____

_____

3 Possible actions that I can take to improve my level of wellness are (try to be as specific as possible):_____

_____

_____

4 Of the actions listed in number 3, the one that I most need to include in an action plan is:_____

_____

_____

5 Factors I need to keep in mind to be successful in my action plan are:_____

_____

_____

Review Questions

1. What are the definitions of obesity and overweight?
2. What evidence exists to support the notion that Americans are obsessed with weight control?
3. What is the pattern of growth of adipose cells from birth through puberty?
4. Do you agree or disagree with the idea that neonatal adiposity is not a good predictor of adult obesity? Defend your answer.
5. What evidence can you use to support the existence of an influential role of heredity in the development of obesity?
6. How effective are diet-only strategies in weight management?
7. What is weight cycling?
8. What is the roll of exercise in weight management?
9. How effective are behavior-modification techniques in weight management?
10. Why does obesity increase morbidity and mortality?
11. How does the distribution of body fat affect health and longevity?
12. What are the symptoms of anorexia and bulimia, and how is each treated?
13. What is essential fat, and why does it differ for each sex?

References

1. Britton AG: Thin is out, fit is in, American Health, pp 66-71, July/August 1988.
2. Willix RD Jr: Risk factor identification, ACSM Reference Guide 2(1-7):7, 1989.
3. Toufixis A: Dieting: the losing game, Time 54-60, Jan 20, 1986.
4. Gortmaker SL et al: Increasing pediatric obesity in the United States, Am J Disabled Child 141:535-539, 1987.
5. Ross JG and Pate RR: The national children and youth fitness study, II: a summary of findings, J Phys Ed Rec Dance 58:51-56, 1987.
6. Poissonnet CM et al: Growth and development of adipose tissue, J Pediatr 113:1-9, 1988.
7. Leibel RL and Hirsch J: Metabolic characteristics of obesity, Ann Intern Med 103:1000-1004, 1985.
8. Wardlaw GM and Insel PM: Perspectives in nutrition, St. Louis, 1990, Times Mirror/Mosby College Publishing.
9. Foster WR and Burton BT, editors: Health implications of obesity: National Institutes of Health development conference, Ann Intern Med, Supp 6, part 2, 103:981-982, 1985.
10. Stunkard A et al: An adaption study of human obesity, N Engl J Med 314:193-198, 1986.
11. Stunkard A et al: A twin study of human obesity, JAMA 256:51-54, 1986.
12. Pochlman ET et al: Genotype controlled changes in body composition and fat morphology following overfeeding in twins, Am J Clin Nutr 43:723-730, 1986.
13. You can lose weight and keep it off, Tufts University Diet and Nutrition Letter 7:1, March 1989.
14. Owen E et al: A reappraisal of caloric requirements in healthy women, Am J Clin Nutr 44:1-19, 1986.
15. Zuti B and Golding L: Comparing diet and exercise as weight reduction tools, Physician Sportsmedicine 4:49-54, 1976.
16. Dieting-induced obesity: a hidden hazard of weight cycling, Environmental Nutrition 10:1, 1987.
17. Moss AJ: Caution: very-low calorie diets can be deadly, Ann Intern Med 102:121-123, 1985.
18. Munnings F: Exercise and estrogen in women's health: getting a clearer picture, Physician Sportsmedicine 16:152-161, 1988.
19. Lamb L: Exercise protects heart during dieting, The Health Letter 31:3, Feb 12, 1988.
20. Myers RJ et al: Accuracy of self-reports of food intake in obese and normal-weight individuals: effects of obesity on self-reports of dieting intake in adult females, Am J Clin Nutr 48:1248-1251, 1988.
21. Wood P: California diet and exercise program, Mountain View, Calif, 1983, Anderson World Books, Inc.
22. Wood PD: Increased exercise level and plasma lipoprotein concentrations: a one-year, randomized controlled study in sedentary middle-aged men, Metabolism 31:31, 1983.
23. Leon AS et al: Effects of a vigorous walking program on body composition and carbohydrate and lipid metabolism of obese young men, Am J Clin Nutr 32:1776-1787, 1979.
24. The Surgeon General's Report on Nutrition and Health, Washington, DC, 1988, U.S. Department of Health and Human Services.
25. Groves D: Is childhood obesity related to TV addiction? Physician Sportsmedicine 16:117-122, 1988.
26. Manson JE et al: Body weight and longevity: a reassessment, JAMA 257:353-357, 1987.
27. Lipnickey SC: Beyond dieting: a preventive perspective on eating disorders, Health 89/90, Guilford, Conn, 1989, The Dushkin Publishing Group, Inc.
28. Love S and Johnson CL: Eating disorders, Dairy Council Digest 56:1-5, 1985.
29. Anderson AE: American Anorexia/Bulimia Association, Inc. Newsletter 9:16, 1986.
30. Bjorntorp P: Regional patterns of fat distribution, Ann Intern Med 103:994-995, 1985.

Annotated Readings

Brownell KD and Steen SN: Modern methods for weight control: the physiology and psychology of dieting, Physician Sportsmedicine 15:122-137, Dec 1987.
Discusses the physiological and psychological factors that influence the regulation of body weight and reviews several approaches to weight loss. The authors propose a comprehensive, multidisciplinary program for weight management.

Chinnici M: Picking the perfect diet, The Walking Magazine 4:40-43,46,48, May/June 1989.
Discusses the futility of rapid weight loss, describes 29 of the most popular diets, and presents the health implications and their positive and negative points.

Dusek DE: Weight management the fitness way, Boston, 1989, Jones & Bartlett Publishers.
Presents a holistic approach to weight management. Systematically illustrates how individuals may set goals suitable for themselves. Offers several exercise, nutrition, and stress-management options that can be incorporated into a healthy lifestyle.

Lamb L, editor: Calorie loss after exercise, The Health Letter 30:1-2, Dec 11, 1987.
Discusses the contribution of the calories expended during recovery from exercise to weight loss.

Long P: What America eats, Hippocrates 3:38-45, May/June 1989.
Shows how American eating patterns have changed in the last few decades and why this has taken place. Convenience is replacing cooking, and sit-down meals in the home are rare.

To lose weight, walk, don't swim, Tufts University Diet and Nutrition Letter 7:2, April 1989.
Presents a rationale for walking for weight loss and discusses the reasons why swimming appears to be ineffective in promoting fat loss.

ASSESSMENT ACTIVITY   4-1

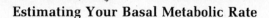

Estimating Your Basal Metabolic Rate

Directions: Study the example below and then calculate your personal total energy expenditure.

The calculations for estimating BMR use different constants for men and women. The constant for men is 1 calorie per kilogram (2.2 lbs) per hour; for women 0.9 calories per kilogram per hour. These constants are referred to as the BMR factor. An example for a 125-pound woman follows:

1. Convert body weight in pounds to kilograms: 125 lbs ÷ 2.2 lbs = 56.8 kg

2. Multiply weight in kilograms by the BMR factor: 56.8 × 0.9 cal/kg/hr = 51.5 calories/hr

3. Multiply calories/hr by 24 hours: 51.1 calories/hr × 24 hrs = 1227.3 calories/24 hrs

4. The BMR is 1227.3 calories/day.

To determine the total daily calories expended, you need to estimate the number of calories used in muscular movement during a typical day. This is a rough approximation at best, but you should be within your range if you follow the guidelines below and select the category that fits you best.

1. Sedentary—Student, desk job, sitting during most of your work and leisure time: add 40% to 50% of the BMR.

2. Light activity—Teacher, assembly line worker, walk two miles regularly: add 55% to 65% of the BMR.

3. Moderate activity—Waitress, waiter, aerobic exercise at about 75% of maximum heart rate: add 65% to 70% of the BMR.

4. Heavy activity—Construction worker, aerobic exercise above 75% of maximum heat rate: add 75% to 100% of BMR.

If our subject determines that her level of activity is in the "light" category, then she will proceed as follows to calculate the range of her daily total calorie expenditure:

1. Multiply BMR by the level of activity
   a. 1227.3 × .55 = 675
   b. 1227.3 × .65 = 797.7

2. Add BMR calories to level of activity calories to get total calories
   a. 1227.3 + 675 = 1902.3 calories/day
   b. 1227.3 + 797.7 = 2025 calories/day

This subject's total calorie expenditure in a day falls between 1902.3 and 2025 calories.

Calculate your BMR by doing the following:

I. Calculate BMR:

   1. Convert body weight (BW) in pounds to kilograms.

      _____ ÷ 2.2 = _____kg
      BW in lbs

   2. Multiply weight in kilograms by the BMR factor for your sex (male factor 1.0, female factor 0.9).

      _____× _____= _____calories/hr
      BMR factor   weight in kg

   3. Multiply _____× 24 hrs = _____calories/24 hrs
          calories/hr

   4. BMR = _____calories/24 hrs

II. Determine your level of physical activity.

   1. Multiply BMR by the level of activity factor

      _____× _____= _____calories/24 hrs
       BMR   Level of activity
                 factor

      _____× _____= _____calories/24 hrs
       BMR   Level of activity
                 factor

   2. Add the number of BMR calories to the level of activity calories to get the range of total calories expended in 24 hrs.

      _____+ _____= _____calories/24 hrs
      BMR calories   Level of activity
                    calories

      _____+ _____= _____calories/24 hrs
      BMR calories   Level of activity
                    calories

   3. Total calories expended range from_____ to _____.

ASSESSMENT ACTIVITY   4-2

Calculating Caloric Expenditure Through Exercise

Directions: The following exercise illustrates the necessary calculations used for determining weight loss through exercise. In the example below a subject weighing 195 lbs. wishes to lose 12 lbs. by exercising 40 minutes per day five times per week. He decides to ride a bike at 13 mph as his form of exercise. We will use Table 4-4 to obtain the appropriate coefficient (0.071) for this activity and 3500 calories in 1 pound of fat. Study this example and then apply it to the problem presented at the end of this assessment to answer the following questions:

1. How many calories are expended per exercise session?
2. How many pounds may be lost per week at this energy expenditure?
3. How long will it take to lose 12 lbs.?

1. Multiply body weight by the appropriate activity coefficient.
    a. 195 lbs $\times$ 0.071 = 13.8 calories for 1 minute.
    b. 13.8 calories/min $\times$ 40 min = 552 calories for 40 min.

2. Multiply the number of calories expended per workout by the number of workouts per week.
    a. 552 calories/40 min $\times$ 5 workouts per week = 2760 calories per week.
    b. $\dfrac{2760 \text{ calories per week}}{3500 \text{ calories per pound of fat}} = 0.79$ pounds of fat per week

3. Divide the total pounds you want to lose (12 lbs) by the number of pounds lost per week.
    $\dfrac{12 \text{ lbs}}{0.79 \text{ lbs of fat per week}} = 15.1$ weeks

    This subject would lose 12 lbs in 15 weeks by riding a bike at 13 mph for 40 min per day five times per week. Your weight-loss goals can be achieved in the same way.

    Now apply your knowledge of energy expenditure through exercise by solving the following problem. Jim weighs 220 lbs and wishes to lose 25 lbs by jogging at 5 mph for 30 min per exercise session 5 days per week. Do the calculations to solve Jim's problem by following the steps below.

1. Multiply body weight by the appropriate activity coefficient from Table 6-4 for jogging 5 mph.
    a. 220 lbs $\times$ _____coefficient = _____calories/min
    b. _____calories/min $\times$ 30 min = _____calories/30 min

2. Multiply the number of calories expended per workout by the number of workouts per week.
    a. _____calories/30 min $\times$ 5 days/week = _____calories/week
    b. _____calories/week $\div$ _____lbs lost/week = _____weeks

3. Divide the total pounds to be lost by the number of pounds lost per week
    25 lbs $\div$ _____lbs lost/week = _____weeks

4. a. How many calories would Jim expend per exercise session?_____
    b. How many pounds will he lose per week at this energy expenditure?_____
    c. How many weeks will it take Jim to lose 25 lbs?_____

ASSESSMENT ACTIVITY   4-3

Are You An Apple or a Pear?

   "Apples" are persons who deposit fat in the abdomen and upper body. This is android deposition and is the characteristic male pattern of fat distribution. Android obesity is associated with a number of metabolic and chronic complications that impair health and longevity, regardless of whether it manifests itself in men or women.

   Pears distribute fat in the hips and thighs. This is gynoid deposition and is the characteristic of female pattern fat distribution. Gynoid obesity is weakly associated with the same diseases as android obesity.

Directions: Are you an apple or a pear? This can be calculated quite easily by determining the waist/hip ratio. Measure the circumference of your waist about one-half inch above the navel and then measure the circumference of the hips at the greatest protrusion of the buttocks. Divide the waist circumference by the hip circumference. If the number is less than 0.75, you are a pear. If it is more than 0.85, you are an apple. Numbers in between these two values are neutral. A waist/hip ratio above 1.0 for men and above 0.8 for women increases the risk of developing Type II diabetes, high blood pressure, coronary heart disease, stroke, and gout.[30] These data suggest that even mild obesity leads to health and longevity when fat is deposited in the male pattern. See Figure 6-17 for an illustration of these two patterns.

Is your fat distributed in a gynoid or android pattern?
To find out, do the following:

1. Measure the circumference of your waist:_____.

2. Measure the circumference of your hips:_____.

3. Divide the waist measurement by the hip measurement:
$$\frac{\text{Waist}}{\text{Hips}} = \underline{\hspace{2cm}}$$

4. Are you an apple or a pear, or are you in the neutral category?

ASSESSMENT ACTIVITY

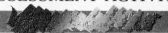

Calculating Desirable Body Weight

Directions: To find your desirable body weight, insert your current weight, percentage of fat, and the desirable body fat that you wish to attain in the appropriate spaces below. Then calculate fat weight, lean weight, and desirable body weight. Then subtract desirable body weight from your current weight. This tells you how much weight you must lose to achieve your desirable percentage of body fat.

_____

Current weight =_____

Current percentage of body fat =_____

Desirable body fat =_____

Desirable body weight =_____

Amount of weight to lose =_____

1. Fat weight = $\dfrac{\text{Body weight} \times \text{percentage of fat}}{100}$

   Fat weight =_____

2. Lean weight = Body weight − Fat weight
   Lean weight =_____

3. Desirable body weight = $\dfrac{\text{Lean weight}}{1.0 - \text{percentage of fat desired}}$

   Desirable body weight =_____

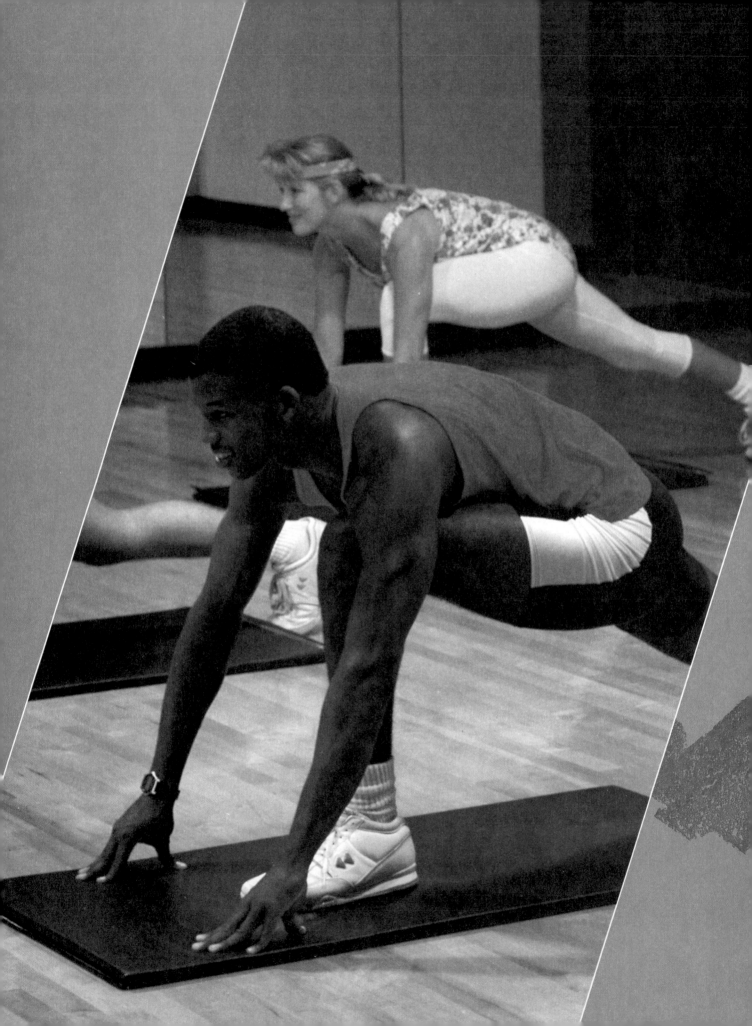

Chapter 5

Cardiovascular Health and Wellness

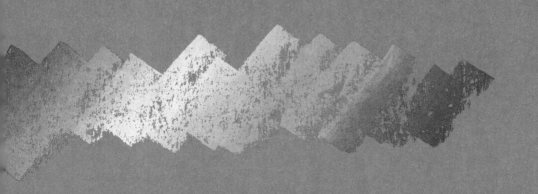

Key terms

aneurysm

atherosclerosis

cerebral hemorrhage

embolus

hypertension

myocardial infarction

thrombus

Objectives

After completing this chapter, you will be able to:

▌ Describe the gross anatomy and function of the heart.

▌ Trace the development of cardiovascular disease during this century in the United States.

▌ Identify and differentiate between several different types of cardiovascular disease.

▌ Identify the risk factors for heart disease and discuss ways to reduce these.

▌ Discuss the lifestyle behaviors that contribute to health promotion and longevity.

Cardiovascular disease includes a group of diseases that affect the heart and blood vessels. The five major forms of cardiovascular disease as classified by the American Heart Association are coronary heart disease, hypertensive disease, rheumatic heart disease, strokes, and congenital heart defects.[1] Cardiovascular disease—the leading cause of death in the United States—accounts for 47% of all deaths. Twenty-five percent of Americans (approximately 66 million people) have one or more forms of heart or blood vessel disease. There have been approximately 1,500,000 heart attacks in each of the last few years and more than 500,000 of these resulted in death. Three hundred thousand, or 60%, of these deaths occurred before the victim reached a hospital emergency room. This is a tragedy that is made even worse because a significant number of these premature deaths could have been avoided with early and proper treatment.

Fifty percent of heart attack victims wait an average of 2 hours before seeking medical attention. Denying the possibility that a heart attack may be in progress is the primary reason for the delay. Denial is reinforced because the symptoms of a heart attack are similar to those of other physical ailments and we are more prone to believe that it is one of the other problems rather than a heart attack.

Although the figures are foreboding, and while there is much that remains to be done in the battle against cardiovascular disease, substantial progress has occurred during the last 3 decades. The death rate for all cardiovascular diseases declined by approximately 23% from 1976 to 1986. During this same 10-year span, the death rate from coronary heart disease, which is responsible for the majority of heart attack deaths, declined by 28%. Deaths from strokes declined by 4% during the same period. The downward trend in the death rate from cardiovascular disease has been attributed primarily to lifestyle changes and more sophisticated medical diagnosis and treatment.

The Fundamentals of Circulation

The Heart, Blood, and Blood Vessels

Circulation is better understood if one is familiar with the basic anatomy and function of the heart. The heart consists of cardiac muscle and weighs between 8 and 10 ounces. It is about the size of a fist and lies in the center of the chest. The heart is divided into two halves, or pumps, by a wall (the septum) and each half is subdivided into an upper chamber (the atrium) and a lower chamber (the ventricle). The right heart, or "pulmonary pump," receives deoxygenated blood from all tissues of the body and then transports it to the lungs so carbon dioxide can be exchanged for a fresh supply of oxygen. From the lungs, the oxygen-rich blood is sent to the left heart, or "systemic pump," so that it can be transported to all of the tissues of the body. Both pumps work simultaneously. The left pump carries the heavier workload of the two and thus has a more muscular ventricular wall. Figure 5-1 illustrates pulmonary and systemic circulation.

The primary function of circulation is to provide a constant supply of blood and nutrients to the cells while removing their waste products. Under ordinary circumstances, the interruption

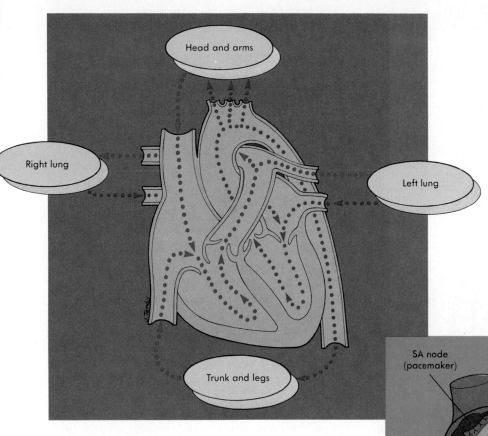

Figure 5-1 Circulation of the pulmonary and systemic pumps.

Figure 5-2 The electrical conduction system of the heart.

of blood flow for as little as 4 minutes can impair the brain and may possibly result in death.

The average heart beats 70 to 80 times per minute at rest. Endurance athletes often have resting heart rates in the 30 and 40 beat range, while some overweight and sedentary smokers have resting heart rates in the nineties. The low heart rates of endurance athletes reflect physiological adaptations to training and represent normal values for this group. The Framingham Heart Disease Study showed that a rapid resting heart rate increased the risk of death from heart attack. Mortality increased progressively with heart rate, especially among male subjects.

The resting heart rate is established by the sinoatrial node (SA node, or pacemaker) located in the right atrium as shown in Figure 5-2. The atria contract, forcing blood into the ventricles as the electrical impulse travels from the SA node to the atrioventricular node (AV node) located between the right atrium and right ventricle. The electrical impulse pauses for one-tenth of a second at the AV node to allow the ventricles to fill with blood and then resumes down the system and spreads throughout the ventricular walls. The ventricles contract during this time, ejecting blood from these chambers.

Blood that enters the chambers of the heart does not directly nourish it. Cardiac muscle receives its nourishment when the heart contracts, sending blood via the aorta (the largest artery in the body) to the coronary arteries that supply it with blood and nutrients. Coronary circulation is illustrated in Figure 5-3. The left coronary artery supplies a major portion of the myocardium with blood, while the right coronary artery services less of it. Both vessels divide and subdivide downstream and eventually culminate in a dense

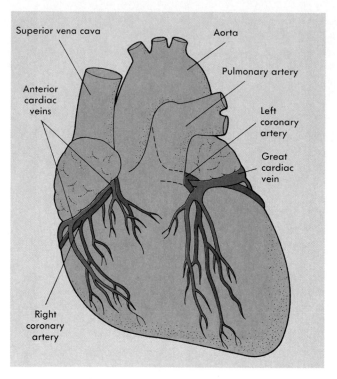

Figure 5-3 The coronary circulation.

network of capillaries (the smallest blood vessels in the body). Blood supply to the myocardium is so important that every muscle fiber is supplied by at least one capillary. The coronary veins return deoxygenated blood to the right atrium so that it can enter pulmonary circulation. The veins bring deoxygenated blood from all tissues of the body back to the right atrium.

Blood plasma is a clear yellowish fluid that carries approximately 100 chemicals. Plasma represents 55% of the blood contents. The remaining 45% consists of blood solids—the erythrocytes (red cells), the leukocytes (white cells), and the blood platelets. The red cells are the most abundant of the blood solids. They carry oxygen and carbon dioxide to and from the tissues of the body attached to hemoglobin, an iron-containing protein. The white cells are an important part of the body's defense system against invading microorganisms and other foreign substances. The blood platelets are involved in the complex processes that lead to the formation of clots for repairing damaged blood vessels.

Cardiovascular Disease: A Twentieth Century Phenomenon

Cardiovascular disease, a relatively rare event 100 years ago, reached epidemic proportions dur-

ing the middle of the twentieth century. The term *angina* pectoris (chest pain) was introduced into the medical literature by William Heberden, a British physician in the latter part of the eighteenth century. He was unable to offer any treatment for this strange malady. It wasn't until 1910 that recurrent episodes of angina pectoris began to be connected to heart disease by physicians. Chest pain and other manifestations of a heart attack were not identified with obstructions of the coronary arteries until the early 1900s. The first accurate description of the events associated with a heart attack by an American physician occurred in 1912. The illness he described, that had occurred to a 55-year old man with no previous evidence of disease, is now a commonplace episode in American life. The man died 3 days after the onset of symptoms. A postmortem examination of the heart revealed the formation of a clot that had occluded, or blocked, one of the major coronary arteries. In 1912, this was a medical rarity.

Coronary heart disease is responsible for the majority of heart attack deaths, but there are other forms of heart disease that contribute to disability and death. *Congenital heart defects* exist at birth and affect approximately 25,000 newborns annually. *Rheumatic heart disease,* caused by a streptococcal infection of the throat or ear, is virtually 100% preventable. Antibiotic treatment during the infection stage will arrest the processes that might lead to rheumatic heart disease. *Congestive heart failure* occurs when the heart muscle is damaged to the extent that it is no longer capable of contracting with sufficient force to pump blood throughout the body. The damage is usually due to long-standing hypertension. Mild to moderate hypertension may be controlled through appropriate lifestyle interventions; severe hypertension requires medication in addition to lifestyle approaches.

Coronary Heart Disease

Coronary heart disease is actually a disease of the arteries that supply the heart with blood and nutrients. A heart attack, or **myocardial infarction,** (death of heart muscle tissue) occurs when an obstruction or spasm disrupts or terminates blood flow to a portion of the heart muscle. The amount of heart muscle damage is determined by the location of the obstruction or spasm and how quickly medical intervention is begun. Heart attacks of any magnitude produce irreversible injury and myocardial tissue death. It usually takes

5 to 6 weeks after a heart attack has occurred for the dead cardiac tissue to form a fibrous scar. This area of dead tissue can no longer contribute to the pumping of blood, resulting in a less efficient heart. Massive heart attacks that cause extensive muscle damage result in death.

Although most heart attacks occur after the age of 65, the processes leading to them often begin prior to adolescence. These processes are insidious and often go undetected until, without warning, a heart attack occurs. The attack is sudden but the processes leading to it are long-standing. In fact, there is considerable evidence that the silent phase of coronary heart disease has pediatric origins.

The ongoing Framingham Study, which began in 1949, identified the risk factors connected with heart disease.[2] Cigarette smoking, high blood pressure, elevated cholesterol, diabetes, overweight, stress, physical inactivity, age, gender, and family history were found to be highly related to heart attack and stroke. As the risks were uncovered, the realization evolved that heart disease was not the inevitable consequence of aging or bad luck, but an acquired disease that was potentially preventable. It took a few years to realize that preventive efforts should begin in childhood and a few more years before researchers investigated the prevalence of these risks among children and adolescents.

An autopsy study of 18-year-olds showed a positive relationship between blood cholesterol levels and the prevalence of fatty streaks on the walls of the coronary arteries and aorta.[3] The evidence indicates that the average cholesterol level in children in overfed, underexercised societies such as our own is too high.

High blood pressure has been reported in children as young as 3 years of age, and there is general agreement that blood pressure levels tend to track into adulthood.[4] Almost 19% of high school seniors smoke cigarettes on a daily basis, and the use of smokeless tobacco products has increased substantially among 17- to 19-year old males.[5] It is estimated that one in five youngsters between the ages of 5 and 17 are substantially overweight; that is, they are a minimum of 20% above their desirable weight.[6]

Autopsy studies of American combat battle casualties, average age of 22 years, in the Korean and Vietnamese wars showed obstructions in the coronary arteries.[7,8] Native Korean and Vietnamese soldiers had clean and open arteries. These obstructions are caused by **atherosclerosis,** which is a slow progressive disease of the arteries that can originate in childhood. It is characterized by the deposition of plaque on the inner lining of arterial walls (See Figure 5-4). Plaque consists of fatty substances, cholesterol, blood platelets, fibrin, calcium, and cellular debris that anchor to a roughened site in the artery. Several theories have been advanced regarding the development of rough spots in arteries, but whatever the trigger, the smooth muscle cells beneath the lining erupt and form a network of connective tissue that eventually becomes plaque. Plaque enlarges over many years, progressively narrowing the arterial channel through which blood must flow and causing the affected heart muscle to become *ischemic* (diminished supply of blood). Eventually the channel narrows to the extent that a clot forms and closes the vessel completely. The heart muscle formerly supplied by the occluded artery dies. The atherosclerotic process is responsible for 80% of the coronary heart disease deaths in the United States.

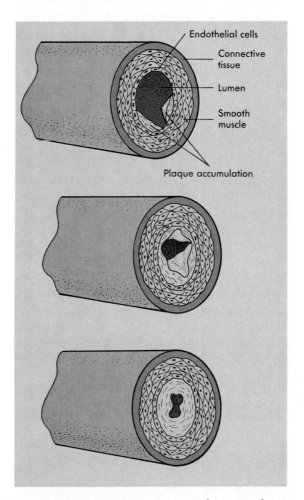

Figure 5-4 Progressive narrowing of a normal coronary artery (atherosclerosis).

Figure 5-5 Signs of a heart attack

The warning signs

▮ Uncomfortable pressure, fullness, squeezing as if a band were being tightened around the chest, or pain in the center of the chest lasting longer than two minutes.

▮ Pain that spreads to the shoulders, arms, or neck. (See the illustration below.)

▮ The above may be accompanied by one or more of the following; dizziness, fainting, sweating, nausea, or shortness of breath.

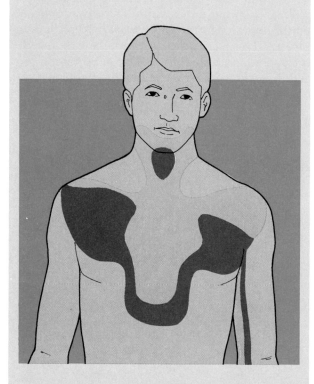

What you should do if these signs appear

If you have chest discomfort lasting more than 2 minutes:

▮ Don't deny what may be occurring.

▮ Call the emergency service or have a friend or family member drive you to the nearest hospital that has 24 hour emergency cardiac care.

▮ Know in advance those hospitals that have such a service.

▮ The telephone number of the emergency rescue service should be prominently displayed and a copy should be carried on your person.

Some heart attacks, quite possibly as many as one-third, are silent and imperceptible to the victim. These events usually involve small areas of the heart muscle and may go unnoticed by the victim unless discovered and verified by an electrocardiogram (EKG). However, the typical heart attack is very noticeable and the symptoms are overt. See Figure 5-5 for the warning signs of a heart attack.

Atherosclerotic lesions are more likely to form where single arteries branch out into two smaller arteries. Vessel diameters reduce where branching occurs. This increases blood turbulence, which produces greater wear and tear at these sites. This combination of events renders these sites more vulnerable to injury and the development of plaque. This phenomenon may occur in the arteries leading to the brain, kidneys, lungs and legs, as well as the heart.

Coronary heart disease may be delayed or prevented by keeping the risk factors associated with heart disease in check. Most of them can be modified and controlled through appropriate lifestyle behaviors. The risks for cardiovascular disease are covered in the next section of this chapter.

Stroke

The majority of strokes (cerebrovascular accidents) follow the same process of events that results in coronary heart disease. A stroke is essentially the result of diseased blood vessels that supply the brain. It shares the same risk factors as coronary heart disease and it takes years to develop.

Strokes are caused by a **thrombus** (a clot that forms and occludes an artery supplying the brain) or an **embolus** (a clot that forms elsewhere in the body and fractures, dislodges, and is transported to one of the cerebral blood vessels that is too small for its passage). **Cerebral hemorrhage** (the bursting of a blood vessel in the brain because of arterial brittleness or aneurysm) is a third cause of stroke. An **aneurysm** is a weak spot in an artery that forms a balloon-like pouch that can rupture. It may be a congenital defect or the result of uncontrolled or poorly controlled hypertension.

On many occasions, but not all, a stroke is preceded by warning signs and signals. These must first be recognized and acknowledged and then acted upon so that prompt medical and lifestyle interventions may be instituted to prevent or delay the advent of a stroke (Figure 5-6).

Strategies intended for the prevention of strokes are similar to those employed in the prevention of coronary heart disease. They include control of blood pressure and cholesterol, smoking cessation, weight management, exercise, and proper nutrition. A study of 22,071 middle-aged male physicians showed that those who took one aspirin every other day had 44% fewer first heart attacks than those who took a placebo, but there was an accompanying increase in the incidence of strokes among the aspirin takers.[2] However, the latest analysis showed that the risk of stroke among the aspirin group was quite small and was far outweighed by the benefits of aspirin in reducing heart attacks.

Management of stroke victims is dependent on the nature and extent of the damage as revealed by a battery of diagnostic tests. In addition to the physical examination, these may include cerebral arteriography, which provides information on the status of the cerebral arteries; computed tomography (CT scan), which enables physicians to examine structures within the body that cannot be observed with conventional x-ray procedures; and the use of the electroencephalograph, which is radiographic imaging of the brain.

Risk Factors for Heart Disease

The risk factors for cardiovascular disease have been categorized by the American Heart Association (AHA) as: (1) major risk factors that can't be changed (increasing age, male sex, and heredity); (2) major risk factors that can be changed (elevated blood cholesterol, high blood pressure, and cigarette smoking); and (3) other contributing factors (obesity, diabetes, stress, and physical inactivity).[1] The AHA is under criticism at the present time for their conservative posture regarding their categorization of the risk factors. Many researchers have suggested that they are moving too slowly in recognizing physical inactivity as a risk factor of major importance in light of current evidence. A case may also be made for upgrading diabetes mellitus, stress, and obesity to major risk factor status. Many in the scientific community are waiting to see how the AHA categorizes these risks in the near future.

Major Risk Factors That Can Not Be Changed

Age. Fifty-five percent of all heart attacks occur to those who are 65 years of age or older. This age group accounts for more than 80% of the fatal heart attacks.

Figure 5-6 Stroke: the warning signs

The American Heart Association suggests that the American public be familiar with the following warning signs:
- Temporary loss of speech, difficulty in speaking or understanding speech.
- Unexplained dizziness, unsteadiness, or sudden falls.
- Temporary dimness or loss of vision, particularly in one eye.
- Sudden, temporary weakness or numbness of the face, arm, and leg on one side of the body.
- A major stroke is often preceded by a series of minor strokes, or transient ischemic attacks (TIA).

These are warning signals that may be experienced days, weeks, or months before a major stroke.

Americans who are 65 years of age and older represent about 12% of the total population, but their health care expenditures are approximately one third of the U.S. total.[10] Cardiovascular diseases, primarily coronary heart disease, is responsible for more than half of the deaths in this age group. With regard to preventing cardiovascular disease, the authors of this article state, "Especially important are the nonpharmacologic therapies, including diet, exercise, and health-promoting lifestyles."[10]

Male sex. Until recently, the incidence of coronary heart disease among women has been largely unexplored. Men have been the primary subjects in the coronary heart disease and risk factor studies because of the high incidence of both among men. But coronary heart disease is also the leading cause of death and disability among women, accounting for almost 250,000 deaths annually.[11] However, women have less heart disease than men, and this is particularly discernible before menopause. After menopause, the heart attack rate among women increases significantly but it does not reach the level observed in men. The reasons advanced for the difference include: (1) the female hormone estrogen protects the coronary arteries from atherosclerosis, and (2) women have higher circulating levels of high density lipoprotein cholesterol, which also protects the arteries. But an alarming trend has sur-

■ TABLE 5-1 Sources of dietary cholesterol and saturated fat

	Cholesterol (in milligrams)*	Saturated fat (in milligrams)*
Meats (3 oz)		
Beef liver	372	2500
Veal	86	4000
Pork	80	3200
Lean beef	56	2400
Chicken (dark meat)	82	2700
Chicken (white meat)	76	1300
One egg	274	1700
Dairy products (1 cup; cheese 1 oz)		
Ice cream	59	8900
Whole milk	33	5100
Butter (1 tbsp)	31	7100
Yogurt (low fat)	11	1800
Cheddar	30	6000
American	27	5600
Camembert	20	4300
Parmesan	8	2000
Oils (1 tbsp)		
Coconut	0	11,800
Palm	0	6700
Olive	0	1800
Corn	0	1700
Safflower	0	1200

	Cholesterol (in milligrams)*	Saturated fat (in milligrams)*
Fish (3 oz)		
Squid	153	400
Oily fish	59	1200
Lean fish	59	300
Shrimp (6 large)	48	200
Clams (6 large)	36	300
Lobster	46.5	75
Other items of interest		
Pork brains	2169	1800
Beef kidney	683	3800
Beef hot dog	75	9900
Prime ribs of beef	66.5	5300
Doughnut	36	4000
Milk chocolate	18	16,300
Green or yellow vegetable or fruit	0	trace
Peanut butter (1 Tbsp)	0	1500
Angel food cake	0	1960
Skim milk (1 cup)	4	300
Cheese pizza (3 oz)	6	800
Buttermilk (1 cup)	9	1300
Ice milk, soft (1 cup)	13	2900
Turkey, white meat (3 oz)	59	900

*1000 mg = 1 gram; 454 grams = 1 lb.

faced in recent years—the incidence of heart attacks in young women has increased because they have been smoking cigarettes for a long enough period of time for it to affect their health, especially when combined with oral contraceptive use.

Heredity. According to the AHA, "A tendency toward heart disease or atherosclerosis appears to be hereditary, so children of parents with cardiovascular disease are more likely to develop it themselves."[1] First-degree relatives (parents, grandparents, and siblings) who have died of coronary heart disease prior to the age of 55 would strongly indicate a familial tendency. It becomes imperative to control the modifiable risk factors if the family history is positive.

Race is also a factor to consider. Because of pervasive hypertension, black Americans are susceptible to stroke and cardiovascular disease.[12] One of every three blacks is hypertensive compared with one of every four adults in the general population. Also, blacks have moderate hypertension twice as often and severe hypertension three times as often as whites. Possible causes for these differences include genetics, salt sensitivity, and psychological stress.[13] Black women are particularly vulnerable to hypertension because of obesity and physical inactivity.

Major Risk Factors That Can Be Changed

Cholesterol. *Cholesterol* is a steroid that is an essential structural component of neural tissue; it is used in the construction of cell walls; and it is necessary for the manufacture of hormones and bile (for the digestion and absorption of fats). A certain amount of cholesterol is required for good health, but high levels circulating in the blood are associated with heart attacks and strokes.

The AHA suggests that Americans reduce

■ TABLE 5-2 Risk of total cholesterol

Cholesterol (mg/dl)	Risk
<200*	Desirable level
200-239	Borderline
≥240†	High level

* < less than
† ≥ equal to or greater than

cholesterol consumption to less than 300 milligrams per day (300 mg/day), and that fat intake be reduced to a maximum of 30% of the total calories consumed and that saturated fat be reduced to no more than 10% of the total calories. Many authorities are convinced that it is more important to limit total fat and saturated fat than to be overly restrictive of cholesterol.

Cholesterol is consumed in the diet (exogenous, or dietary cholesterol) but it is also manufactured by the body from saturated fats (endogenous). We manufacture 1000 to 2000 mg/day and typically consume 500 to 600 mg/day. See Table 5-1 for some common foods that contain cholesterol and saturated fat.

A number of population studies during the last 20 years have indicated a positive relationship between serum cholesterol (the level of cholesterol circulating in the blood) and the development of coronary heart disease. Values of serum cholesterol above 200 mg/dl (milligrams per deciliter of blood) are higher than the average risk. The ideal value for adults has been determined to be somewhere between 130 and 190 mg/dl.[14] Table 5-2 presents the manner in which cholesterol is categorized and the risks associated with each.

An important collaborative study involving 12 research centers throughout the United States provided clinical evidence implicating cholesterol as a culprit in coronary heart disease.[15] Half of a group of 3,806 subjects was given a cholesterol-lowering drug, and the other half was given a placebo (a substance that looked like the drug but had no medicinal properties). The subjects were followed for approximately 7.4 years, at which time the data indicated that the drug group reduced their cholesterol by 13%, suffered 19% fewer heart attacks, and experienced 24% fewer fatal heart attacks. There was also a significant reduction in coronary bypass surgery and angina. The researchers concluded that each 1% reduction in cholesterol level would result in a 2% reduction in the risk of coronary heart dis-

Figure 5-7 Does oat bran lower cholesterol?

The results of a study in the New England Journal of Medicine (January, 1990) raised serious questions about the effectiveness of oat bran in lowering serum cholesterol. In this study, wheat fiber performed almost as well as oat bran in lowering serum cholesterol. The researchers concluded that oat bran functioned indirectly in lowering cholesterol by replacing some of the fatty foods that the subjects would have normally eaten.

This was a small study (20 subjects) of short duration (6 weeks). The subject's average serum cholesterol at the beginning of the study was 186 mg/dl, which was in the desirable range. Furthermore, the subjects were also atypical in that they habitually consumed 23 grams of fiber daily (twice the American average). Many of the earlier studies that reported the beneficial effects of oat bran used subjects that had high cholesterol levels (above 250 mg/dl) who were consuming a less than healthful diet. A change to a high-fiber diet should and actually did significantly help these subjects.

Of course, oat bran is just one of many foods that are high in soluble fiber, and soluble fiber is just one type of fiber. While increasing daily intake of fiber is important, lowering the intake of total fat, saturated fat, and cholesterol remain the major lifestyle changes in reducing serum cholesterol. At the very least, oat bran and other foods high in complex carbohydrates may lower serum cholesterol by leaving less room for foods high in fats and calories. Yet, the possibility still exists that oat bran may contain inherent properties that directly lower serum cholesterol, as earlier studies had indicated. More study is needed, but regardless of the fiber effect on cholesterol, one must remember that oats and other grains are low in calories and fat and high in vitamins and minerals. Oat bran and other fibers are good food.

ease. These results were independently corroborated by the Helsinki Heart Study, in which 23,531 middle-aged men were evaluated over a 5-year period.[16] During the last 3 years of the study, the incidence of coronary heart disease decreased by more than 50% in the drug versus the placebo group.

Strategies for lowering the total amount of cholesterol in the blood include (1) reduction in dietary cholesterol and saturated fat; (2) increase in the consumption of soluble fiber (the kind found in oats, beans, fruits, and vegetables, see Figure 5-7(3) reduction of body weight; and (4) quitting the cigarette habit.

The amount of total cholesterol circulating in the blood accounts for only a part of the cholesterol story. Unlike sugar or salt, cholesterol does not dissolve in the blood, so it is transported by protein packages, which facilitate its solubility. These transporters are the lipoproteins. They include the chylomicrons, very low-density lipoprotein (VLDL), intermediate-density lipoprotein (IDL), low-density lipoprotein (LDL), and high-density lipoprotein (HDL). Dietary cholesterol enters the body from the digestive system attached to the chylomicrons.[14] The chylomicrons shrink in size as they give up their cholesterol to the cells of the body. The fragments that remain are removed by the liver and used to manufacture and secrete VLDLs, which are triglyceride-rich lipoproteins. The triglycerides represent 99% of the stored fats in the body.[17] The VLDLs are degraded as their cargo of triglycerides are either used by the cells for energy or stored in adipose cells. The VLDL remnants may be removed by the liver or converted to LDLs.[14]

Low-density lipoproteins are the primary transporters of cholesterol and the most capable of producing atherosclerosis. Michael S. Brown and Joseph L. Goldstein won a 1985 Nobel Prize in Medicine and Physiology for discovering that liver cells have receptor sites which bind LDLs and remove cholesterol from the blood.[18] When LDL concentrations are excessive, the liver sites become saturated and further removal of them from the blood is significantly impeded. As a result plasma levels of cholesterol rise, leading to the formation and/or exacerbation of atherosclerotic plaque. Figure 5-8 is a schematic drawing of how the lipoproteins are made and what each does.

Heart attacks are rare when LDL values in the blood are below 100 mg/dl. A national panel of experts has developed guidelines for safe and unsafe levels of LDL, and these appear in Table 5-3. A high circulating level of LDL cholesterol is positively related to cardiovascular disease. Weight loss, a diet low in saturated fat and total fat, exercise, and medication, if needed, will lower LDL levels in the blood.

High-density lipoproteins are involved in "re-

TABLE 5-3 Risk of LDL cholesterol

LDL cholesterol (mg/dl)	Risk
<130	Desirable level
130-159	Borderline—high risk
>160	High risk

verse transport," that is, they accept cholesterol from the blood and tissues and transfer it to VLDLs and LDLs for transport back to the liver, where it can be degraded, disposed of, or recycled.[14] High-density lipoproteins protect the arteries from atherosclerosis because they clear cholesterol from the blood. Cardiovascular health is substantially dependent upon low levels of total cholesterol and LDLs and a high level of HDLs. Cigarette smoking, diabetes, elevated triglycerides, and anabolic steroids lower HDL, while physical exercise, weight loss, and moderate alcohol consumption raise it. However, before reaching for a beer, it should be noted that alcohol does not increase the sub-fraction of HDL that protects the arteries. It increases HDL3, which has no effect on heart disease.

Assessing the cholesterol risk requires the measurement of total cholesterol, HDL and LDL because it is quite conceivable that someone with desirable total cholesterol could be at substantial risk if the HDL value is low. Men whose HDL is below 25 mg/dl and women whose HDL is below 40 mg/dl are at three times the risk for heart disease.[16] The ratio between total cholesterol and HDL (TC/HDL) should also be considered when interpreting the risk. This ratio is determined by dividing TC by HDL, and the risk levels are found in Table 5-4. The average value for men is 45 mg/dl, and for women it is 55 mg/dl. This bio-

TABLE 5-4 Ratio of total cholesterol to HDL cholesterol

Risk	Male	Female
Very low (½ average)	Under 3.4	Under 3.3
Low risk	4.0	3.8
Average risk	5.0	4.5
Moderate risk (2 × average)	9.5	7.0
High risk (3 × average)	Over 23	Over 11

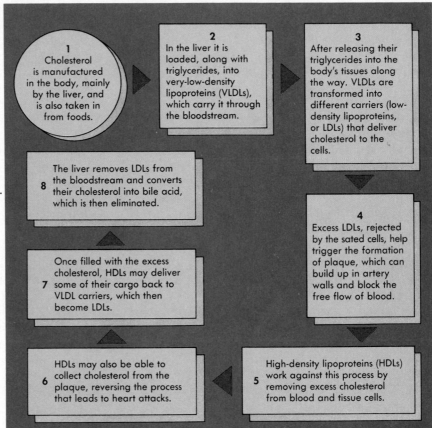

Figure 5-8 The cholesterol carriers.

logical difference in HDL between the sexes partly accounts for the lower incidence of heart disease in women as compared with men.

Over the years, a few medical investigators have challenged the validity of cholesterol as a primary risk for heart disease. The latest challenge comes from a science writer, Thomas Moore, whose book *Heart Failure* has created a stir in the scientific community. His assertions include the following: (1) diet has little effect on blood cholesterol level; (2) drugs that lower cholesterol may have serious and possible fatal consequences; and (3) there is no evidence that lowering cholesterol lengthens life. He also raises questions regarding the motives of the researchers who directed the long-term clinical trials that generated the evidence indicting cholesterol. He raises serious questions regarding the objectivity of the researchers due to conflict of interest since many of them were consultants to the pharmaceutical companies.

This latest assault on cholesterol has some merit, and Moore presents the case articulately, but there are some exaggerations and omissions of pertinent data. Possibly his watchdog critique will stimulate future researchers to tighten their

designs and to approach the problems associated with long-term research in innovative and productive ways. In the meantime, the preponderance of evidence indicates that high levels of TC and LDL, and low levels of HDL represent a blood profile that is highly related to cardiovascular disease. Don't give up your low fat, low cholesterol ways of eating just yet.

Blood pressure. Blood pressure, which is recorded in millimeters of mercury (mm Hg) is the force exerted against the walls of the arteries as blood travels through the circulatory system. Pressure is created when the heart contracts and pumps blood into the arteries. The arterioles (smallest arteries) offer resistance to blood flow and if the resistance is persistently high the pressure rises and remains high. The medical term for high blood pressure is **hypertension.**

Hypertension is a silent disease that has no characteristic signs or symptoms, so it should be checked periodically. Blood pressure can be measured quickly with a sphygmomanometer. A rubber cuff is wrapped around the upper arm and inflated with enough air to compress the artery, temporarily stopping blood flow. A stethoscope is placed on the artery below the cuff so that the sound of blood coursing through the artery can be heard when the air is released. The first sound represents the systolic pressure (the maximum pressure of blood flow when the heart contracts) and the last sound heard is the diastolic pressure (the minimum pressure of blood flow between heart beats). A typical pressure for young adults is 120/80. Pressures of 140/90 or greater are considered to be hypertensive.[1] The lower limit of normal is 100/60.[20] From a health perspective, it is advantageous to have a low-normal blood pressure and to maintain it as long as possible.

Approximately 60 million American adults and children have high blood pressure, and 30,000 people die of its complications annually. Ninety percent of the time the cause of high blood pressure is not known—this is referred to as *essential hypertension*. "Essential" is a medical term that means of unknown origin or cause. Essential hypertension cannot be cured but it can be controlled. The other 10% of the cases of hypertension have a specific cause. If the cause can be determined and eliminated, blood pressure will return to normal.

The heart is adversely affected by uncontrolled or undiagnosed hypertension of long duration. Pumping blood for years against high resistance in the arteries increases the workload of the heart so that it hypertrophies in response.

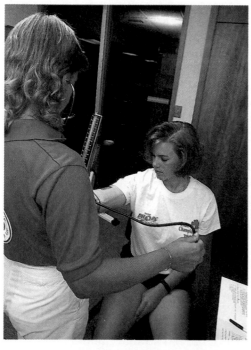

Periodic blood pressure checks can help determine whether dietary or other changes may be needed to help control hypertension.

The heart receives inadequate rest because the resistance to blood flow is consistently high, and this produces muscle fibers that become overly stretched. They progressively lose their ability to snap back. The end result is that they contract less forcefully. At this point, the heart loses its efficiency and becomes weakened. If intervention does not occur early in the process, congestive heart failure is inevitable. High blood pressure also damages the arteries and accelerates atherosclerosis.

Treatment for hypertension may include all or some of the following: weight loss, salt and alcohol restriction, calcium and potassium supplementation, voluntary relaxation techniques, exercise, and medication. Excess body weight increases the work of the heart because it must meet the nutrient demands of the extra tissue.

Americans consume approximately 6 to 18 grams (1 to 3½ teaspoons) of salt daily. Table salt, composed of sodium and chloride, accounts for most of the daily consumption because it is added to many foods as a flavor enhancer and an inexpensive preservative. The real culprit in table salt is sodium, which accounts for about 40% of its make-up. There are 5 grams of salt in one teaspoon, 2.2 grams of which are sodium. Based on total salt consumption, the average American ingests 4.4 to 8.8 grams of sodium per day. The recommended daily allowance for sodium is 1.1 to 3.3 grams (½ to 1½ teaspoons). Excessive salt intake has been implicated as an important factor in the development of high blood pressure. It appears that high salt intake increases the blood pressure in those who are salt sensitive. It is imperative for such people to lose the salt shaker and abstain from salt-laden foods. Salt is an acquired taste, and it is prudent for all people to reduce their intake to the recommended amount.

Some calcium-deficient hypertensives may normalize their blood pressure by taking calcium supplements. However, calcium supplementation does not work for all calcium-deficient hypertensives, and it does not work for hypertensives who are not calcium deficient.

Yoga, meditation, hypnotherapy, biofeedback and other relaxation techniques may help to alleviate tension and anxiety and beneficially affect high blood pressure. Exercise is also an effective relaxation therapy whose effects on blood pressure are discussed in Chapter 6. Many people drink alcohol because it makes them feel relaxed, among other things, but more than 2 ounces per day raises the blood pressure of some people.

Medications have been developed that are effective in controlling blood pressure. However, they have side effects that include weakness, leg cramps, stuffy nose, occasional diarrhea, heartburn, drowsiness, anemia, depression, headaches, joint pain, light headedness, impotence, skin rash, and others. The type of side effect is unique to the class of drug being used to control blood pressure. In spite of these side effects, many people find it easier to take the medicine than to make the difficult lifestyle changes that lower blood pressure. It is wise to make the effort to control blood pressure without medication but if it is needed, that does not negate the importance of controlling those lifestyle factors that contribute to the problem. Medicine and lifestyle efforts are not mutually exclusive—each makes a contribution in blood pressure management.

Cigarette smoking. Many medical authorities consider cigarette smoking to be the most potent of the preventable risk factors associated with chronic illness and premature death.[21] Forty percent of the male smokers and 28% of the female smokers die prematurely. Smokers have twice the risk of having a heart attack and they are two to four times more likely to die suddenly from a heart attack than non-smokers.[1] High blood pressure results from peripheral resistance to blood flow, and cigarette smoking contributes to peripheral resistance by constricting the arterioles. Smoking significantly exacerbates the effects of high blood pressure. Although cigarette smoking is on the decline, 26.5% of Americans over the age of 20 continue to smoke.[21]

Two products in cigarette smoke, carbon monoxide and nicotine, have a devastating effect on the heart and blood vessels. Carbon monoxide, a noxious gas that is a by-product of the combustion of tobacco products, displaces oxygen in the blood because it has a greater affinity for hemoglobin. The diminished oxygen-carrying capacity of the blood is partly responsible for the shortness of breath that smokers experience with mild physical exertion.

Nicotine is a powerful stimulant that[22]:

1. Increases LDL and lowers HDL.
2. Causes the platelets to aggregate, which increases the probability of arterial spasms.
3. Increases the oxygen requirement of cardiac muscle.
4. Constricts blood vessels.
5. Produces cardiac arrhythmias (irregular heart beat).
6. Up to 30% of all coronary heart disease deaths are related to smoking.

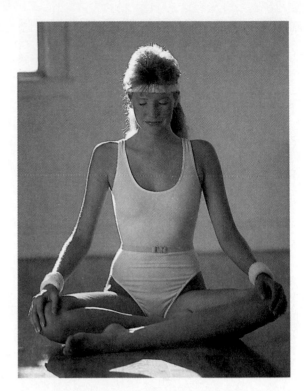

Relaxation techniques may help to reduce stress and lower blood pressure.

The harmful effects of cigarette smoking are insidious and take time to appear. The medical profession measures the damage from smoking in pack years. For instance, smoking one pack of cigarettes per day for 15 years is equal to 15 pack years (15 years × 1 pack per day = 15 pack years). Two packs per day for 15 years is equal to 30 pack years (15 × 2 = 30). Twenty-five to thirty pack years represents a threshold beyond which medical problems become evident.

To quit the tobacco habit, one must first break the addiction to nicotine, and second, break the psychological dependence on smoking. This involves a change in behavior as well as effective ways to deal with the social and situational stimuli that promote the desire to smoke. Males have been more successful than females in quitting smoking. Since 1964, 21.4% of the males have quit compared with 5.8% of the females.[22] Today more young women than young men are smoking—this represents a reversal of a long-standing trend.[23] The increasing number of young female smokers, coupled with the number of years that women have been smoking has reversed another

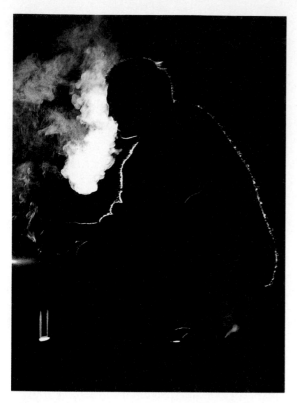

There are no known physiological benefits to cigarette smoking.

trend—breast cancer has been replaced by lung cancer as the leading cause of cancer death among women.

Complicating the effort to quit, particularly among young women, is the fear of gaining weight. Approximately 65% of these who quit do gain weight, but the physiological adaptations that occur may only account for a 3- to 4-pound weight gain. The physiological mechanisms responsible are probably associated with a slowing of metabolism and increased transit time of food in the digestive system so that more is absorbed by the body. Weight gain beyond 4 pounds is probably due to altered eating patterns rather than physiology. Food smells and tastes better, it may substitute for a cigarette, especially during social activities, it may provide some of the oral gratification previously obtained from smoking, and it may relieve tension. Weight gain can be avoided by eating sensibly and exercising moderately and frequently. An often-seen combination is the link-up between cigarette smoking and caffeine intake. See Figure 5-9 for some information on the caffeine/nicotine connection.

As a group, smokers are 7% lighter than non-smokers, but smokers tend to distribute more fat in the abdominal area.[24] The waist-to-hip ratio (WHR) is greater in smokers even though they are lighter. Fat distributed in this manner is not only esthetically unappealing but also predisposes to coronary heart disease, diabetes, stroke, and gout.

Involuntary or passive smoking (inhaling the smoke of others) is associated with premature disease and death. Studies in the United States and several other countries have indicated that non-smoking spouses of smokers are two to four times more likely to contract and die from lung cancer as compared with non-smoking couples.[25] Furthermore, nonsmoking spouses are three times more likely to die of a heart attack if their mate smokes.[26] Passive smoking aggravates and may precipitate angina and it also induces small airway dysfunction in adults.

An alarming trend is the escalating sale of smokeless tobacco products. Chewing tobacco and dipping snuff have become very popular among high school- and college-age males. The World Health Organization (WHO) has described the growing use of smokeless tobacco as a new threat to society. Nicotine is an addictive drug regardless of the method of delivery and its effects are similar whether it is inhaled, as in smoking, or absorbed through the tissues of the oral cavity, as in dipping and chewing. The incidence of oral cancer may be 50 times higher among long-term users of smokeless tobacco products than among non-users. Smokeless tobacco is addictive and deadly. Assessment Activity 5-1 at the end of this chapter will assist you in clarifying your perceptions of the effects of smoking.

Other Contributing Risk Factors

Physical inactivity. Physical inactivity *(hypokinesis)* is debilitating to the human body. A couple of weeks of bed rest or chair rest produces muscle atrophy, bone demineralization, and decreases in aerobic capacity and maximal ventilatory capacity. Our bodies were constructed for and thrive upon physical exertion. The American College of Sports Medicine has established guidelines for the development and maintenance of physical fitness. Issues remain that concern the amount of physical activity needed to improve and maintain good health and how much is needed to affect longevity. Results from a number of studies have shown that people who regularly engage in moderate physical activities have significantly less heart attacks and experience fewer deaths from all causes than people who exercise little or not at all. In these studies, walking one to two miles per day (five to ten miles per week) was categorized as a moderate level of ac-

Figure 5-9 The caffeine/nicotine connection

It is very difficult to stop smoking and even more difficult to give up coffee and cola drinks at the same time. Why should smokers attempt to tackle both simultaneously? Smokers metabolize caffeine more quickly than nonsmokers, so they experience its stimulating effects for a much shorter time. Four days of nonsmoking normalizes the response to caffeine so that the caffeine now remains in the blood as long as it does for any nonsmoker. The enhanced effect causes former smokers to suffer from the caffeine jitters at a time when the tensions associated with withdrawal from smoking are occurring. Two cups of coffee at this time have the same effect of five cups when the individual was a smoker. In other words it takes less to induce the coffee "buzz."

Coffee- and cola-drinking smokers who are quitting the smoking habit need to be aware of their heightened sensitivity to caffeine and that the jitters and crankiness they are experiencing are due to the effects of the caffeine plus nicotine. The obvious solution is to reduce or eliminate caffeinated drinks and other caffeine-containing substances. One can substitute caffeine-free coffee and cola drinks and in this manner get the same taste and consistency as the caffeinated substances without the jitters.

tivity. The greatest health benefits for the time and effort invested accrued to those who expended 2000 calories per week (20 to 22 miles of walking) in physical activity.[27] Sallis and co-workers[28] found that while moderate physical activity did not produce measurable improvement in cardiorespiratory endurance, it did produce healthful changes in the coronary risk factors.[28] Researchers at the Centers for Disease Control, after to an extensive review of the literature, have suggested that physical inactivity is a risk factor equal in importance to cigarette smoking, hypertension, and elevated cholesterol in the development of cardiovascular disease.[29] Blair and his associates[30] at the Dallas Aerobics Center added further validity to the effectiveness of moderate exercise as an attenuating factor in cardiovascular disease. Their epidemiological study showed that physically fit people with cholesterol levels equal to or greater than 280 mg/dl were three

times less likely to die prematurely of heart disease than unfit people whose cholesterol was in the desirable range. Also, physically fit hypertensives had less chance of dying from coronary heart disease then physically unfit normotensives (people with normal blood pressure). In other words, it is better to be fit with elevated cholesterol and high blood pressure than to have normal levels of both and be unfit. Blair found that the amount of activity to obtain this degree of protection from cardiovascular disease could be acquired by "walking."

For most sedentary people, the thought of exercise conjures up pain and sweating, and neither of these prospects is appealing. Actually, physical activities selected by the health enthusiast should not be painful. Those who dislike exercise can take some comfort in the fact that the health benefits may also be obtained with everyday activities as opposed to fitness activities such as jogging, swimming, and cycling. Activities such as walking, climbing stairs, carrying one's packages from the store, mopping and vacuuming floors, mowing the lawn (without a riding or self-propelled mower), gardening, substituting some physical activity for coffee and doughnuts at the break, and so on, may contribute minimally to physical fitness, but their cumulative effect will positively affect a person's health status. These activities along with others should be viewed as opportunities to exercise and not as chores that have to be done. Developing and cultivating this attitude and the resultant behavioral changes that accompany it will provide many health and cosmetic benefits—and it might make a person happier. It is important to note that these activities will not contribute to good health and fitness if participation is sporadic. It is also important to note that activities that develop cardiorespiratory and muscular fitness (such as jogging, swimming, cycling, cross-country skiing) produce health benefits such as weight loss, lower serum cholesterol, higher HDL-cholesterol, and lower blood pressure and do it more effectively than everyday activities. Those who are willing to expend the effort will receive optimal benefits. Today we recognize that there is exercise for physical fitness and exercise for health. Exercise for physical fitness will produce fitness and health benefits; exercise for health produces health benefits with some improvement in physical fitness.

Obesity. According to deVries,[31] "There are very few, very fat, very old people around. Your own observations—and the national statistics—

Figure 5-10 Dietary fat versus dietary carbohydrate

Dietary fat promotes fat storage in the body. The body expends only 3 calories to convert an extra 100 calories of dietary fat to storage fat.[37] Fat storage is accelerated if dietary fat is combined with simple sugar in the same meal, such as a hamburger with a sugared cola drink. Sugar triggers the release of extra insulin. Insulin, in turn, activates fat cell enzymes that promote movement of fat from the blood to the fat cells. On the other hand, the ingestion of an extra 100 calories of complex carbohydrates requires that the body expend 23 calories to convert it to fat for storage. The conversion process for carbohydrates is more costly than that for fats and provides another reason for reducing fat consumption and increasing carbohydrate consumption.

clearly show that long life does not mean survival of the fattest." Obesity is a strain on the heart, and it co-exists with and is a precursor for many of the modifiable risk factors that promote cardiovascular disease. The National Institutes of Health (NIH) has summarized the data that was collected before 1985 on the relationship between obesity and health. The results indicated that obesity is highly related to increased sickness and death. Studies since 1985 have confirmed the NIH results. This section will concentrate on the relationship between obesity and cardiovascular disease because other hazards associated with obesity were covered in Chapter 4.

The incidence of high blood pressure is three times greater among the obese than among normal-weight people.[32] The same relationship was observed in schoolchildren.[33] Obese children and adults are more likely to have higher levels of blood cholesterol and triglycerides.[32] More of their cholesterol is in the form of LDL and less in HDL. The risk factors for heart disease are more prevalent among the obese, and mortality is higher and occurs earlier.[34] Estimates indicate that there would be 25% less coronary heart disease, 35% less congestive heart failure, and 35% less strokes if all Americans were at optimal weight.[35] The prevalence of type II diabetes (non-insulin dependent) is three times greater among the obese than among normal-weight people.[36]

Poorly controlled diabetes has a devastating effect on the blood vessels. Weight loss by type II diabetics results in predictable improvement in their insulin and blood glucose levels and it alone often normalizes these values.

The risks to health associated with obesity are reversible with weight loss. The strategies for weight loss were covered in Chapter 4 but one more piece of information needs to be included in the weight loss equation. See Figure 5-10 for more information.

Diabetes mellitus. Diabetes mellitus has numerous long-range complications that are often difficult to explain. Primarily, these involve degenerative disorders of the blood vessels and nerves. Diabetics who die prematurely are usually the victims of cardiovascular lesions and accelerated atherosclerosis. The incidence of heart attacks and strokes is higher among diabetics than nondiabetics.

The arteries supplying the kidneys, eyes, and legs are particularly susceptible to atherosclerosis. Kidney failure is one of the long-term complications of diabetes, and diabetes is the second-leading cause of blindness in the United States. Impaired delivery of blood to the legs may lead to gangrene, resulting in amputation of the affected tissues. In addition to circulatory problems, degenerative lesions in the nervous system lead to multiple neuropathies that result in dysfunction of the brain, spinal cord, and peripheral nerves. Unfortunately, medical science has been unable to identify the biological mechanisms responsible for these long-term vascular and neural complications. However, the good news is that these complications can be mitigated by leading a balanced, well-regulated life, thereby keeping diabetes under control. Control includes dietary manipulation, exercise, weight control, rest, and medication if needed.

Stress. Stress is difficult to define and quantify. Authorities agree that distress or chronic stress produces a complex array of physiological changes in the body (these are covered in Chapter 7). Stress per se probably does not cause disease but it predisposes a person to illness and it may hasten the process of subclinical disease.

The mechanisms through which stress weakens the body are not well understood but it appears that there is immune system involvement. Chronic stress may depress the immune system for weeks, months, or years. Under chronic stress, the body secretes above normal amounts of hormones, the catecholamines, that circulate at high levels in the bloodstream. The catecholamines, which ready the body for physical action, are metabolized and efficiently removed from the bloodstream when a physical response is made. Blood levels remain elevated if no physical action is forthcoming. Circulating catecholamines constrict the arteries and increase the workload of the heart.

It is the individual's reaction to stress rather than the stressor itself that presents the problem. Two people may react differently to the same stressor. One might perceive a stressor as an exciting challenge to overcome while the other views the same stressor as anxiety producing and threatening. Obviously the perceptions of the latter need to be changed. This is not an easy task. Possibly a course in stress management and the utilization of stress reduction techniques—exercise and voluntary relaxation—should help to mitigate the stress response.

Now that you have a good foundation of knowledge of the risk factors for cardiovascular disease, turn to Assessment Activity 5-3 at the end of this chapter. Read the case study and answer the questions pertaining to it.

The Contributions of Medical Science

Lifestyle changes commensurate with positive health behaviors are the cornerstone of health promotion. But for many reasons—familial, genetic, and environmental—most people will require the services of the medical profession at some time in their lives. Great strides have been made in the diagnosis and treatment of disease. We will concentrate on cardiovascular disease and the innovations that have dramatically improved the quality of life with some improvement in quantity as well.

Diagnostic Techniques

Diagnosing cardiovascular disease is becoming more sophisticated every day. Diagnosis begins with a medical examination and patient history. This procedure may be supplemented with a variety of tests that might confirm or refute the physician's suspicions of the presence of cardiovascular disease. Exercise stress tests using a motor driven treadmill with the patient hooked to an EKG have gained popularity in the last ten years or so. It is a noninvasive test employing surface electrodes on the chest that are sensitive to the electrical actions of the heart. Mechanical anomalies of the heart produce abnormal electrical impulses that are displayed on the EKG strip.

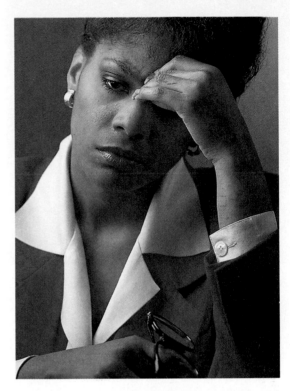

Chronic stress will eventually erode one's health.

These are read and interpreted by the physicians.

The treadmill is a device that actually "road-tests" the heart as it works progressively harder to meet the increasing oxygen requirement as the exercise protocol becomes more physically demanding (Figure 5-11). This test is more accurate for men than women. The gender difference in response to the treadmill test is not completely understood, but it is believed that women's breasts and extra fat tissue interfere with the reception of electrical impulses by the chest electrodes.

In some cases a thallium treadmill test is required because it is a more sensitive test; however, it is also a much more expensive test. This involves the injection of radioactive thallium during the final minute of the treadmill test. Thallium is accepted, or taken-up, by normal heart muscle but not by ischemic heart muscle. This can be seen on a television monitor. The thallium stress test increases diagnostic sensitivity to cardiovascular disease to approximately 90%.

Echocardiography is a safe, noninvasive technique that uses sound waves to determine the size of the heart, the thickness of the walls, and the function of its valves. *Cardiac catheterization*

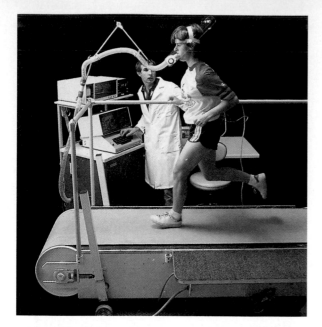

Figure 5-11 The treadmill test may be used as a diagnostic tool and it may also be used to measure aerobic capacity.

is an invasive technique in which a slender tube is threaded from a blood vessel in an arm or leg into the coronary arteries. Areas of blockage can be seen on a television monitor.

Medical Treatment

A variety of drugs have been developed that lower blood pressure and cholesterol, minimize the likelihood of blood clotting, dissolve clots during a heart attack, and so on. Even the common aspirin seems to play a significant role in preventing a second heart attack or an initial heart attack.[9] Remember, all drugs, including aspirin, should be prescribed by a physician based on patient need.

Surgical techniques have also affected the treatment of cardiovascular disease. *Coronary artery bypass surgery* is designed to shunt blood around an area of blockage by sewing one end of a leg vein into the aorta and the other end into a coronary artery below the blockage, thereby restoring blood flow to the heart muscle (Figure 5-12).

Balloon angioplasty uses a catheter with a doughnut-shaped balloon at the tip. The catheter is positioned at the narrow point in the artery and the balloon is inflated to compress the fatty deposits against the arterial walls. The channel is opened, and blood flow is enhanced (Figure 5-13). A laser beam (a powerful light beam) precisely directed can dissolve clots in blood vessels. This technique has great potential for treating cardiovascular disease if it can be perfected. *Coronary artherectomy,* one of the newest techniques, utilizes a specially tipped catheter

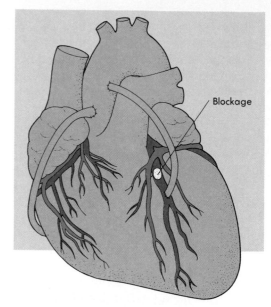

Figure 5-12 Coronary bypass graft.

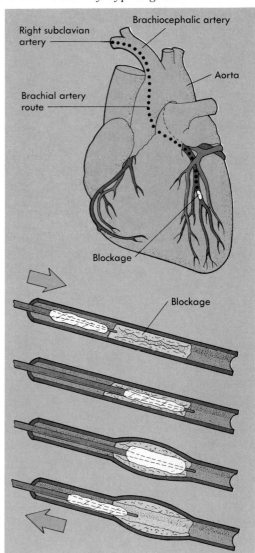

Figure 5-13 Balloon angioplasty.

equipped with a high-speed rotary cutting blade to shave off plaque.

Artificial valves have been developed to replace defective heart valves, and these work quite well. On the other hand, artificial, or mechanical, hearts have not performed up to expectation because modern technology is yet to produce a surface smooth enough to simulate the natural interior of the human heart. Blood clotting continues to occur at the valves in these devices.

Heart transplants have prolonged the lives of a number of recipients. The outlook for patients has improved considerably because of the development and use of cyclosporine, an antirejection drug.

Prevention remains the best course of action and this cannot be overemphasized. Prevention includes regular exercise, maintenance of optimal body weight, sound nutritional practices, abstinence from tobacco products, use of alcohol in moderation, or better yet, not at all, abstinence from drugs, dealing with stress in constructive ways, removing oneself, as much as possible, from destructive and disease-producing environmental conditions, and having periodic preventive-style medical examinations. It is much better

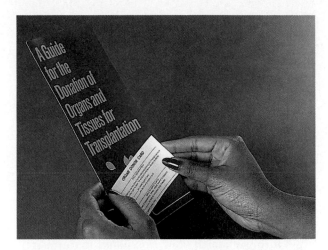

Heart transplantation can be a life-saving procedure for people with severe heart damage who depend on donor hearts.

physically, psychologically, and economically to make the effort now to enhance health rather than to reject or ignore health promotion principles and treat disease later. The choice is yours. Turn to Assessment Activity 5-2 at the end of this chapter. Answer the questions honestly and then interpret your results according to the directions.

Summary

- There are approximately 1,500,000 heart attacks each year, and 500,000 of these result in death.
- From 1976 to 1986, the death rate from coronary heart disease declined by 28%.
- The heart is actually two pumps in one: the "pulmonary pump," which sends deoxygenated blood to the lungs, and the "systemic pump," which sends oxygenated blood to all tissues of the body.
- Blood plasma is a clear yellowish fluid that makes up about 55% of the blood. The remaining 45% consists of blood solids—red cells, white cells, and blood platelets.
- Strokes are caused by a thrombus, an embolus, or a hemorrhage.
- Coronary heart disease is actually a disease of the coronary blood vessels that bring nourishment and oxygen to the heart.
- Many of the risk factors for heart disease have their origin in childhood.
- The treatment of heart disease includes the development of appropriate lifestyle habits and medical intervention.
- The major risk factors that can't be changed are age, male sex, and heredity.
- The major risk factors that can be changed are elevated cholesterol, hypertension, and cigarette smoking.

- The other contributing risk factors are physical inactivity, obesity, diabetes mellitus, and stress.
- Cholesterol is a steroid that is essential for many bodily functions, but too much circulating in the blood is a risk for cardiovascular disease.
- Low-density lipoproteins are associated with the development of atherosclerotic plaque.
- High-density lipoproteins protect the arteries from the formation of plaque.
- Blood pressure is the force exerted against the walls of the arteries as blood is pumped from the heart and travels through the circulatory system.
- *Hypertension* is the medical term for high blood pressure.
- Cigarette smoking may be the most potent of the risk factors associated with chronic illness and premature death.
- Involuntary, or passive, smoking is associated with premature disease and death.
- Physical inactivity is considered by some to be a major factor of equal importance to cholesterol, blood pressure, and cigarette smoking.
- Obesity often co-exists with many of the other risk factors for cardiovascular disease.
- Diabetes mellitus must be controlled to reduce the cardiovascular complications that accompany it.
- Stress predisposes a person to illness and it may hasten the process of subclinical disease.

Action plan for personal wellness

An important consideration in assuming responsibility for your own quality of life is utilizing information. After reading this chapter, answer the following questions and determine an action plan for enhancing your own lifestyle.

1 Based on the information presented in this chapter, along with what I know about my family's health history, the health problems/issues that I need to be most concerned about are:_____
_____
_____

2 Of those health concerns listed in number 1, the one I most need to act on is:_____
_____
_____

3 The possible actions that I can take to improve my level of wellness are (try to be as specific as possible):_____
_____
_____

4 Of those actions listed in number 3, the one that I most need to include in an action plan is:___
_____
_____

5 Factors I need to keep in mind to be successful in my action plan are:_____
_____
_____

Review Questions

1. Define pulmonary pump and systemic pump and discuss the function of each.
2. Describe the advent of heart disease in this country.
3. Identify and describe the causes of stroke.
4. What is coronary heart disease? Discuss the treatment options that are available.
5. What are the risk factors for heart disease and how are they categorized by the AHA?
6. What is cholesterol? LDL? HDL?
7. What is the relationship between total cholesterol and HDL?
8. What is essential hypertension?
9. What are the ingredients in cigarettes that increase the risk for cardiovascular disease? Describe their effect on the heart and blood vessels.
10. What is the risk associated with smokeless tobacco products?
11. Defend the proposition that a moderate level of exercise improves health and increases longevity.
12. What are the cardiovascular complications of diabetes mellitus?
13. How may stress contribute to cardiovascular disease?

References

1. American Heart Association: 1989 Heart facts, Dallas, Texas, 1988, American Heart Association.
2. Kannell WB et al: Epidemiology of acute myocardial infarction: the Framingham study, Medicine Today 2:50-57, 1968.
3. Kirk B: Child cholesterol levels, a medical controversy, Med J 45:5, Sept 1986.
4. Task Force on Blood Pressure Control in Children: Report of the second task force on blood pressure control in children—1987, Pediatrics 79:1-25, January 1987.
5. US Dept of Health and Human Services: The health consequences of smoking, Washington, DC, 1988, US Government Printing Office.
6. Long P: Kids with a lot to lose, Hippocrates 2:72-78, Nov/Dec 1988.
7. Enos WF et al: Coronary disease among United States soldiers killed in action in Korea: preliminary report, JAMA 152:1090-1093, 1953.
8. McNamara JJ et al: Coronary artery disease in combat casualties in Vietnam, JAMA 216:1185-1187, 1971.
9. For men over 50 only, The Johns Hopkins Medical Letter—Health After 50, 1:1, October 1989.
10. Van Camp SP, and Boyer JL: Cardiovascular aspects of aging, Physician Sportsmedicine Vol 17, No. 4:121-130, April, 1989.
11. Bush TL: Influence on cholesterol and lipoprotein levels in women, Cholesterol and Coronary Disease—Reducing the Risk 2(6):1-5, Feb. 1990.
12. Lubell A: Can exercise help treat hypertension in black Americans: Physician Sportsmedicine, 16:165-168, Sept. 1988.
13. Lubell A: Prescribing exercise to black Americans, Physician Sportsmedicine, 16:169-174, Sept. 1988.
14. Grundy SM: Cholesterol and coronary heart disease, JAMA 256:2849-2858, 1986.
15. The lipid research clinics coronary primary prevention trial results: I. reduction in the incidence of coronary heart disease, JAMA 251:351-364, 1984.
16. Manninen V et al: Lipid alterations and decline in the incidence of coronary heart disease in the Helsinki heart study, JAMA 260:641-651, 1988.
17. Wardlaw G and Insel P: Perspectives in Nutrition, St. Louis, 1990, Times Mirror/Mosby College Publishing.
18. Brown MS and Goldstein JL: A receptor-mediated pathway for cholesterol homeostasis, Science 232:34-47, 1986.
19. Casstelli WP et al: Incidence of coronary heart disease and lipoprotein cholesterol levels, JAMA 256:2835-2838, 1986.
20. Sherwood L: Human physiology, St. Paul, Minn, 1989, West Publishing Co.
21. American Cancer Society: Cancer facts and figures—1989, New York, 1989, American Cancer Society, Inc.
22. Lamb LL, editor: Cigarettes and women, The Health Letter 31:4, 1988.
23. Manley M: Smoke damage—the health effects of tobacco, Annual Editions–Health 89/90, Guilford, Conn, 1989, The Dushkin Publishing Group, Inc.
24. The health consequences of smoking—nicotine addiction, a report of the Surgeon General, Rockville, Md, 1988, U.S. Department of Health and Human Services.
25. Chandler WU: Banishing tobacco, Annual Editions-Health 89/90, Guilford, Conn, 1989, The Dushkin Publishing Group, Inc.
26. Lamb LL, editor: Passive smoking causes heart attacks, The Health Letter, 29:4, March, 1987.
27. Paffenbarger RS et al: Physical activity, all cause mortality, and longevity of college alumni, N Engl J Med 314:605-613, 1986.
28. Sallis JF et al: Moderate-intensity physical activity and cardiovascular risk factors: the Stanford five-city project, Prevent Med 15:561-568, 1986.
29. Powell KE: Physical activity and the incidence of coronary heart disease, Annu Rev Pub Health 8:253-260, 1987.
30. Blair SN: Low physical fitness and increased risk of death and disability, Speech delivered at SDAAHPERD Convention, Chattanooga, TN, Feb 24, 1989.
31. de Vries HA: Health Science, Santa Monica, Calif, 1979, Goodyear Publishing Co.
32. Hubert HB et al: Life-style correlates of risk factor change in young adults: an eight year study of coronary heart disease risk factors in the Framingham offspring, Am J Epidemiol 125:812-831, 1987.
33. Jequier E: Energy, obesity, and body weight standards, Am J Clin Nutr 45:1035-1047, 1987.
34. Hamm P et al: Large fluctuations in body weight during young adulthood and twenty-five year risk of coronary death in men, Am J Epidemiol 129:312-318, 1989.
35. Bray GA and Gray DS: Obesity. part I pathogenesis, 149:429-441, 1988, West J Med.
36. National Institutes of Health Consensus Development Conference Statement, Health Implications of Obesity, February 11-13, 1985, Ann Intern Med 103:981-1077, 1985.
37. Sims EAH and Danforth E, Expenditure and storage of energy in man, J Clin Invest 79:1019-1025, 1987.

Annotated Readings

Shell ER, Kids, catfish and cholesterol, Am Health, 52-57, January/February, 1988.

Presents the results of the Bogalusa Heart Study, which has been in operation for 16 years. Its major purpose is to determine the extent that lifestyle in childhood can contribute to heart disease later in life. The results indicate that millions of children should exercise and watch their diet.

You can reduce your risk for coronary artery disease, Annual Editions Health 89/90, Guilford, Conn, 1989, The Dushkin Publishing Group, Inc.

The risk factors for coronary artery disease are identified and discussed. An instrument for the assessment of cardiovascular risk is presented with guidelines for interpretation.

Not just what to do for heart health but how to do it, Tufts University Diet and Nutrition Letter, 7, no. 1: 3-8, March 1989.

Discusses the relationship between diet and heart health. Presents a sample of menus designed to increase nutrient density while lowering fat, cholesterol, and salt intake.

The diet/exercise link: separating fact from fiction, Tufts University Diet and Nutrition Letter, 6, no. 12: 3-6, February 1989.

Presents selected exercise and nutrition myths, discusses why they are not true, and presents the facts as supported by current evidence.

Blood pressure monitoring devices, Mayo Clinic Health Letter, 7, No. 11: 3, November, 1989.

Briefly discusses blood pressure as a risk for coronary heart disease. Identifies three different types of blood pressure monitoring devices that provide the most accurate readings. Discusses the importance of having these devices calibrated at regular intervals.

ASSESSMENT ACTIVITY   5-1

Clarifying Your Perceptions of the Effects of Smoking

Directions: For each statement circle the number that shows how you feel about it. Do you strongly agree, mildly agree, mildly disagree, or strongly disagree? It is important to answer every question.

	Strongly agree	Mildly agree	Mildly disagree	Strongly disagree
a. Cigarette smoking is not nearly as dangerous as many other health hazards.	1	2	3	4
b. I don't smoke enough to get any of the diseases that cigarette smoking is supposed to cause.	1	2	3	4
c. If a person has already smoked for many years it probably won't do him much good to stop.	1	2	3	4
d. It would be hard for me to give up smoking cigarettes.	1	2	3	4
e. Cigarette smoking is enough of a health hazard for something to be done about it.	4	3	2	1
f. The kind of cigarette I smoke is much less likely than other kinds to give me any of the diseases that smoking is supposed to cause.	1	2	3	4
g. As soon as a person quits smoking cigarettes he begins to recover from much of the damage that smoking has caused.	4	3	2	1
h. It would be hard for me to cut down to half the number of cigarettes I now smoke.	1	2	3	4
i. The whole problem of cigarette smoking and health is a very minor one.	1	2	3	4
j. I haven't smoked long enough to worry about the diseases that cigarette smoking is supposed to cause.	1	2	3	4
k. Quitting smoking helps a person live longer.	4	3	2	1
l. It would be difficult for me to make any substantial change in my smoking habits.	1	2	3	4

Continued.

How to score:

1 Enter the numbers you have circled above in the spaces below by putting the number you have circled for question a over line a; to question b over line b, and so on.

2 Total the three scores on each line to get your totals. For examples, the sum of your scores over lines A, E, and I gives you your score on *Importance*—lines B, F, and J give the score on *Personal Relevance*, and so on.

Totals

_____ + _____ + _____ = _____
    a   e   i   Importance

_____ + _____ + _____ = _____
    b   f   j   Personal relevance

_____ + _____ + _____ = _____
    c   g   k   Value of stopping

_____ + _____ + _____ = _____
    d   h   l   Capability for stopping

Scores can vary from 3-12. A score of 9 and above is *High*; a score of 6 and below is *Low*. A low score on any of the factors may truly reflect your attitude regarding smoking behavior or it may be due to lack of knowledge. In either case it would be profitable to read once again the section on cigarette smoking. Further information regarding tobacco usage can be obtained from the American Heart Association.

ASSESSMENT ACTIVITY

5-2

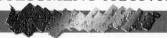

Arizona Heart Institute Cardiovascular Risk Factor Analysis

Directions: Indicate the points that you have scored in the column on the right for each of the following risk factors. When you finish, total your points and compare that with the results at the end of the activity.

Risk Factors	Score	
1. Age	Age 56 or over	1
	Age 55 or under	0 _____
2. Sex	Male	1
	Female	0 _____
3. Family history	If you have:	
	Blood relatives who have had a heart attack or stroke at or before age 60	12
	Blood relatives who have had a heart attack or stroke after age 60	6
	No blood relatives who have had a heart attack or stroke	0 _____
4. Personal history	50 or under: If you had either a heart attack, a stroke, heart or blood vessel surgery	20
	51 or over: If you had any of the above	10
	None of the above	0 _____
5. Diabetes	Diabetes before age 40 and now on insulin	10
	Diabetes at or after age 40 and now on insulin or pills	5
	Diabetes controlled by diet, or diabetes after age 55	3
	No diabetes	0 _____
6. Smoking	Two packs per day	10
	Between one and two packs per day or quit smoking less than a year ago	6
	If you smoke 6 or more cigars a day or inhale a pipe regularly	6
	Less than one pack per day or quit smoking more than one year ago	3
	Never smoked	0 _____
7. Cholesterol (If cholesterol count is not known answer 8)	Cholesterol level—276 or above	10
	Cholesterol level—between 225 and 275	5
	Cholesterol level—224 or below	0 _____
8. Diet (If you have answered 7, do not answer 8)	Does your normal eating pattern include:	
	One serving of red meat daily, more than seven eggs a week, and daily consumption of butter, whole milk, and cheese	8
	Red meat 4-6 times a week, 4-7 eggs a week, margarine, low fat dairy products and some cheese	4
	Poultry, fish, little or no red meat, three or fewer eggs a week, some margarine, skim milk, and skim milk products	0 _____
9. High blood pressure	If either number is:	
	160 over 100 (160/100) or higher	10
	140 over 90 (140/90) but less than 160 over 100 (160/100)	5
	If both numbers are less than 140 over 90 (140/90)	0 _____

10. Weight

Ideal Weight Formula:
Men = 110 lbs. plus 5 lbs. for each inch over 5 feet
Women = 100 lbs. plus 5 lbs. for each inch over 5 feet

25 pounds overweight	4
10 to 24 pounds overweight	2
Less than 10 pounds overweight	0 _____

11. Exercise

Do you engage in any aerobic exercise (brisk walking, jogging, bicycling, racketball, swimming) for more than 15 minutes:

Less than once a week	4
1 to 2 times a week	2
3 or more times a week	0 _____

12. Stress

Are you

Frustrated when waiting in line, often in a hurry to complete work or keep appointments, easily angered, irritable	4
Impatient when waiting, occasionally hurried, or occasionally moody	2
Comfortable when waiting, seldom rushed, and easygoing	0 _____

Total points _____

Score Results

PLEASE NOTE: A high score does not mean you will develop heart disease. It is merely a guide to make you aware of a potential risk. Since no two people are alike, an exact prediction is impossible without further individualized testing.

With answer to question 9		Without answer to question 9	
High risk	40 and above	High risk	36 and above
Medium risk	20-39	Medium risk	19-35
Low risk	19 and below	Low risk	18 and below

ASSESSMENT ACTIVITY   5-3

A Case Study on Bill M.

Directions: To determine your understanding of cardiovascular health and wellness, read the following case study, and respond to the accompanying questions.

Bill, a 38-year-old male who is 5′8″ tall and weighs 205 lbs., has the following history:

1 Father died of a heart attack at age 48; grandfather died of a heart attack at age 52

2 Cholesterol level is 256 mg/dl; LDL is 172 mg/dl; HDL is 40 mg/dl

3 Blood pressure is consistently in the 150/95 range

4 Smokes one pack of cigarettes per day

5 Drinks six to eight brewed cups of coffee daily

6 Eats two eggs with bacon or sausage and buttered toast daily

7 Meat is a major part of supper; he skips lunch

8 Favorite snacks are ice cream, buttered popcorn, and salted peanuts

9 Occasionally plays tennis on Sunday afternoons

10 Owns his own business and often works 55 to 60 hours per week

Answer the following:

1 What are his risk factors for coronary heart disease?_____
_____

2 Which of these can he control?_____
_____

3 What suggestions can you give him regarding his current diet?_____
_____

4 What effect may a change in diet have upon his coronary risk profile?_____
_____

5 What suggestions can you make regarding his need for exercise and how might a change in his activity level affect his coronary risk profile?_____
_____

6 What are the risks associated with obesity?_____
_____

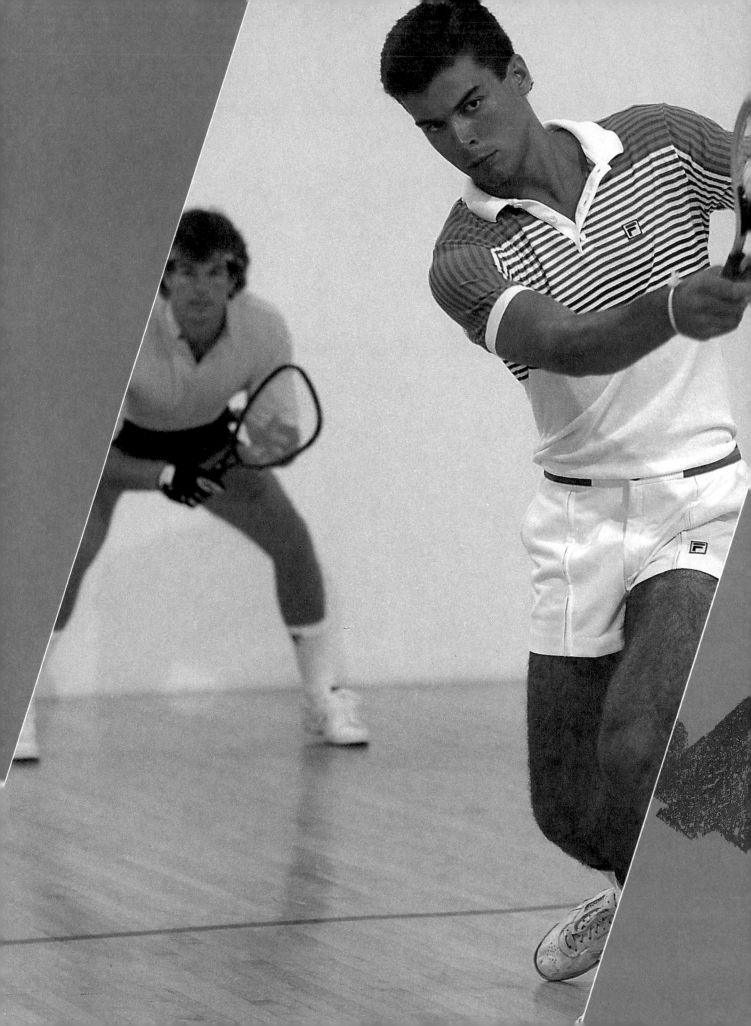

Chapter 6

Exercise for Fitness and Leisure

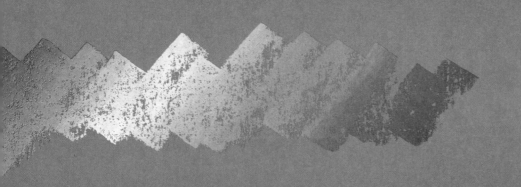

Key terms

aerobic

aerobic capacity

anaerobic

body composition

cardiorespiratory endurance

flexibility

muscular endurance

muscular strength

Objectives

After completing this chapter, you will be able to:

▌ Identify and define the health-related components of physical fitness

▌ Discuss the principles of conditioning

▌ Calculate your target heart rate for exercise by two different methods

▌ Identify and discuss the health benefits of consistent participation in exercise

▌ Describe the problems associated with exercise in hot and cold weather

A major change in American life has been the effect that science and technology have had in increasing productivity while simultaneously reducing, and in some cases eliminating, the amount of physical work required by the labor force. As a result, physical fitness can no longer be attained on the job, and leisure hours represent the only viable time for its development. During leisure time, choices are available from literally dozens of activities that are sufficiently different from each other so that almost anyone can find a physical activity that is enjoyable and challenging. This chapter focuses on the principles and concepts required to develop and maintain a physical fitness program.

The Components of Physical Fitness

Authorities have yet to agree on a definition of physical fitness, but most have endorsed the dichotomous concept of *performance-related* and *health-related* fitness. Performance-related fitness, or sports fitness, consists of the following components: speed, power, balance, coordination, agility, and reaction time. These are essential for the execution of sports skills but they may or may not contribute significantly to those activities performed for health enhancement.

The health-related components of fitness are cardiorespiratory endurance, muscular strength, muscular endurance, flexibility, and body composition. Since wellness is the theme of this text, the exercise emphasis will be on health-related fitness. Performance-related and health-related fitness, though separate, are not mutually exclusive. For example, competitors may find that the

health-related components of their sport or activity are essential for success. Racquetball, tennis, basketball, soccer, handball, and so on all require one or more of the health-related components. Conversely, health enthusiasts may engage in physical activities that require some or all of the performance-related components. However, it is necessary to understand that the development and maintenance of health-related fitness is not dependent on athletic ability nor does it rely on activities that are high in the performance components. Fitness for health purposes can be achieved with minimal psychomotor ability when activities such as walking, jogging, cycling, hiking, backpacking, orienteering, swimming, rope jumping, weight training, and so on are selected.

Remember the old adage, "no pain, no gain"? Well, **forget it!** Trying to comply with this bit of nonsense has done more harm than good to sedentary people who are attempting to become physically active. While this may be one of the cardinal principles of athletic competition, it is likely to result in injury and negativity in those who wish to exercise for health enhancement. The health benefits of exercise occur when exercise is somewhat uncomfortable rather than painful. Only the most dedicated health enthusiasts, competitors, and masochists can face exercise that produces pain week after week. While exercise for the purpose of health enhancement should stress cardiorespiratory development, the other components of fitness should not be neglected. Flexibility exercises should be a part of the warm-up and cool down procedures. Resistance/strength training plays an important role and should be an integral part of a well-rounded fitness program. The American College of Sports Medicine (ACSM) recognized the necessity of resistance/strength training for the average person in their revised position statement on exercise.[1] They reported that runners who did no resistance training over a 10-year period suffered muscle atrophy in their upper body while maintaining muscle size in their legs. Their arms decreased in circumference but their legs did not. When one reflects on the importance of maintaining the integrity of the muscular system for weight management and for performing daily physical chores without becoming fatigued, one can appreciate the significance of resistance training.

Cardiorespiratory Endurance

Cardiorespiratory endurance is the ability to take in, deliver, and extract oxygen for physical work. It is the ability to persevere at a physical task, and it improves with regular participation in aerobic activities such speed walking, jogging, cycling, swimming, and cross-country skiing. The term **aerobic** literally means "with oxygen" but when applied to exercise, it refers to activities whose oxygen demand can be supplied continuously by individuals during performance. Aerobic performance depends on a continuous and sufficient supply of oxygen to burn the carbohydrates and fats needed to fuel such activities. In other words, the intensity or the energy requirement is within the capacity of the performer to sustain it for longer than a couple of minutes.[2] Cardiorespiratory endurance is also referred to as **aerobic capacity,** or maximum oxygen consumption (Vo_2 max). From a health perspective, cardiorespiratory endurance is the most important component of physical fitness, and it

is the foundation for the development of total fitness.

The physiological changes that result from cardiorespiratory training are referred to as the long-term, or *chronic, effects of exercise.* The effects of training are measurable and predictable.

Heart rate. A few months of aerobic training will lower the resting heart rate by 10 to 25 beats per minute. It will also lower the heart rate for a given workload. For example, a slow jog might produce a heart rate of 165 beats per minute prior to training and 140 beats per minute after a few months of training. The trained heart is a stronger, more efficient pump that is capable of delivering the required oxygen with fewer beats.

Stroke volume. *Stroke volume* is the amount of blood that the heart can eject in one beat. Aerobic training increases the stroke volume by (1) increasing the size of the cavity of the ventricles, which results in greater filling of the heart with blood and (2) by increasing the contractile strength of the ventricular wall so that contraction is more forceful and a greater amount of blood is ejected from the ventricles (Figure 6-1).

Cardiac output. *Cardiac output* is the amount of blood ejected by the heart in 1 minute. Cardiac output (Q) is the product of heart rate (HR) and stroke volume (SV). Cardiac output increases with aerobic training during maximal effort—it does not increase at rest or during submaximal exercise.

The average cardiac output at rest is 4 to 6 liters of blood per minute. During maximal exertion, cardiac output reaches values of 20 to 25 liters of blood per minute for the average person, but may reach as much as 40 liters per minute for large, well-conditioned athletes. To put this in

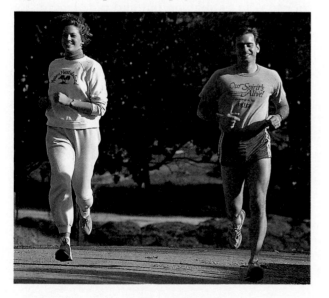

Achieving health-related fitness is not dependent on athletic ability.

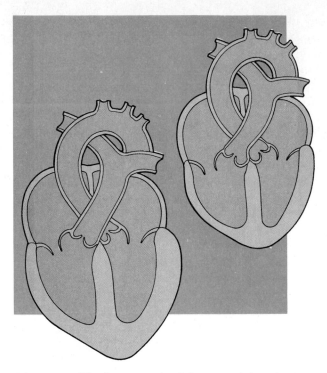

Figure 6-1 The heart on the left exemplifies the results of aerobic training. The ventricles are larger than the non-athletic heart on the right and the walls are slightly thicker.

perspective, imagine 10 to 20 2-liter drink bottles filled with liquid; that's the amount of blood the heart is capable of pumping in 1 minute during exercise of maximal intensity.

Blood volume. Aerobic training increases blood volume, and to a lesser extent, the number of red blood cells that transport oxygen and carbon dioxide to and from the cells. The increase in the ratio of blood volume or plasma to the red blood cells is an adaptation to exercise that lowers the viscosity, or stickiness, of the blood. Decreased viscosity results in an increase in the liquid volume of the blood, allowing it to flow more easily through the circulatory system.

Blood is automatically shunted by the body to areas of greatest need. At rest, a significant amount is sent to the digestive system and kidneys but during vigorous exercise as much as 90% of the blood is sent to the working muscles with a considerable reduction to the digestive and urinary systems.[3]

Heart volume. The muscles of the body respond to exercise by growing larger and stronger and the heart, as a muscular pump, is no exception. The volume as well as the weight of the heart increase with endurance training. Training that lowers the resting heart rate stimulates greater filling of the ventricles, whose muscle fi-

bers respond to the increased pool of blood by stretching. This produces a recoil effect in the muscle fibers that results in a stronger contraction with more blood ejected per beat. Continued training causes the ventricles to enlarge and grow stronger so that the weight as well as the size of the heart increases. The hypertrophied (enlarged) heart is a normal response to endurance training that has no long-term detrimental effects. In fact, while it is beneficial to maintain this effect for life, several months of inactivity will reduce heart weight and size to pretraining levels. The atrophy (wasting away) associated with physical inactivity is inevitable.

Respiratory responses. The chest muscles that support breathing improve in both strength and endurance. There is an increase in *vital capacity* (the amount of air that can be expired after a maximum inspiration) and a decrease in *residual volume* (the amount of air remaining in the lungs after expiration). Ventilation (the amount of air moved in and out of the lungs in 1 minute) increases substantially during maximal effort.

Metabolic responses. Endurance training improves aerobic capacity by 15% to 30% in previously untrained healthy adults. The improvement is due to several physiological adaptations that combine to increase the body's production of energy. First, *ATP* (adenosine triphosphate), the actual unit of energy for muscular contraction, is increased because organelles within the cells that use oxygen to produce ATP increase in number and size. These organelles are the *mitochondria* that are often referred to as the cell's powerhouse. Second, there is an increase in the enzymes located within the mitochondria that accelerate the production of ATP. Third, there are increases in cardiac output and blood perfusion of the muscles performing the work. Fourth, training facilitates and increases the extraction of oxygen by the exercising muscles. These are some of the major adaptations that combine to enhance aerobic endurance.

Aerobic capacity is limited by heredity and is finite. Reaching one's aerobic potential can only occur through aerobic endurance training. High genetic potential plus diligent and knowledgeable training result in the performance of amazing feats of endurance. Many people have participated in marathons, ultramarathons, triathalons, cross-country runs, long-distance swims, and long-distance bike races. Most people are average in aerobic ability and cannot compete with the specially endowed, but all people can achieve their aerobic potential with endurance training.

Aerobic capacity reaches a peak with 6 months to 2 years of steady endurance training. At this point it levels off and remains unchanged for a number of years even if training is intensified. However, aerobic performance continues to improve with harder training since a higher percentage of the aerobic capacity can be maintained for a longer period of time. For example, 6 months of appropriate training might allow one to jog 3 miles at 60% of the aerobic capacity. Another year of harder training might allow this same individual to run 3 miles at 85% of capacity. Capacity has not changed during this time, but physiological adaptations have occurred that enable the body to function at progressively higher percentages of maximum.

Aerobic capacity does decrease with age, but an excellent longitudinal study indicated that it declines more slowly in physically active subjects compared to sedentary subjects.[4] The subjects were middle-aged men whose average age at the inception of the study was 45 years. They were involved in consistent physical training for the next 23 years and, at the end of that time, they experienced only one third of the aerobic decline that was measured in a nonexercising control group. Additionally, their body weight decreased by an average of 8 pounds, and blood pressure did not increase with age, as is so often the case among sedentary people.

The effects of training persist as long as training continues. Fitness developed with years of continuous training can be lost in a matter of months if training is interrupted or discontinued. Subjects who suspended training for 84 days after 10 years of active participation experienced a significant decline in aerobic capacity after 3 weeks of inactivity and returned to pretraining levels in most fitness parameters by the end of the study.[5] The exceptions to complete reversal were muscle capillary density and mitochondrial enzymes that remained 50% higher than levels measured in sedentary control subjects.[6] This study indicated that the results of inactivity are variable and affect some systems more quickly than others. Physical decline cannot be prevented with physical inactivity.

A relatively quick and effective way to measure your level of cardiorespiratory fitness is to take the Rockport Fitness Walking Test, found at the end of this chapter.

Cardiorespiratory endurance and wellness. Most Americans believe that exercise is good for them but the majority cannot explain how or why. This section will provide some of the how's and why's.

Consistent participation in exercise is necessary if it is to improve health status. Sporadic exercise does not promote physical fitness nor does it contribute to health enhancement. In fact, infrequent participation increases the risk of sudden death during the time that one is exercising.[7] Those who exercise regularly and vigorously have a slightly elevated chance of dying suddenly during exercise, but the long-term compensatory health advantages gained from training

TABLE 6-1 A summary of selected health related benefits associated with regular aerobic exercise

Reduces the risk of cardiovascular disease

1. Increases HDL-cholesterol
2. Decreases LDL-cholesterol
3. Favorably changes the ratios between total cholesterol and HDL-C, and between LDL-C and HDL-colesterol
4. Decreases triglyceride levels
5. Promotes relaxation; relieves stress and tension
6. Decreases body fat and favorably changes body composition
7. Reduces blood pressure especially if it is high.
8. Blood platelets are less sticky
9. Less cardiac arrhythmias
10. Increases myocardial efficiency
    a. Lowers resting heart rate
    b. Increases stroke volume
11. Increase oxygen-carrying capacity of the blood

Helps control diabetes

1. Cells are less resistant to insulin
2. Reduces body fat

Develops stronger bones that are less susceptible to injury

Promotes joint stability by

1. Increasing muscular strength
2. Increasing strength of the ligaments, tendons, cartilage, and connective tissue

Contributes to fewer low back problems

Acts as a stimulus for other lifestyle changes

Improves self-concept

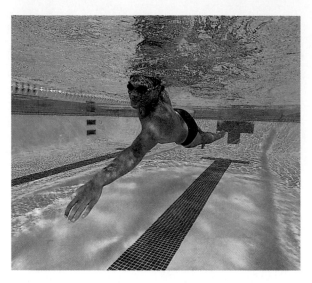

Regular participation in an aerobic activity such as swimming improves cardiorespiratory endurance.

clearly outweigh the minimal risk. Some selected health benefits of regular exercise that are supported by research evidence appear in Table 6-1.

Regular participation in aerobic exercise reduces many of the risks associated with cardiovascular disease. The risk imposed by cholesterol can be reduced through exercise. The primary effect of exercise is on the high density lipoprotein (HDL) fraction. HDL is the only lipoprotein that is involved in reverse transport; that is, it acts as a scavenger by picking up cholesterol from the blood and tissues and transferring it to other lipoproteins for delivery to the liver. The liver degrades and recycles or removes cholesterol from the body. The higher the level of HDL the better. Exercise, particularly of the aerobic type, is the primary way to increase HDL.

Total cholesterol (TC) and low-density lipoproteins (LDL) are affected indirectly by exercise. LDL is harmful because it sloughs off cholesterol in the bloodstream where it can be used to formulate the plaque that, if unchecked, narrows and eventually closes arterial vessels, leading to heart attacks and strokes. Exercise effectively promotes weight loss that results in a reduction in both TC and LDL.

Triglyceride levels in the blood may also be reduced by lifestyle changes. Intervention programs designed to lower triglyceride levels in the blood include smoking cessation, alcohol restriction, a diet low in fat and cholesterol, weight loss, and exercise. Aerobic exercise suppresses triglycerides for 48 to 72 hours, so it is important to exercise at least every other day to maintain lower levels in the blood.

Hypertension, the medical term for high blood pressure, is another of the major risk factors that can be changed. Aerobic exercise is one of several nonmedical approaches that are effective in lowering the blood pressure. Exercise reduces the blood level of circulating epinephrine and norepinephrine. These two hormones are vasoconstrictors; that is, they constrict the arterioles (the smallest arteries) and decrease their diameters. In one study, 16 weeks of aerobic exercise decreased the blood levels of both hormones and reduced blood pressure.[8] Other investigators examined the effect of aerobic exercise on plasma norepinephrine and peripheral resistance.[9] Peripheral resistance, which is the resistance to blood flow, is one of the major contributors to high blood pressure. Aerobic exercise reduced peripheral resistance, plasma norepinephrine, and blood pressure.

Cigarette smoking is the third and possibly the most important of the major risk factors that can be changed. There are many methods, suggestions, and support systems for quitting the cigarette and tobacco habit, but the majority of users find it difficult to extinguish the habit. Exercise is one of many alternatives that has met with some degree of success. Cigarette smoking seriously limits one's ability to perform in endurance events, so exercisers who smoke learn early that they must quit in order to maximize the results of training. Also, those who make the transition from a sedentary to an active lifestyle may be more amenable to quitting because participation in physical activity shows an inclination toward making healthful changes.

Diabetes mellitus is a risk factor for cardiovascular disease. Diabetics who are particularly at risk are those whose condition is either not controlled or is poorly controlled. Aerobic exercise contributes to the control of diabetes in the following ways: (1) it reduces the insulin requirement; (2) the lower the insulin dosage the more normal the body's physiology, resulting in less of a "roller coaster" effect and more effective control; (3) it reduces blood platelet adhesiveness for about 24 hours afterward; and (4) it has a mitigating effect on most of the risk factors associated with coronary artery disease.

Stress is another risk factor that can be managed. Crews and Landers[10] examined the relationship between aerobic or cardiorespiratory fitness and psychosocial stress by reviewing 34 relevant studies. Their study indicated that fit subjects were less negatively affected by any of the stressors and recovered more quickly from stress than unfit subjects. The effects of anaerobic activities (such as weight training, and sprinting) on stress reduction are inconclusive because some studies found these to be stress reducing while others show no such benefit. However, Howard's longitudinal study[11] has shown that any exercise, aerobic or anaerobic, is beneficial to the mind and body. Exercise is a readily identifiable, concrete stressor that replaces ambiguous or nonspecific stress. In addition, it is an excellent outlet for the release of excess energy and stuffed emotions. Exercise is an important coping mechanism because it reduces the severity of the stress response, shortens recovery time, reduces stress-related vulnerability to disease, and gives one a sense of control, at least in this segment of life.

Muscular Strength

Muscular strength is the maximal force that a muscle or muscle group can exert in a single contraction. It is developed best by some form of progressive resistance exercise. Weight training with free weights (barbells and dumbbells) or single and multistation machine weights fit the bill very nicely. Some of the exercises commonly employed to develop the major muscle groups of the body are demonstrated in Figures 6-2 to 6-9. Check the anatomical charts in Figures 6-10 and 6-11 for the location of the muscles that are stressed in each exercise.

These exercises are demonstrated on appropriate devices because of their convenience and allure but they can also be performed with free weights with minor modifications. The exercises in these figures are dynamic because the muscles change in length as they contract. If the resistance is constant but the speed of contraction is not, the muscle contraction is *isotonic* (literally meaning equal tension), but if the speed of contraction is constant and the resistance changes to accommodate the application of force, the contraction is *isokinetic* (literally meaning same motion). Isokinetic exercises are dynamic and require special devices that maximally load the muscles throughout the full range of motion. Both isotonic and isokinetic exercises develop strength throughout the full range of movement.

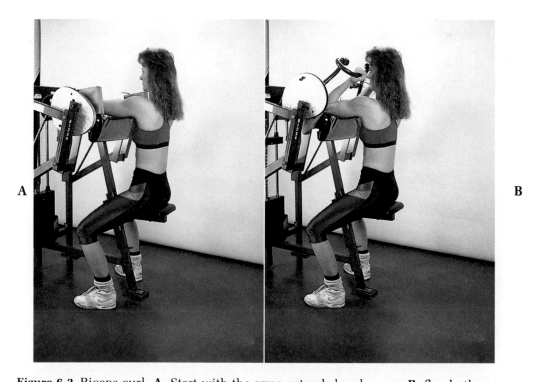

Figure 6-2 Biceps curl. **A,** Start with the arms extended, palms up; **B,** flex both arms and slowly move the weight through a full range of motion and return to the starting position. Prime movers: biceps brachii.

Text continues on p. 150.

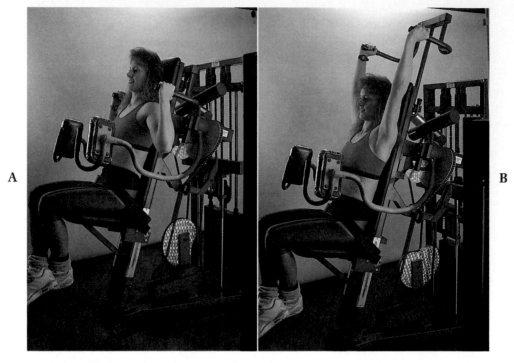

Figure 6-3 Overhead press. **A,** Sit upright with hands approximately shoulder width apart. **B,** Slowly press the bar upward until the arms are fully extended and lower to starting position. Avoid excessive arch in the low back. Prime movers: triceps and deltoid.

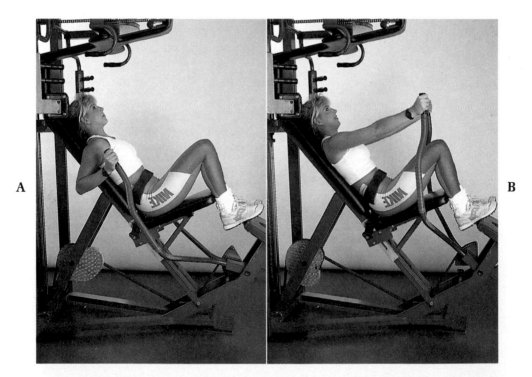

Figure 6-4 Bench press. **A,** Lie on your back with knees bent and the feet flat on the bench to prevent arching of the back. **B,** Slowly press the bar overhead, fully extending the arms and return to the starting position. Prime movers: pectoralis major, triceps, and deltoid.

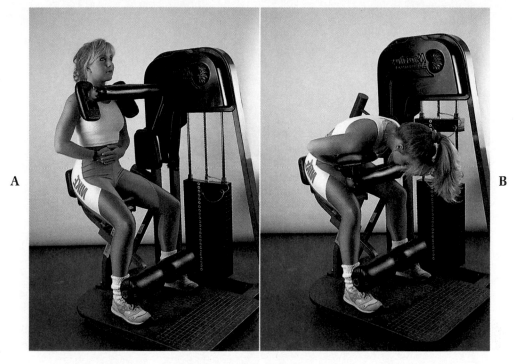

Figure 6-5 Abdominal crunch **A,** Sit upright with the chest against the pads, hands folded across the stomach. **B,** Slowly press forward through a full range of motion and return to the starting position. Prime movers: rectus abdominis.

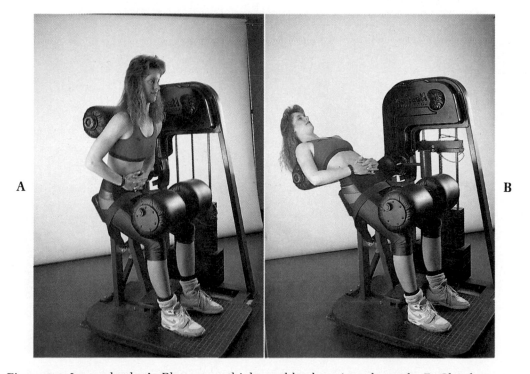

Figure 6-6 Lower back. **A,** Place your thighs and back against the pads. **B,** Slowly press backward until the back is fully extended and return to the starting position. Prime movers: erector spine and gluteus maximus.

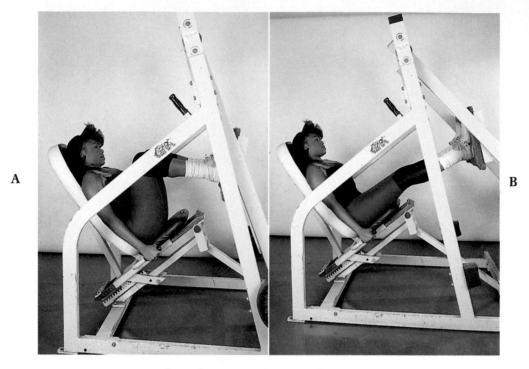

Figure 6-7 Leg press. **A,** Adjust the seat so that your legs are bent at approximately 90°. **B,** Slowly extend your legs fully and return to the starting position. Prime movers: quadriceps groups, gluteus maximus.

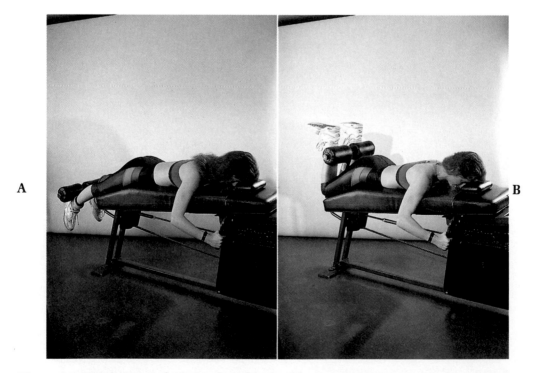

Figure 6-8 Hamstring curl. **A,** Lie face down with your lower legs under the pads. **B,** Curl the weight approximately 90° and return to the starting position. Prime Movers: hamstring group.

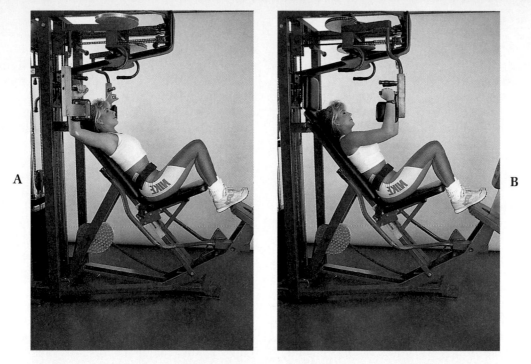

Figure 6-9 Chest press. **A,** Upper arms are parallel to the floor, elbows bent at 90°, hands on handles. **B,** Slowly push the bars until the elbows are pointing forward and return to the starting position. Prime movers: pectoralis major, deltoid.

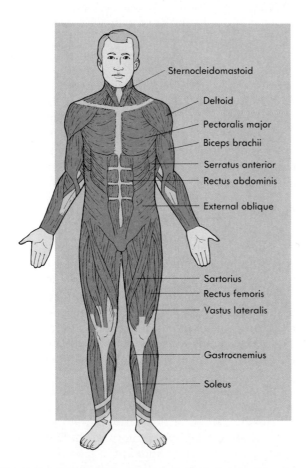

Figure 6-10 Anatomical chart. Selected muscles of the body—front view.

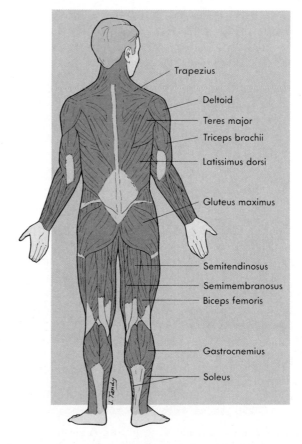

Figure 6-11 Anatomical chart. Selected muscles of the body—rear view.

Isometric (literally means equal length) or static contractions may also be employed to develop strength. These are not dynamic because the exercising muscles cannot overcome the resistance, resulting in no change in muscle length and no muscular movement. See Figure 6-12 for an example of an isometric contraction.

Isometrics are not recommended because they increase the blood pressure disproportionately and they develop strength in the muscles only at the angle of contraction, plus or minus a few degrees. The hectic pace of life in contemporary America compels people to make the most of each minute. This attitude impinges on exercise time as people strive to get the greatest return from their time and effort. Dynamic systems of resistance training yield the greatest return from the effort invested. Additionally, since human movement is essentially dynamic, there is greater transferability to daily activities. Because isometrics contribute little to health enhancement and because they simulate to a lesser extent the movements that humans perform in their daily lives, they will not be treated further in this text. On the other hand, dynamic exercises contribute to the development of strength, muscle endurance, and health enhancement, and there is transferability between strength developed dy-

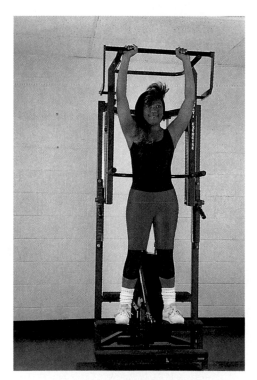

Figure 6-12 Isometric contraction. A static contraction against an immovable object.

namically and the activities of daily living. Consequently, this is the preferred approach to strength enhancement.

Resistance training increases strength by increasing muscle size and total muscle mass and by causing neural adaptations (recruitment of motor units). A motor unit is a nerve and all of the muscle fibers that it stimulates. According to Brooks,[12] "old men and women of all ages seem to increase strength mainly by neural adaptation (with some hypertrophy), whereas young men rely more on increases in muscle size."

The difference in strength between males and females prior to puberty is inconsequential but after puberty it becomes significant as the average male can generate 30% to 40% more force than the average female. The difference is greatest in upper body strength and least for leg strength. One of the major factors responsible for the strength differential between the sexes after puberty is the increased production of testosterone in males. Testosterone stimulates the protein-synthesizing mechanisms and is responsible for the muscle hypertrophy that is unique to males. Females also produce testosterone but in much lower quantities and this primarily accounts for their diminished capacity to develop muscle. However, research has shown that females can improve considerably in strength without developing large muscles.[13] For the average female the development of large muscles with resistance training is virtually impossible. The masculinizing effect of resistance training on women is a myth that continues to persist although there is much evidence to the contrary. To increase muscle size, some female body builders and other sports participants have resorted to using *anabolic steroids*. See Figure 6-13 for a discussion of this topic.

Anabolic steroid use by nonathletes is on the rise. This is particularly true for young males. A nationwide survey of 3,403 male high school seniors indicated that 6.6% of this group were current users or had previously been users of steroids and that 25% of the current users showed signs of dependency.[14] According to this report, the improvement in physical appearance that is reputed to occur with steroid use accompanied by peer approval of those physical changes functioned as a powerful reinforcer for continued use.

Heavy steroid users were more likely than light users to take two or more steroids concomitantly and they were more apt to take these drugs by injection rather than in pill form. Injection as a method of delivery is highly characteristic of

Figure 6-13 You be the judge: are athletes who use steroids to gain competitive advantage really winners or losers?

The testing of athletes for drugs and the exclusion from competition of those found to be using substances outlawed by sports federations has stirred considerable controversy and has been much publicized. One such group of drugs are *anabolic androgenic steroids* (anabolic means "build up of tissues"; androgenic means "male producing"; steroids are a class or hormone). These agents are closely related to testosterone, the natural male sex hormone that is responsible for promoting the increased muscle mass characteristic of males.

Before their use was outlawed, these agents were taken by many athletes who specialized in power events such as weight lifting and sprinting in the hopes of increasing muscle mass and, accordingly, increasing muscle strength in an attempt to gain a competitive edge. Both male and female athletes have resorted to using these substances. The adverse effects of these drugs, however, outweigh any benefits derived. In males, who already have an abundance of their own naturally produced testosterone, sought-after increases in muscle mass, strength, and body weight are not well demonstrated. Small, variable gains occur only in conjunction with a regular muscle-building exercise program and are not experienced by all who take the agents. In fact, some suggest that the changes that do occur are largely due to the exercise alone. In females, who lack potent androgenic hormones, the effect of promoting "male type" muscle mass and strength is readily demonstrated when these agents are used. However, these drugs also "masculinize" females in other ways, such as by inducing growth of facial and overall body hair and by lowering the voice.

These are but a few of the side effects of using anabolic steroids. In both males and females, these agents adversely affect the liver and the reproductive and cardiovascular systems.

Adverse effects on the reproductive system

In males, testosterone secretion and sperm production by the testes are normally controlled by hormones released from the anterior pituitary gland. In negative-feedback fashion, testosterone inhibits secretion of these controlling hormones so that a constant circulating level of testosterone is maintained. The anterior pituitary is similarly inhibited by androgenic steroids taken as a drug. As a result, because the testes do not receive their normal stimulatory input from the anterior pituitary, sperm production decreases, the testes atrophy, and testosterone secretion declines.

In females, inhibition of the anterior pituitary by the androgenic drugs results in repression of the hormonal output that controls ovarian function. The result is failure to ovulate, menstrual irregularities, and decreased secretion of female sex hormones. Since the latter are "feminizing hormones," their decline results in diminution in breast size and other female characteristics.

Adverse effects on the liver

Liver dysfunction is not uncommon with high steroid intake, perhaps because the liver, which normally inactivates steroid hormones and prepares them for urinary excretion, is overloaded by the excess steroid intake.

Adverse effects of the cardiovascular system

Use of anabolic steroids induces several changes in the cardiovascular system that increase the risk of developing atherosclerosis, which in turn is associated with an increased incidence of heart attacks and strokes. Among these adverse cardiovascular effects are (1) a reduction in high-density lipoproteins (HDL), which are the "good" cholesterol carriers that help remove cholesterol from the body, and (2) an elevation in blood pressure. Furthermore, damage to the heart muscle itself has been demonstrated in animal studies.

Adverse effects on behavior

Although still controversial, anabolic steroid use appears to promote aggressive, even hostile behavior.

For health reasons, not even taking into account the ethical issues involved, athletes should not use anabolic steroids in an attempt to gain a competitive advantage. Despite these potential dangers, however, some athletes continue to illegally use these drugs and seek measures to mask their use from testing procedures.

drugs that involve addiction. The steroid "hook" is insidious and powerful, so much so that 30% of the heavy users vowed that they would not discontinue steroid use even if it were proved that they caused liver cancer; 31% said they would not stop even if they proved to cause heart attacks; and 39% said they would not stop using steroids even if they caused infertility.[14]

Although hard evidence of the long-term effects of steroid use is as yet unavailable, the potential for long-term harm is certainly real. It is impossible to predict how and when the effects of steroids will be manifested because people respond individually to these drugs due to differences in body chemistry. The steroid effect is complicated further because "black market" preparations contain additives and some preparations are contaminated. The potential for harm is readily discernible because 80% to 90% of all steroids used are purchased through the black market. Table 6-2 presents a synopsis of some of the known and some of the possible effects of steroid use.

Strength differences between the sexes essentially disappear when it is expressed by cross-sectional area of muscle tissue. Each sex is capable of generating 3 to 4 kilograms of force per centimeter of muscle tissue squared (kg/cm^2).[15] The quality of muscle for both sexes is equal and does not account for strength differences. Males may have as much as 50% more muscle tissue than females and this does account for the difference.

Calisthenics are not as effective as weight training in the development of strength because overload is more difficult to apply. In calisthenic-type exercises the body weight is the resistance, and this cannot be conveniently changed as participants become stronger. Calisthenics rather quickly lose their effectiveness in developing strength and become more associated with promoting muscle endurance.

Strength development exercises are **anaerobic.** Anaerobic literally means "without oxygen" and when applied to exercise it refers to high intensity physical activities whose oxygen demand is above that which can be supplied during performance. Short-term supplies of fuel that are stored in the muscles provide the energy for anaerobic activities. As a result, these can only be sustained for a matter of seconds. Sprinting 100 yards, lifting a heavy weight, and running up two or three flights of stairs are some examples of anaerobic activities.

TABLE 6-2 Anabolic steroids in a nutshell

Effects	Male	Female	Reversible
Increase in aggressive, hostile, and violent behavior	x	x	x
Dependence and potential addiction	x	x	x
Psychotic episodes	x	x	x
Hair growth on body and face		x	
Male pattern baldness		x	
Acne	x	x	x
Sexual dysfunction	x	x	x
Increased libido	x	x	x
Menstrual irregularities		x	x
Testicular atrophy and sterility	x		Unclear for long term use
Deepening of the voice		x	
Decreased breast size		x	x
Increased breast size (gynecomastia)	x		Unclear for long term use
Acceleration of atherosclerosis	x	x	x
High blood pressure	x	x	x
Decrease in HDL cholesterol	x	x	x
Liver damage	x	x	Some disorders are reversible; some are not
Prostrate cancer	x		
Muscle growth	x	x	x
Affects ultimate height attained when use begins in adolescence	x	x	

Evidence has been accumulating during the last decade that shows a positive relationship between dynamic resistance training and health enhancement. It is weight training (exercising the major muscles of the body at an intensity level of 70% to 90% of maximum strength) rather than weight lifting (lifting maximum loads in power, or Olympic style) that has produced these changes.[16] Very recent studies have shown that cardiac patients can benefit from appropriately planned weight training programs. Although weight training had always been considered too dangerous for cardiac patients, 25 cardiac patients engaged safely in 3 years of circuit weight training. As a group they had a 24% increase in strength and a 12% increase in cardiorespiratory endurance.[17] A summary of the wellness benefits of resistance training that are supported by research appear in Figure 6-14.

Figure 6-14 Muscle development and wellness

Exercises such as weight training that develop the muscular system produce the following beneficial health and wellness effects:
1. Increases muscle tissue and decreases fat tissue—this change enhances body composition and speeds up metabolism. The results of this change are a more aesthetic physical appearance and a greater likelihood of controlling one's body weight.
2. Develops strong abdominal and back muscles that improve posture and decrease the likelihood of sustaining low back problems.
3. Strengthens the *tendons* (tendons attach muscle to bone), *ligaments* (attach bone to bone), cartilage, and connective tissue producing more stable joints that resist injury.
4. Strengthens and maintains the integrity of the skeletal system, thereby resisting the advent of bone demineralization and osteoporosis.
5. Increases HDL cholesterol—the "good" cholesterol.

Increasing one's level of strength has practical advantages as well since the chores of daily living become easier. Changing a flat tire, rearranging furniture, carrying packages from the store, raking leaves, etc., all become easier as one becomes stronger.

The principles of exercise—intensity, frequency, duration, overload, progression, and specificity—apply to resistance training as well as aerobic training. For muscular development and health enhancement, the intensity of resistance training may be set by selecting a weight (through trial and error) that can be lifted at least eight times but no more than twelve times. This weight would probably represent 70% to 80% of a maximal effort.[16] Each of these lifts is called a repetition. The duration of resistance training is determined by the number of repetitions of each exercise and the number of sets completed. Eight to twelve repetitions of an exercise constitutes one set of that exercise.

The new ACSM guidelines for resistance training for healthy adults include the following: (1) the program should consist of eight to ten, exercises designed to stress the major muscle groups; (2) the exercise program should be repeated a minimum of twice weekly; and (3) the exercise program should consist of a minimum of one set of 8 to 12 repetitions to near fatigue.[1] These must be regarded as minimum standards that will produce approximately 75% of the gain documented with resistance programs featuring three sets of each exercise 3 days per week. Resistance programs following the ACSM guidelines do not produce optimal results but are excellent adjuncts to the cardiorespiratory component and appropriate when time is a factor.

Except for very advanced participants, resistance exercises should be performed no more than every other day. This type of training produces microscopic muscle tears that result in delayed muscle soreness and requires 48 hours of rest between each exercise session.

Overload may be applied by progressively increasing the amount of weight lifted or the number of repetitions performed or by decreasing rest time between sets. An increase in the number of repetitions leads to increases in muscle endurance; an increase in the amount of weight lifted leads to an increase in muscle strength; and a decrease in rest time increases muscular and aerobic endurance.

Muscular Endurance

Muscular endurance is the application of repeated muscular force. Inflating a tire with a bicycle pump, walking five flights of stairs, lifting a weight 20 times, and doing 50 sit-ups are some examples of muscular endurance. It is developed by many repetitions against resistances that are considerably less than maximum. Absolute muscular endurance is dependent on one's level of strength, but strength is not dependent on muscle endurance.[2] On the basis of limited data, significant muscle endurance may be developed in most people with a weight training program featuring 12 to 15 repetitions at 70% of maximal strength.[18] Exercises for endurance should be performed every other day.

Flexibility

Flexibility refers to the range of motion at a joint, such as the elbow, shoulder, or knee. It is specific to each joint; that is, one may be quite flexible in the shoulders but inflexible in the lower back. The flexibility of one joint cannot be predicted by measuring another. Therefore, several measurements at different sites are necessary to assess this component of fitness.

Motion is limited at a given joint by its bony structure, muscles, tendons, ligaments, and connective tissue. Additionally, the skin may be involved in resistance to movement. Improvement in flexibility is accomplished primarily by increasing the elasticity of the muscles, tendons, and ligaments.

Flexibility of the hamstring muscles (a group of muscles in the back of the thighs) and the low back muscles along with abdominal strength, good posture, and normal body weight are indispensable to a healthy back. Active individuals are usually more flexible than their sedentary counterparts.

Flexibility decreases with age, but there appears to be no evidence that the biological processes associated with aging are responsible for the decline. Loss of flexibility is more likely the result of diminishing physical activity that accompanies aging. All systems of the body deteriorate from lack of use. The range of motion for most movements begins to decline in the mid-twenties for males and about 30 years of age for females.

Flexibility can be improved by exercises that promote the elasticity of the soft tissues. Figures 6-15 through 6-22 present some selected exercises that have the capacity to maintain and improve the flexibility of the major body sites. These exercises can be done every day, both before and after exercise and also during days of rest from exercise. They can be performed while watching television, while listening to music, or at any 10-minute block of free time.

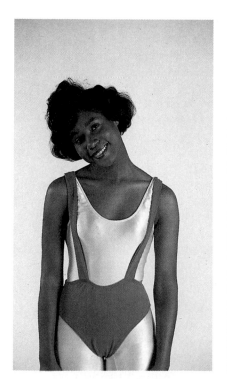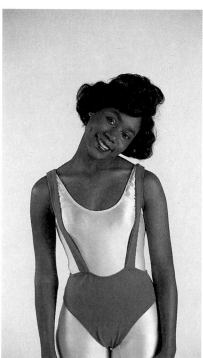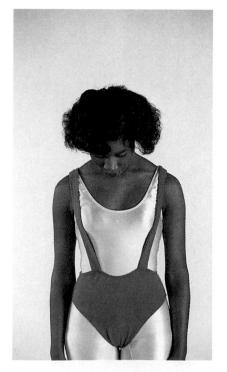

Figure 6-15 Neck stretches. Slowly bend your neck from side to side and front to back. Do not do head circles.

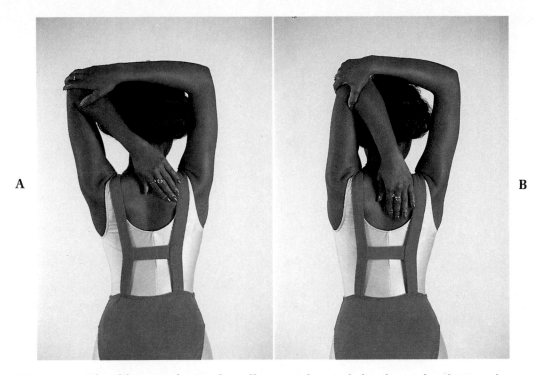

Figure 6-16 Shoulder stretch. Gently pull your right arm behind your head **(A)** and hold for 15 to 30 seconds **(B)**. Repeat with the other arm.

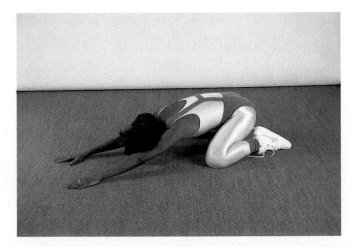

Figure 6-17 Chest and shoulder stretch. Stretch your arms to full extension with both palms on the floor **(A)** and press your chest down to the floor **(B)**. Hold 15 to 30 seconds and slowly release.

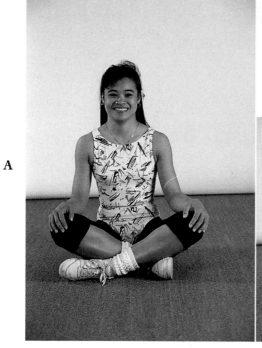

A

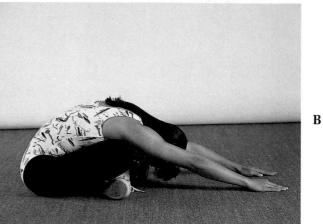

Figure 6-18 Back stretch. Cross your legs and lean forward **(A)**, extending the arms to the front **(B)**. Hold for 15 to 30 seconds and slowly release.

B

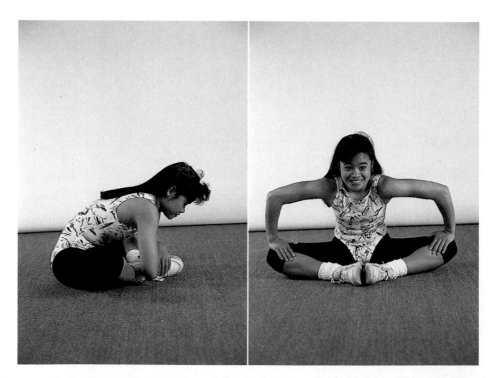

A   B

Figure 6-19 Groin stretch. **(A),** Place the soles of your feet together and lean forward **(B)**. Hold 15 to 30 seconds. Variation: Push down gently on both knees and hold for 15 to 30 seconds.

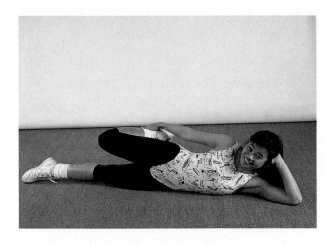

Figure 6-20 Quadriceps stretch. Lie on your side as shown. Bend the knee of the top leg, grasp the ankle with the free hand, and slowly pull the heel toward the buttocks until the stretch is felt in the muscles in the front of the thigh. Hold 15 to 30 seconds, roll over to the other side, and repeat with the other leg.

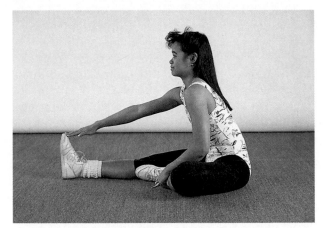

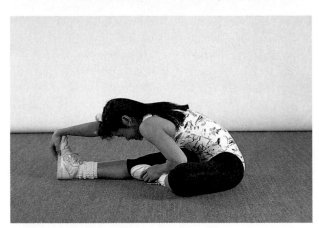

Figure 6-21 Hamstring stretch. Place the sole of the left foot against the thigh of the extended right leg. Lean forward without bending the knee of the extended leg. Hold for 15 to 30 seconds and repeat with the other leg.

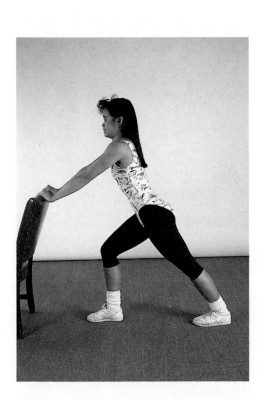

Figure 6-22 Calf and achilles tendon stretch. Assume the position shown above. Be sure the the heel of the extended leg remains in contact with the floor and that both feet are pointed straight ahead. Slowly move your hips forward until you feel the stretch in the calf of the extended leg. Hold 15 to 30 seconds and repeat with the other leg.

Flexibility is an important component of a fitness program designed to improve total fitness. Stretching exercises do improve flexibility but may not be effective in reducing injury from exercise. Muscle soreness and injury are possible when tight muscles are subjected to strenuous physical activity. Therefore it is intuitively appealing to associate lack of stretching with an increased potential for injury but there is little evidence in the literature to support this idea.

Muscles must contract for movement to occur. The contracting muscles are called *agonists* and they are the prime movers. For an agonist to contract and shorten there must be a reciprocal lengthening of its *antagonists* or movement will not occur. For example, when the biceps muscle of the upper arm contracts, its opposite, the triceps muscle, must relax and lengthen. In this case the biceps is the agonist and the triceps is the antagonist. The triceps become the agonist for movements that require it to contract, in which case the biceps become the antagonist. Understanding these concepts is necessary to understand stretching techniques.

Ballistic stretching utilizes dynamic movements to stretch muscles. Each time a muscle is stretched in this manner, the myotatic reflex (stretch reflex) located in that muscle is also stretched. It responds by sending a volley of signals to the central nervous system that orders the muscle to contract, thus resisting the stretch. This is not only counterproductive—the muscle is forced to pull against itself—but it can lead to injury because the elastic limits of the muscle may be exceeded. Dynamic stretching is not recommended.

Static stretching involves slowly moving to desired positions that are held for 15 to 30 seconds and then are slowly released. This method of stretching does not activate the myotatic reflex so that the muscle is essentially stretched without opposition. These positions should produce a feeling of mild discomfort but not pain. Static stretching (Figures 6-15 to 6-22) results in little or no muscle soreness, has a low incidence of injury, and requires little energy.

The following guidelines should be followed for safe and effective stretching:

▮ Warm-up for a few minutes prior to stretching by walking, slow jogging, and light calisthenics.
▮ Stretch to the point of discomfort.
▮ Stretching should not be painful.
▮ Hold each stretch for 15 to 30 seconds.

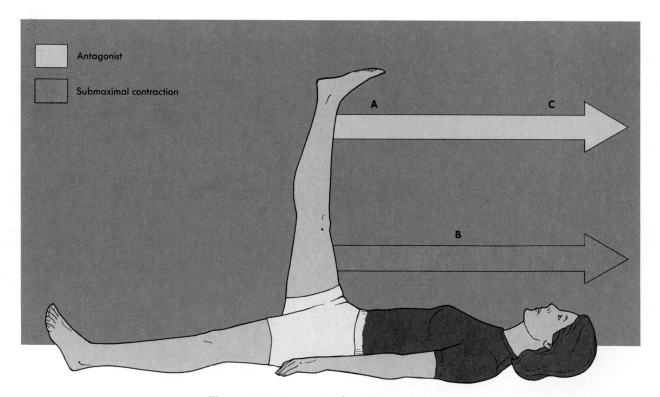

Figure 6-23 Contract-relax (CR) technique.

■ Move slowly from position to position.

■ Perform each stretch at least twice.

■ Stretch after the workout—this may actually produce the greatest benefit because the muscles are warm and are more amenable to stretching.

■ Stretching exercises may and probably should be performed daily.

Proprioceptive neuromuscular facilitation (PNF) is another effective and acceptable stretching technique. It is more complex than most of the methods of stretching, but it is the most effective.[19] By combining slow passive movements (the force for passive movement is supplied by a partner) with maximal voluntary isometric contractions, it becomes possible to bypass the myotatic reflex stimulation that accompanies changes in muscle and tendon length.

There are several variations of PNF stretching, all of which require a partner and some combination of passive stretching and isometric contractions. Two of the common PNF methods, contract-relax (CR) as seen in Figure 6-23 and slow-reversal-hold-relax (SRHR), Figure 6-24 are presented. For comparison, both figures exemplify stretching the hamstring group (muscles in the back of the thigh). The hamstrings are the antagonist muscle group and the quadriceps muscles (muscles in the front of the thigh) are the agonists. The contract-relax method is performed in the manner shown in Figure 6-23:

a. A partner gently pushes the upraised leg in the direction of arrow "a." This movement passively stretches the antagonist (hamstrings).

b. The subject follows this with a 6-second submaximal contraction of the agonist (quadriceps).

c. This is followed by another passive stretch of the hamstrings. This is repeated twice with a few seconds rest between sequences.

The slow-reversal-hold-relax (SRHR) method is performed in the following manner shown in Figure 6-24:

a. A partner gently pushes the upraised leg in the direction of arrow "a."

b. Then the subject performs a 6-second maximal voluntary isometric contraction (MVIC) of the antagonists (hamstrings) against resistance supplied by the partner.

c. The subject follows this with a 6-second submaximal contraction of the agonists (quadriceps).

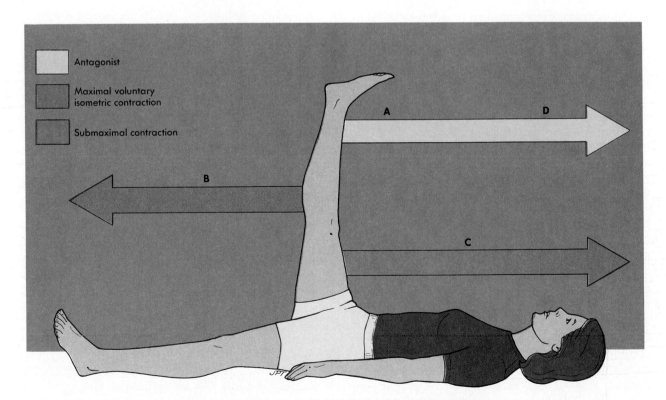

Figure 6-24 Slow-reversal-hold relax (SRHR) technique.

Figure 6-25 Flexibility and wellness

The major contribution of flexible muscles to wellness is in the maintenance of low back health. A healthy low back is dependent on abdominal strength, good posture, and flexibility of the hamstring and back extensor muscles. Flexibility of those structures decreases with age but there appears to be no evidence that the biological processes associated with aging are responsible. Inactivity rather than age seems to be associated with the loss of flexibility because muscles and other soft tissues lose their elasticity when they are not used.

Figure 6-26 Hazards of obesity

Obesity is a negative influence in the attainment of high level wellness. In addition to being a disease, it is the forerunner of and co-exists with the chronic diseases and it complicates the risks associated with these diseases.
1. There is a positive correlation between obesity and Type II diabetes, high blood pressure, and cholesterol level.
2. Obese women are more likely to suffer from cancer of the uterus, breast, ovaries, and gallbladder; obese men are more apt to contract cancer of the rectum, prostate, and colon.
3. The relationship between obesity and cardiovascular disease is well established.
4. Obesity leads to early death.
5. Obesity contributes to negative body image and self-concept.

d. This is followed by another passive stretch of the hamstrings. This is repeated twice with a few seconds of rest between sequences.

While PNF appears to be the most effective of the stretching methods for enhancing flexibility, it has some limitations. It requires a partner, it produces more pain and muscle stiffness, it takes more time, and the risk of injury is increased, particularly when novices use this technique. In a practical sense, it is more convenient to stretch statically because it does not require assistance nor does it take much time. For those interested in learning more about PNF stretching, we recommend *Modern Principles of Athletic Training* by Daniel Arnheim.[20]

As a component of health-related fitness, flexibility contributes to wellness in several ways. See Figure 6-25 for the major contributions.

Body Composition

Body composition refers to the percentage of lean versus fat tissue in the body. Fat includes essential and storage fat; the lean component includes all other tissues of the body. Body composition significantly affects wellness, longevity, and quality of life as we have learned in this chapter. It is favorably affected by appropriate aerobic and anaerobic activities. Exercise stimulates and develops the muscular system while reducing storage fat. Muscle development enhances the BMR, is esthetically appealing, and

improves self-concept. Its antithesis, obesity, is a health hazard (Figure 6-26).

Principles of Conditioning

It is necessary to become familiar with the principles of exercise to maximize the results of a physical fitness program. One's objectives can be met through the appropriate manipulation of the principles of intensity, frequency, duration, overload, progression, and specificity. Setting objectives, warm-up, cool-down, and type of activity are important elements that add to the enjoyment and effectiveness of exercise.

Intensity

Intensity refers to the degree of vigorousness of a single bout of exercise. The intensity level recommended by the American College of Sports Medicine (ACSM) is 60% to 90% of the maximum heart rate (HR_{max}).[1] Maximum heart rate can be measured by a physical work capacity test on a treadmill or cycle ergometer. Because most people don't have access to such tests, HR_{max} can be estimated by subtracting age from 220. A 20-year-old person has an estimated HR_{max} of 200 beats per minute (220 − 20 = 200). This formula predicts rather than measures HR_{max}; therefore there is some measurement error associated with its use. The error is estimated to be approximately plus or minus 10 beats per minute.

After the HR_{max} has been determined, the target for exercise may be calculated. The target zone for exercise provides the desirable heart rate for the development of physical fitness. For the 20-year old whose HR_{max} is 200 beats per minute, the target zone for exercise is calculated as follows:

$$\begin{array}{r} 200 \ (\text{estimated } HR_{max}) \\ \times \ .60 \quad (60\% \text{ of } HR_{max}) \\ \hline 120 (\text{lower limit target}) \end{array}$$

$$\begin{array}{r} 200 \ (\text{estimated } HR_{max}) \\ \times \ .90 \quad (90\% \text{ of } HR_{max}) \\ \hline 180 (\text{upper limit target}) \end{array}$$

This 20-year old should exercise at a heart rate between 120 and 180 beats per minute, depending on his or her objectives and level of fitness. The target for one whose level of fitness is average would be 150 to 160 beats per minute for exercise. The training effect occurs at heart rate levels below the maximum, and this rather nicely dispels the cherished myth that exercise must be painful to be beneficial.

Another method for calculating exercise heart rate, the Karvonen formula, takes fitness level and resting heart rate into account.[21] The training heart rate is calculated with this formula by utilizing a percentage of the *heart rate reserve*, which is the difference between the maximum and resting heart rates. The best way to determine the resting heart rate for this method is to count the pulse rate for 15 seconds while in the sitting position at the side of the bed after waking up in the morning. Repeat this for 4 to 5 consecutive days and average the readings for a rela-

tively accurate representation of resting heart rate. Next, estimate your level of fitness based on your exercise habits. Use this estimate to select a category from Table 6-3 to determine the appropriate exercise intensity level. If you cannot decide which category is the most appropriate then take the Rockport Fitness Walking Test (Assessment Activity 6-1 at the end of this chapter). This test should place you in the appropriate fitness category.

As an example, the Karvonen calculations for a 25-year old with a resting heart rate of 75 beats per minute and an average fitness level is as follows:

1. Calculate the max HR

$$\begin{array}{r} 220 \\ - \ 25 \\ \hline 195 \ \text{max HR} \end{array}$$

2. The Karvonen formula is:
   $$THR = (MHR - RHR) \times TI\% + RHR$$
   where

   $$THR = \text{Training heart rate}$$
   $$MHR = \text{Max HR}$$
   $$RHR = \text{Resting heart rate}$$
   $$TI\% = \text{Training intensity (see Table 6-3)}$$
   therefore
   $$THR = (MHR - RHR) \times TI\% + RHR$$
   $$= (195 - 75) \times .70 + 75$$
   $$= 120 \times .70 + 75$$
   $$= 84 + 75$$
   $$THR = 159$$

The training heart rate for this 25-year old subject is 159 beats per minute. Assessment Activity 6-2 is provided at the end of the chapter for you to determine your target heart rate for exercise.

Learning to take pulse rate quickly and accurately is necessary if you are going to monitor exercise intensity by heart rate. Two of the sites most commonly used for taking pulse rate are the radial artery at the thumb side of the wrist and the carotid artery at the side of the neck. Figure 6-27 illustrates the location of both of these sites. Use the first two fingers of the preferred hand to palpate the pulse. At the wrist, the pulse is located at the base of the thumb with the hand held palm up. For the carotid pulse, slide your fingers downward at the angle of the jaw below the ear-

---

TABLE 6-3 Guidelines for selecting exercise intensity level

Fitness level	Intensity level %
Low	60%
Fair	65%
Average	70%
Good	75%
Excellent	80-90%

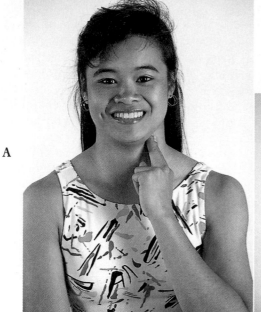

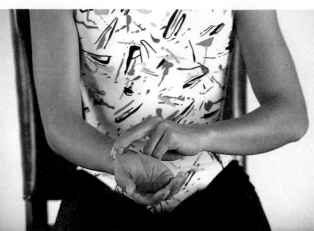

Figure 6-27 A, Location for taking pulse at the carotid artery. **B,** Location for taking pulse at the wrist (radial artery).

lobe to the side of the neck. Apply only enough pressure to feel the pulse, particularly at the carotid artery. Excessive pressure at this point stimulates specialized receptors that automatically slow the heart rate, leading to an underestimation of the heart rate actually achieved during exercise. The wrist is the preferred site for the *palpation* (examination by touch or feel) of the pulse rate. The carotid pulse should be used if the pulse cannot be felt at the wrist.

It is important to locate and count the pulse rate immediately after exercise stops. Count the beats for 10 seconds and multiply by 6 to get beats per minute. The first beat takes a count of zero. Some practice is required to locate the pulse quickly and to count accurately.

Another method for monitoring the intensity of exercise is by rating your subjective perception of the effort. Some days exercise seems easier than normal and other days it may seem more difficult. The "perceived exertion scale" in Figure 6-28 may be used to quantify the effort. The intensity level of exercise for the majority of people should fall in the categories of 11 to 15 and this should correspond approximately to the target heart rate. In other words, if you are in the appropriate target heart rate zone, the perceived exertion will probably be between 11 and 15.

Frequency

The *frequency* of exercise refers to the number of days of participation each week. The ACSM recommends that exercise be pursued 3 to 5 days per week for optimal results. Less than 3 days is an inadequate stimulus for developing fitness and, conversely, more than 5 days per week represents a point of diminishing returns from exercise and increases the likelihood of sustaining an injury.[1] Of course these guidelines can be used with some degree of flexibility. For example, exercise may be pursued more than 5 days per week if (1) low-intensity exercises of moderate duration (20 to 40 minutes), such as walking, are the preferred forms of activity, (2) one engages in cross-training (participating in different activities each day or per each exercise session), and (3) weight loss is the objective.

One can overdo exercise—too much results in staleness or overtraining. The signs of overtraining include:

▮ A feeling of chronic fatigue and listlessness.
▮ Inability to make further fitness gains or the level of fitness may regress.
▮ Sudden loss of weight.
▮ An increase of five beats per minute in resting heart rate.
▮ Loss of enthusiasm for working out.

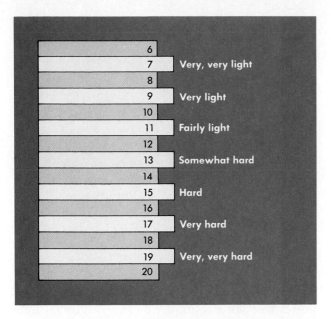

Figure 6-28 The perceived exertion scale.

Treatment requires that the individual cut back on training or stop completely for 1 to 2 weeks. When exercise is resumed it must be of lower intensity, frequency, and duration. The exerciser must rebuild and regain fitness gradually. Prevention is the best treatment for overtraining.

Duration

Duration refers to the length of each exercise session. Intensity and duration are inversely related—the more intense the exercise, the shorter its duration. Intensity is always an important consideration for the development of physical fitness but for health enhancement purposes it is best to reduce the intensity somewhat while increasing the frequency and duration. The ACSM recommends 20 to 60 minutes of continuous or noncontinuous aerobic activity.[1] Another way to monitor duration is by the number of calories expended per exercise session. The ACSM recommends 300 to 500 calories per session. Check Table 4-4 in Chapter 4 to determine how long you need to exercise in the activities of your choice to achieve this goal.

Progression, Overload, and Specificity

As people attain a level of fitness that meets their needs and further improvement is not desired, the program switches from the development of fitness to the maintenance of fitness. At this point, the principles of overload and pro-

gression may be set aside but both are necessary for the improvement phase of fitness. *Overload* involves subjecting the body to unaccustomed stress, while *progression* implies that overload is applied systematically and gradually and only when the individual is ready to accept a new challenge. The body adapts and physical fitness improves by the knowledgeable application of overload and progression.

The principle of *specificity* of training suggests that the body adapts according to the specific type of stress placed on it. The muscles involved in any given activity are the ones that adapt, and they do so in the specific way in which they are used. For example, jogging prepares one for jogging but it is poor preparation for cycling. Cycling does not prepare one for swimming. Although these activities all stress the cardiorespiratory system, they are sufficiently different from each other so that there is little fitness carry-over between them.

The principle of specificity is of paramount importance for competitive athletes. Competitors are attempting to maximize the returns from their training effort, therefore runners must train by running, swimmers must swim, and cyclists must cycle. The focus is on maximum improvement in one activity so the body is trained in the specific manner in which it is to perform. This locks athletes into regimented training programs, but people who exercise for health reasons are not under such constraints. They can vary activities and avert the boredom and tedium of participating in the same activity week after week. Cycling, jogging, swimming, racquetball, cross-country skiing, weight training, and the like may be employed in any combination or order for the development of physical fitness.

Setting Objectives

Identifying goals, or what one hopes to accomplish, will provide some direction for the activity selected and how the principles of exercise are to be manipulated to increase the probability of success. Only one or two major goals should be selected, and these should be articulated as specifically and clearly as possible so that an effective exercise program may be devised. Without specific objectives, the exercise program might become an exercise in frustration if activities, objectives, and principles do not match. This might be analogous to sightseeing in Los Angeles with a map of San Francisco: right state;

wrong city. You may reach your destination, but the odds are against it.

Warming Up For Exercise

Warming up prepares the body for physical action. The process involves stretching exercises and physical activities that gradually heat the muscles and elevate the heart rate. Refer to Figures 6-15 to 6-22 for some typical stretches that are appropriate to use during the warm-up. A slow jog, jogging or hopping in place, and rope jumping are some activities that will raise the heart rate and increase muscle temperature. Participants should break out in a sweat during the warm-up. This indicates that body temperature has increased to some extent and the individual is ready for more vigorous activity.

It is most important to increase the heart rate gradually during the warm-up period. This allows the circulatory system to adjust to the load. If the heart rate is allowed to elevate suddenly, circulation cannot adjust rapidly enough to meet the oxygen and nutrient demand of the heart muscle. The effects of this lag time are abolished in about 2 minutes, but this practice can be potentially hazardous, particularly for those with compromised circulation due to latent or subclinical heart disease. Even the healthy heart may be affected by eliminating this important phase of warm-up. One study showed that each of 44 healthy male subjects, ages 21 to 52, had normal EKG responses to running on a treadmill when they were allowed a warm-up consisting of 2 minutes of easy jogging. However, 70% of the group developed abnormal EKG responses to the same exercise when they were not allowed to warm-up.

Warm-up may be specifically tailored to the activity that is to be performed. For example, joggers may warm-up by slowly jogging the first ½ to ¾ of a mile, gradually speeding up to the desired pace. Cyclists, swimmers, cross-country skiers, rope skippers, and others may employ the same approach.

Cooling Down From Exercise

The cool-down is as important as the warm-up except that the process is reversed and the body is allowed to slow down gradually. Cool-down should last 8 to 10 minutes and consists of two phases. The first phase involves approximately 5 minutes of walking or other light activities to prevent blood from pooling in the muscles that have been working. Light activity causes rhythmical contractions of the muscles, which in turn act as a stimulus to circulate blood from the muscles to the heart for redistribution throughout the body. This boost to circulation following exercise, often referred to as the "muscle pump," is essential for recovery and shares with the heart some of the burden of circulation. The muscle pump effect does not occur if a period of inactivity follows exercise. This forces the heart to work at a high rate to compensate for the reduced volume of blood returning to it because of blood pooling in the muscles. The exerciser runs the risk of dizziness, fainting, and perhaps more serious consequences associated with diminished blood flow.

Light physical activity following exercise also speeds the removal of lactic acid that has accumulated in the muscles. *Lactic acid* is a fatiguing metabolite resulting from the incomplete breakdown of sugar. It is produced by exercise of high intensity or of long duration.

The second phase of cool-down should focus on the stretching exercises that were performed during the warm-up. Most participants find that stretching after exercise is more comfortable and quite possibly more effective because the muscles are heated and more elastic.

Type of Activity

Many activities contribute to one or more of the components of health-related physical fitness. Activity selections should be based on objectives, skill level, availability of equipment, facilities, instruction, climate, and interest. The President's Council on Physical Fitness and Sports (PCPFS) enlisted the aid of 7 experts to evaluate 14 popular physical activities for their contribution to physical fitness and general well-being. Although this assessment occurred several years ago, the ratings are equally as valid today as when they were originally conceived. A summary of these appear in Table 6-4.

Selected sports have been evaluated for their contribution to the health-related components of physical fitness. These appear in Table 6-5. Lifetime sports (such as tennis, badminton, and racquetball) are more conducive in a practical sense for the development of fitness than team sports (such as volleyball, soccer, softball, and basketball) because fewer players are needed. Ideally, fitness should be developed and maintained primarily through self-paced activities (jogging, cycling, walking, or swimming) but the challenge inherent in sports participation may be necessary to sustain the fitness program for some people. Lifetime sports are challenging and fun and they

TABLE 6-4 Rating 14 sports and exercises

	Jogging	Bicycling	Swimming	Skating (ice or roller)	Handball/squash	Skiing—nordic	Skiing—alpine	Basketball	Tennis	Calisthenics	Walking	Golf	Softball	Bowling
Physical fitness														
Cardiorespiratory endurance (stamina)	21	19	21	18	19	19	16	19	16	10	13	8	6	5
Muscular endurance	20	18	20	17	18	19	18	17	16	13	14	8	8	5
Muscular strength	17	16	14	15	15	15	15	15	14	16	11	9	7	5
Flexibility	9	9	15	13	16	14	14	13	14	19	7	9	9	7
Balance	17	18	12	20	17	16	21	16	16	15	8	8	7	6
General well-being														
Weight control	21	20	15	17	19	17	15	19	16	12	13	6	7	5
Muscle definition	14	15	14	14	11	12	14	13	13	18	11	6	5	5
Digestion	13	12	13	11	13	12	9	10	12	11	11	7	8	7
Sleep	16	15	16	15	12	15	12	12	11	12	14	6*	7	6
Total	148	142	140	140	140	139	134	134	128	126	102	66*	64	51

The ratings are on a scale of 0-3; thus a rating of 21 is the maximum score that can be achieved (a score of 3 by all 7 panelists). Ratings were made on the following basis: Frequency = 4 times per week minimum; duration = 30 to 60 minutes per session.
*Golf rating was made on the basis of using a golf cart or caddy. If you walk the course and carry your clubs the values improve.

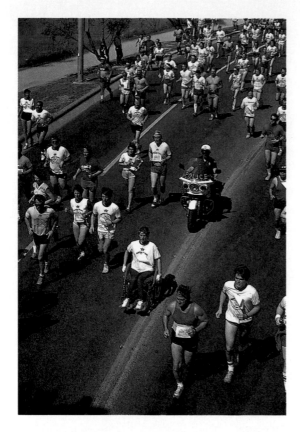

inject variety into the program. However, fitness attained from these activities is dependent on skill level and a willingness to exert maximal effort ·in singles competition. The orthopedic demands of these activities may be greater than a sedentary beginner can tolerate. Quick stops and starts, bursts of high-intensity activity, sudden changes of direction, and rapid twists and turns place a great deal of stress on the musculoskeletal system. The physically fit are able to handle the aerobic and musculoskeletal requirements of active sports. Attempting to play yourself "into shape" is a mistake. First, become physically fit, then play the games.

Now that you have completed the sections on the principles of exercise, warm up, cool down, and the contribution of various physical activities to physical fitness, you are ready to attempt Assessment Activity 6-3, designing an exercise program, at the end of this chapter.

Exercise and Selected Chronic Conditions

Osteoporosis

Osteoporosis is a chronic disease in which the mineral content of the bones progressively decreases so that the bones become brittle and sub-

The physically fit can meet many aerobic and musculoskeletal challenges.

ject to breakage. It is responsible for approximately 1.2 million bone fractures annually— 530,000 involve the vertebral bones in the spinal column and another 227,000 are fractures of the hip.[22]

The primary risk factors for osteoporosis include female gender, white or Oriental race, slender body type, and early menopause. The secondary risks include alcohol and tobacco abuse, calcium deficiency, family history, sedentary lifestyle, anticonvulsant medication use, and thyroid hormone use.

Type I osteoporosis affects eight times as many women as men and the effects are seen during the first 2 years after menopause.[23] The fractures in order of prevalence in type I are vertebral crush fractures and fractures of the arm above the wrist. Accelerated bone loss after menopause due to estrogen deficiency contributes significantly to these fractures. Type II osteoporosis occurs later in life, about age 70, and affects twice as many women as men. Fractures of the hips are the most frequent events. Estrogen deficiency is only one of many possible causes in type II osteoporosis. Other contributing causes include calcium deficiency, fluoride deficiency, and lack of exercise.

Bone is living organic tissue that responds to physical stress. It is continuously undergoing remodeling, but osteoporosis accelerates bone loss so that replacement cannot keep pace; and this results in weakened and brittle bone. Inactivity and the absence of gravitational force (weightlessness) contribute to the process. Conversely, physical exercise forces bone to adapt to the stresses imposed on it and it hypertrophies, as

■ TABLE 6-5 Rating of selected sports*

Sport	Cardiorespiratory endurance	Muscular strength/endurance		Flexibility	Body composition
		Upper	Lower		
Badminton	M-H	L	M-H	L	M-H
Football (touch)	L-M	L-M	M	L	L-M
Ice hockey	H	M	H	L	H
Racquetball	H	M	H	M	H
Rugby	H	M-H	H	M	H
Soccer	H	L	H	M	H
Volleyball	M	M	M	L-M	M
Wrestling	H	H	H	M-H	H

*H = High; M = medium; L = low. The values in this table are estimates that will vary according to the skill and motivation of the participants.

other tissues do, in response. Bones atrophy when they are unstressed.

The development of the muscular system is essential to the development and maintenance of bone mass. Athletes have greater bone density than age-matched nonathletes. Unilateral athletes, those who use one limb extensively, and vigorously such as tennis players and baseball pitchers, have larger and thicker muscles and bones in the dominant arm compared with their nondominant arm. Weight-bearing activities, such as jogging, racquetball, and weight training, are more effective activities for the development and maintenance of the skeletal system than non-weight-bearing activities such as swimming and cycling.

Mild to moderate exercises have been effective in promoting bone strength in the elderly. Studies whose subjects were 60 to 95 years of age suggest that exercise effectively arrests bone loss and/or increases bone mineral content well into old age.

People with osteoporosis can and should exercise but the type of physical activity and the intensity of exercise must be carefully selected. Forceful contractions of muscles or high-impact activities should be avoided because they may stress the bones beyond their breaking point. Swimming, water aerobics, stationary cycling, walking, and light weight training are good starting activities for those with osteoporosis.

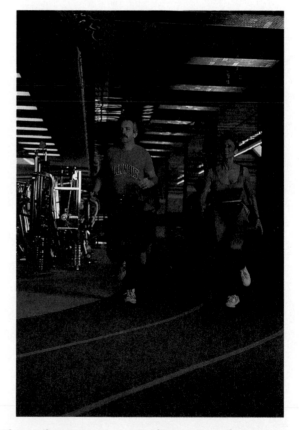

Physical activity promotes bone strength, especially important for women who are at higher risk of developing osteoporosis.

Low Back Pain

It is estimated that 8 of every 10 Americans will suffer a back injury sometime during their lives.[24] It is the most common symptomatic complaint for both sexes in the 25 to 60 year-old group who visit a physician's office.[25] Low back pain costs business and industry $250 million in worker's compensation and approximately $1 billion in lost output annually.

The high incidence of low back pain may be primarily attributed to "mechanical factors."[24] These include overweight, poor posture, and lack of physical fitness. Most low back pain involves muscle and ligament strain and inflamed joints along the vertebral column. Some injuries involve discs that herniate or tear so that the jell-like inner substance escapes and exerts pressure on the spinal nerves. Back pain also occurs as a result of injuries sustained from accidents, falls, lifting objects incorrectly, and participation in sports. Arthritis and osteoporosis also cause low back pain.

Ninety percent of all back problems occur in the lumbar region (low back) of the spine. The spinal column consists of 33 bones (the vertebrae) and represents the only bony connection between the upper and lower halves of the body. Located between the bones of the spine are rings of tough fibrous tissue, the discs, that act as shock absorbers and that keep the vertebrae from rubbing against each other. The spinal column is S-shaped and consists of three naturally occurring curves. When these three curves are in balance, the body weight is evenly distributed and movement occurs fluidly. The fact that the bones are not stacked on each other in a straight line increases susceptibility of the injury especially to the lower back, which must bear the brunt of the weight of the torso. Misalignment in this region applies substantial stress to the concave, or inner side of the exaggerated curve. The more pronounced the curve, the greater the stress because of the uneven distribution of weight on the bones and discs.

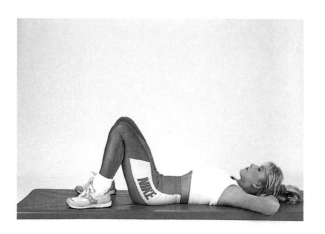
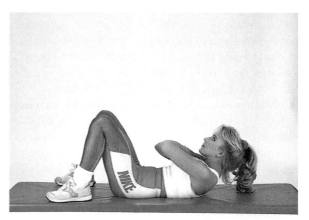
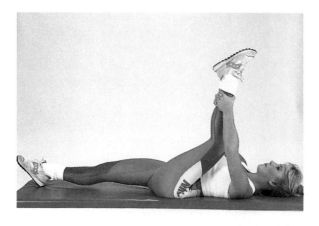
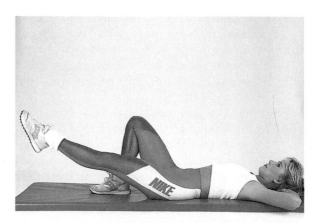

Figure 6-29 Maintaining a healthy back.

Overweight is a stressor of the low back because the excess weight pulls the spinal column forward, accentuating the lumbar curve and putting pressure on the discs. Research supports the notion that weak abdominal muscles combined with lack of flexibility in the lower back and hamstring muscles promotes fatigue and poor posture.[26] Fatigue causes the pelvis to tilt forward, increasing stress on the spinal column and its supporting structures. High-heeled shoes tilt the pelvis forward, and many wearers of this footwear experience discomfort and/or pain in the low back at the end of the day.

Stress may be a factor in inducing or prolonging low back pain. Muscles that are under constant tension result in tightness and fatigue in the low back. Exercises that develop and strengthen the abdominal muscles as well as those that stretch the low back and hamstrings are invaluable in preventing low back pain. See Figure 6-29 for commonly performed exercises for the maintenance of a healthy back. Exercise also contributes to weight control, is an excellent stress reducer generally and specifically for the muscles that are exercised, and develops the antigravity muscles—the calves, front and back of the thighs, hips, back, and abdominals, thereby contributing to correct posture. Also, be sure to lift objects correctly. See Figure 6-30 for lifting techniques that minimize the potential for injury.

Should a back problem occur, consult a physician for treatment. Surgery may be suggested. If so, get a second opinion. Be sure to explore alternative treatments. Many back problems can be treated with Williams flexion exercises[27] and McKenzie's extension exercises.[28] The selection of either depends on the type of problem being experienced, and the selection should be made by a health care professional. For more information regarding the Williams and McKenzie exercises, refer to references 27 and 28 at the end of this chapter.

Osteoarthritis

Osteoarthritis is a degenerative joint disease characterized by the deterioration of articular cartilage in the joints. The weight bearing joints—knees, hips, and ankles—are particularly affected. Osteoarthritis, often referred to as a "wear and tear" disease, is the most common joint disease in the United States.[29] It is a progressive disease of unknown origin that worsens with age and ultimately affects most people to some extent. Thirty-five percent of adult Americans exhibit clinically identifiable osteoarthritis

of the knee. The weight bearing joints of most 40- to 50-year olds are affected, and 85% of 75-year olds have diagnosable osteoarthritis.

Does jogging, with its constant pounding, cause the early onset of osteoarthritis? The research evidence emphatically indicates that it does not. In fact, there is growing evidence that suggests that jogging may slow musculoskeletal aging. Hundreds of runners who were followed for several years visited a physician less often and had less physical disability than age-matched nonrunners, and osteoarthritis seemed to be developing more slowly among them.[30] Runners, age 50 to 72, had 40% more bone mineral content in the vertebral bones of the spinal column than age-matched nonrunners, and there was no difference between the two groups in the clinical manifestations of osteoarthritis.[31] Thirty-five years of data collected by the Framingham investigators showed that obesity rather than running was the major cause of osteoarthritis of the knee.[32] Even high mileage running (average of 28 miles per week for 12 years) was not associated with the premature development of osteoarthritis.[33]

Weight-bearing activities such as jogging do expose the joints to substantial forces. Compared to walking, the forces generated by jogging are twice as great at the hip, six times greater at the knee, and twice that at the ankle.[34] The forces developed by the weight bearing, impact-loading activities such as jogging can be accepted by the body usually without permanent detriment because the joints are capable of dissipating these forces through their supporting elastic structures. Secondly, all movement is buffered by compressible shock-absorbing cartilage whose surfaces articulate in an essentially friction-free environment. The soft tissues of the joints—muscles, tendons, ligaments, connective tissue, and cartilage—respond to exercise by becoming thicker and stronger. This is important in delaying osteoarthritis and for protecting the joints from injury.

Cancer

Researchers are currently investigating the role of aerobic exercise in the prevention of cancer. The Harvard Alumni Study, where 17,000 men were followed for more than 20 years, showed that cancer mortality was highest in those who exercised least, even after age and cigarette smoking were controlled.[35] The risk of colon cancer in 1.1 million Swedish men was 1.3 times greater for subjects in sedentary occupa-

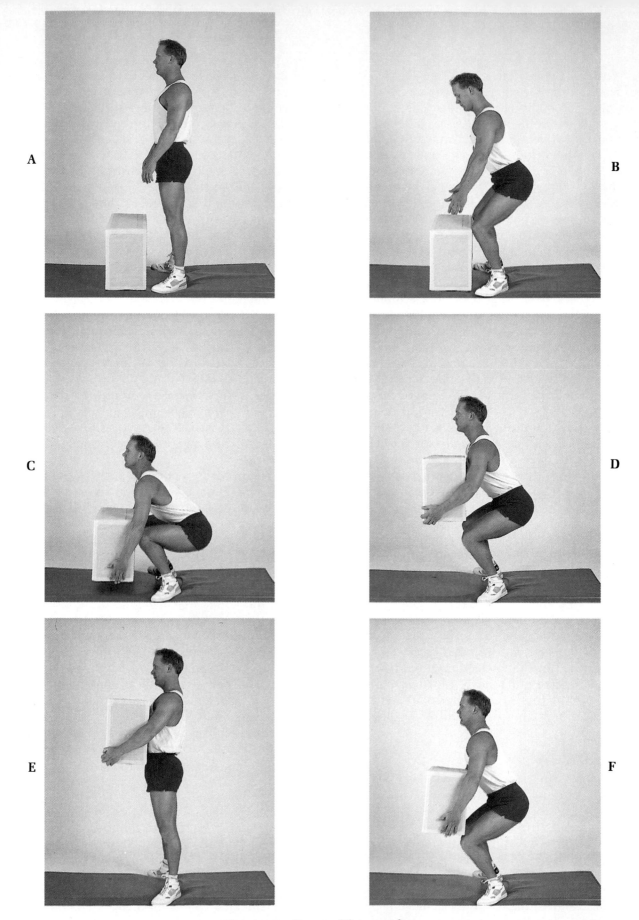

Figure 6-30 How to lift properly.

Continued.

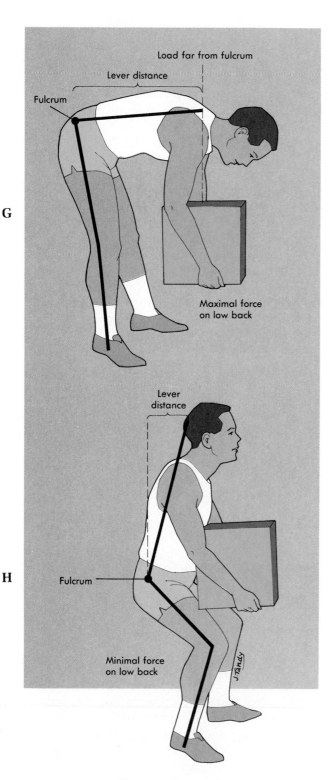

G

Lever distance

Load far from fulcrum

Fulcrum

Maximal force
on low back

H

Lever
distance

Fulcrum

Minimal force
on low back

J. Tandy

Figure 6-30, cont'd.

tions compared with men in active occupations.[36] American women doing sedentary jobs had a higher risk for breast and colon cancer than women in active occupations and men in sedentary jobs had twice the risk of colon cancer than men in active jobs.[37]

The evidence of a relationship between physical inactivity and cancer is mounting, but it falls short of cause and effect. Several hypotheses have been advanced to explain the mechanisms through which exercise may operate to prevent cancer. The first of these involves the effect of exercise in reducing body fat. Because the amount of body fat is positively correlated with the incidence of cancer, and because exercise is one of the most effective methods for reducing fat, it seems reasonable to conclude that this may be one of the possible mechanisms contributing to the prevention of cancer. Secondly, several studies have indicated that exercise may augment or stimulate the body's immune system in several ways, the end result being that cancerous cells are recognized and destroyed early in their development.[38] Exercise received official recognition in 1985 when the American Cancer Society began recommending it to protect against cancer.[39]

Environmental Conditions

Human beings work and exercise in a variety of environmental conditions. Hot and cold weather produce unique sets of problems for people who function out-of-doors. Their safety and comfort depend on their knowledge of how the body reacts to physical activity in different climate conditions.

Heat is produced in the body as a by-product of metabolism. Physical activities significantly increase metabolism, so more heat than normal is generated. The problem becomes one of dissipating the heat effectively or the heat build-up may result in illness and possible death. *Heat exhaustion* is a serious condition but not an imminent threat to life. It is characterized by dizziness, fainting, rapid pulse, and cool skin. Treatment includes immediate cessation of activity and moving the victim to a cool shady place. The victim is then placed in a reclining position and given cool fluids to drink.

Heat stroke is a medical emergency and a threat to life. It is the most severe of the heat-induced illnesses. The symptoms include a high temperature (106° or above) and dry skin because sweating has stopped. These symptoms are accompanied by some or all of the following: delirium, convulsions, and loss of consciousness. The early warning signs include chills, nausea, head-ache, and general weakness. Victims of heat stroke should be rushed immediately to the nearest hospital for treatment.

Heat is lost from the body by conduction, radiation, convection, and evaporation of sweat. Evaporation of sweat is the major avenue of heat loss during exercise, and this process is most effective when the humidity is low. High humidity significantly impairs the evaporative process because the air is very saturated and cannot accept much moisture. If both temperature and humidity are high, it becomes difficult to lose heat by any of these processes. Under these adverse conditions, it may be best to adjust the intensity and duration of exercise or to move indoors where the climate can be controlled.

Exercise in hot and humid conditions forces the body to divert more blood than usual from the working muscles to the skin in an effort to carry the heat that is accumulating in the deeper recesses to the outer shell. The net result is that the exercising muscles are deprived of a full complement of blood and cannot work as long or as hard. Exercise is more difficult in hot and humid weather.

Heat loss by evaporation is seriously impeded when participants wear nonporous garments such as rubberized and plastic exercise suits. These garments encourage sweating but their nonporous nature does not allow sweat to evaporate. This practice is dangerous because it may easily result in heat build-up and *dehydration* (excessive water loss), leading to heat stress illnesses. One should dress for hot-weather exercise by wearing shorts and a porous top. A mesh baseball-type cap is optional. It is effective in blocking the absorption of radiant heat if one exercises in the middle of the day because the sun's rays are vertical. Wearing a cap is not necessary if exercise occurs in the cooler parts of the day or if the sun is not shining.

Guidelines for exercising in heat and humidity have been developed for road races but these can be applied to any strenuous physical activity performed outdoors during the warm weather season. Ambient conditions are considered safe when the temperature is below 70° F (Fahrenheit) and the humidity is below 45%. Caution should be used when the temperature is greater than 70° F or the humidity is over 45%. People who are sensitive to heat and humidity should carefully consider whether or not to exercise when the temperature is greater than 75° F or the humidity is more than 50%.[40] People who are trained and

heat acclimated can continue to exercise in these conditions but they should be aware of the potential hazards and take precautions to prevent heat illness.

The key to exercising without incident in hot weather is to maintain the fluid level in the body. Dehydration from profuse sweating is to be avoided because hyperthermia and heat stress illnesses are positively correlated with fluid loss. Heat illness can be avoided by following a few guidelines.

▌ Liberally drink water or a noncarbonated beverage that is low in sugar and salt prior to the workout. Continue to drink fluids (preferably water) approximately 8 to 12 ounces every 15 to 20 minutes during the workout. Drink all you can hold after the workout. Get into the habit of drinking even when not thirsty because our thirst mechanisms and tissue needs are not in good accord. Drink refrigerated water because this will absorb some of the heat.

▌ Do not ingest salt during exercise because it slows the absorption of water by the tissues from the gastrointestinal tract. Only small quantities of salt are lost in sweat and this will probably be replaced during the next meal.

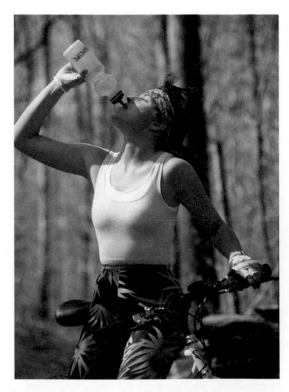

In hot and humid conditions, drinking water and wearing loose clothing will help avoid hyperthermia and heat stroke illnesses.

■ Do not take salt tablets at any time. They are stomach irritants; they attract fluid to the gut; they sometimes pass through the digestive system undissolved; and they may perforate the stomach lining.

■ Potassium is lost in sweat but not in large quantities. However, it is a good idea to consume potassium-rich foods everyday. Citrus juices, potatoes, dates, bananas, and meats are excellent sources of potassium.

■ Modify the exercise program by (1) working out during the cooler times of the day; (2) choosing shady routes where water is available; (3) slowing the pace and/or shortening the duration of exercise on particularly oppressive days; and (4) wearing light, loose porous clothing to facilitate the evaporation of sweat.

Problems related to exercise in cold weather include frostbite and *hypothermia* (abnormally low body temperature). Frostbite can lead to permanent damage or loss of a body part due to gangrene. This can be prevented by adequately protecting exposed areas such as fingers, nose, ears, facial skin, and toes. Gloves, preferably mittens or thick socks, should be worn to protect the fin-

gers, hands, and wrists. A stocking hat is preferable for two reasons: (1) blood vessels in the scalp do not constrict effectively so a significant amount of heat is lost if a head covering is not worn, and (2) a stocking type hat can be pulled down to protect the ears. In very cold or windy weather participants may use surgical or ski masks and scarves to keep facial skin warm and to moisten and warm inhaled air. All exposed or poorly protected flesh is vulnerable to frostbite when the temperature is low and the windchill high. Use Table 6-6 as a safety guide for working and exercising in cold windy weather.

People often experience a hacking cough for a minute or two following physical exertion in cold weather. This is a normal response and one that should not cause alarm. Very cold dry air may not be fully moistened when it is inhaled rapidly and in large volumes during exercise, so the lining of the throat dries out. When exercise is discontinued, the respiratory rate slows down and the volume of inhaled air decreases, allowing enough time for the body to fully moisturize it. Coughing stops within a couple of minutes as the linings are remoistened.

■ **TABLE 6-6 Wind chill index**

Wind speed (in MPH)	Actual thermometer reading (°F)											
	50	40	30	20	10	0	−10	−20	−30	−40	−50	−60
	Equivalent temperature (F)											
Calm	50	40	30	20	10	0	−10	−20	−30	−40	−50	−60
5	48	37	27	16	6	−5	−15	−26	−36	−47	−57	−68
10	40	28	16	4	−9	−21	−33	−46	−58	−70	−83	−95
15	36	22	9	−5	−18	−36	−45	−58	−72	−85	−99	−112
20	32	18	4	−10	−25	−39	−53	−67	−82	−96	−110	−124
25	30	16	0	−15	−29	−44	−59	−74	−88	−104	−118	−133
30	28	13	−2	−18	−33	−48	−63	−79	−94	−109	−125	−140
35	27	11	−4	−20	−35	−49	−67	−82	−98	−113	−129	−145
40*	26	10	−6	−21	−37	−53	−69	−85	−100	−116	−132	−148

Little danger (for properly clothed person) ... Increasing danger—Cover up fully (hands, ears, face, head, etc.) ... Great danger— Exercise Indoors

*Wind speeds greater than 40 MPH have little additional effect.

Summary

- Physical fitness is defined in terms of performance-related and health-related fitness.
- Cardiorespiratory endurance is the most important component of health-related fitness.
- The long-term effects of physical training include modifications in heart rate, stroke volume, cardiac output, blood volume, heart volume, respiration, and metabolism.
- Aerobic capacity is finite, improves by 15% to 30% with training, and decreases with aging but more slowly in those who are physically fit.
- The training effect is lost in stages if exercise is interrupted or discontinued.
- Muscular strength can be improved statically or dynamically. From the standpoint of effectiveness and practicality, dynamic approaches are preferred.
- The principles of exercise include intensity, frequency, duration, overload, progression, and specificity. Participant objectives are met by the appropriate manipulation of these principles.
- Regular exercise promotes health enhancement by reducing the risks associated with the chronic diseases.
- Exercise affects cholesterol, blood pressure, triglycerides, diabetes mellitus, stress, and is an alternative method for quitting the use of tobacco products.
- Osteoporosis is a chronic disease that results in brittle bones that are susceptible to fracture.
- Low back pain is caused by poor level of fitness, poor posture, overweight, accidents, lifting objects incorrectly, and sports participation.
- Osteoarthritis is a "wear and tear" disease of unknown origin that affects most people to some extent.
- The development of physical fitness may have a role to play in protecting people from cancer.
- Evaporation of sweat is the major mechanism of ridding the body of heat that develops during exercise.

 Action plan for personal wellness

An important consideration in assuming responsibility for one's own quality of life is utilizing information. After reading this chapter, answer the following questions and determine an action plan for enhancing your own lifestyle.

1 Based on the information presented in this chapter, along with what I know about my family's health history, the health problems/issues that I need to be most concerned about are:_____

_____

_____

2 Of those health concerns listed in no. 1, the one I most need to act on is:_____

_____

_____

3 The possible actions that I can take to improve my level of wellness are (try to be as specific as possible):_____

_____

_____

4 Of those actions listed in no. 3, the one that I most need to include in an action plan is:_____

_____

_____

5 Factors I need to keep in mind in order to be successful in my action plan are:_____

_____

Review Questions

1. What are the physiological changes that occur from regular participation in aerobic exercise?
2. What are the health benefits that occur from regular participation in aerobic training; resistance training; and flexibility training?
3. What are the differences between isometric, isotonic, and isokinetic training?
4. Name and define the principles of conditioning.
5. Identify and define the mechanisms

References

1. American College of Sports Medicine: The recommended quantity and quality of exercise for developing and maintaining cardiorespiratory and muscular fitness in healthy adults, Medicine and Science in Sports and Exercise 22(2):265-274, 1990.
2. Wilmore JH and Costill DL: Training for sport and activity, Dubuque, Iowa, 1988, William C Brown, Publishers.
3. Eddington DW and Edgerton VR: The biology of physical activity, Boston, 1976, Houghton Mifflin Co.
4. Kasch FW et al: The effect of physical activity and inactivity on aerobic power in older men (a longitudinal study), Physician Sportsmedicine 18:73-83, April, 1990.
5. Coyle EF et al: Time course of loss of adaptations after stopping prolonged intense endurance training, J Appl Physiol 57:1857-1864, 1984.
6. Coyle EF Effects of detraining on responses to submaximal exercise, J Appl Physiol 59:853-859, 1985.
7. Siscovick DS et al: The incidence of primary cardiac arrest during vigorous exercise, N Engl J Med 311:874-877, 1984.
8. Duncan, JJ et al: The effects of aerobic exercise on plasma catecholamines and blood pressure in patients with mild essential hypertension, JAMA 254:2609-2613, 1985.
9. Nelson, L et al: Effect of changing levels of physical activity on blood pressure and hemodynamics in essential hypertension, Lancet 8491:473-476, 1986.
10. Crews, DJ and Landers, DM, A meta-analytic review of aerobic fitness and reactivity to social stressors, Med Sci Sports Exercise, 19, supplement: 5114-5119, 1987.
11. Howard, JH et al: Physical activity as a moderator of life events and somatic complaints: a longitudinal study, Can J Appl Sports Sc 9:194-201, 1984.
12. Brooks GA and Fahey TD: Exercise physiology, New York, 1984, John Wiley & Sons.
13. Cureton KJ et al: Muscle hypertrophy in men and women, Med Sci Sports Exercise, 20:338-344, 1988.
14. Buckley, WE, et al: Estimated prevalance of anabolic steroid use among male high school seniors, JAMA 260:3441-3445, 1988.
15. Fleck SJ and Kraemer WJ: Resistance training: physiological responses and adaptations, Physician Sportsmedicine 16:63-76, 1988.
16. Fleck SJ and Kraemer WJ: Resistance training: basic principles (part 1 of 4), Physician Sportsmedicine 16(3):160-171, March, 1988.
17. Strong body, strong heart, The Johns Hopkins Medical Letter, 2(4): 1-2, June, 1990.
18. Pollock ML: Wilmore JH, and Fox SM: Exercise in health and disease, Philadelphia: W.B. Saunders Company, 1984.
19. Nieman DC: Fitness and sports medicine: an introduction, Palo Alto, Cal, 1990, Bull Publishing Company.
20. Arnheim D: Modern principles of athletic training, St. Louis, 1989, Times Mirror/Mosby College Publishing.
21. Davis AJ et al: A comparison of heart rate methods for predicting endurance training intensity, Med Sci Sports 7:295-298, 1975.
22. Riggs BL and Melton LJ III: Involutional osteoporosis, N Engl J Med 314:1676-1685, 1986.
23. Johnston CC and Slemeda C: Osteoporosis: an overview, Physician Sportsmedicine, 15:64-68, 1987.
24. Low back pain, Mayo Clinic Health Letter 7:4 Feb, 1989.
25. Mayer, TG, et al: A prospective two-year trial of functional restoration in testing industrial low back injuries JAMA 258:1763-1767, 1987.
26. Golding LA, Myers CA, and Snining WE: The Ys way to physical fitness, Champaign, Ill, 1989, Human Kinetics, Publishers, Inc.
27. Williams PC: Low back and neck pain: causes and conservative treatment, Springfield, Ill, 1974, Charles C Thomas Publishers.
28. McKenzie RA: The Lumbar spine, mechanical diagnosis and pain, Waikkanae, New Zealand, 1981, Spinal Publications.
29. Moskowitz RW: Primary osteoarthritis: epidemiology, clinical aspects, and general management, Am J Med 83:5-10, 1987.
30. Lane NE et al: Aging, long-distance running and the development of musculoskeletal disability, JAMA 82:772-780, 1987.
31. Lane NE et al: Long distance running, bone density and osteoarthritis, JAMA 255:1147-1151, 1986.
32. Felson DT: Obesity and knee osteoarthritis. The Framingham study, Ann Intern Med 109:18-24, 1988.

33. Panush RS et al: Is running associated with degenerative joint disease? JAMA 255:1152-1154, 1986.

34. Pascale M and Grana WA: Does running cause osteoarthritis? Physician Sportsmedicine 17:147-154, 1989.

35. Paffenbarger RS et al: A natural history of athleticism and cardiovascular health, JAMA 252:491-495, 1984.

36. Gerhardsson M et al: Sedentary jobs and colon cancer, Am J Epidemiol 123:775-779, 1986.

37. Vena JE et al: Occupational exercise and risk of cancer, Am J Clin Nutr 45:318-327, 1987.

38. Simopoulous AP: Obesity and carcinogenesis: historical perspective, Am J Clin Nutr 45:271-276, 1987.

39. Fauthier MM: Can exercise reduce the risk of cancer? Physician Sportsmedicine 14:170-178, 1986.

40. Noble HB and Bachman D: Medical aspects of distance race planning, Physician Sportsmedicine, 7(6):78-86, June, 1979.

Annotated Readings

Boosting good cholesterol, University of California, Berkeley Wellness Letter 6:1-2, October, 1989.
Discussion of the effect of exercise and diet over total serum cholesterol and the sub-fractions that are the components of total cholesterol.

The diet/exercise link: separating fact from fiction, Tufts University Diet and Nutrition Letter 6:3-6, February, 1989.
Presents many of the popular myths associated with diet and exercise and presents the facts as they are known today.

Hubbard RW and Armstrong LE: Hypertermia: new thoughts on an old problem, Physician Sportsmedicine 17:97-113, June, 1989.
Reviews the causes and treatment of the heat stress illnesses—heat cramps, heat exhaustion, and heat stroke. The effectiveness of cooling methods are discussed and guidelines for prevention are presented.

Lamb L (editor): About fast walking, The Health Letter 30:1-2, July 10, 1987.
Answers the questions: Which is best, walking or jogging? Discusses the benefits and advantages of walking. Also discusses guidelines for determining the intensity needed for significant benefits to occur when walking is the mode of exercise.

Lamb L (editor): Eat less and exercise to protect against cancer, The Health Letter 32:3, Oct. 7, 1988.
Discusses the effect of caloric intake on the development and growth of cancerous tumors. This article also discusses the research on the relationship of exercise and the formation and growth of cancerous tumors.

Zamula E: Back talk: advice for suffering spines, FDA Consumer, 23, No. 3: 28-35, April, 1989.
Discusses the anatomy of the spinal column, causes of back problems, treatment modalities, and prevention techniques.

ASSESSMENT ACTIVITY   6-1

The Rockport Fitness Walking Test

Directions: This walking test estimates aerobic capacity based upon the variables of age, sex, time required to walk one mile, and the heart rate achieved at the end of the test. The guidelines for taking the test are as follows:

1. Heart rate is counted for 15 seconds and multiplied by four to get beats per minute.

2. The course should be flat and measured, preferably a 440 yard track.

3. Be sure to use a stop watch or a watch with a second hand.

4. Warm up for 5 to 10 minutes prior to taking the test. Preparation for the test should include a one-quarter mile walk followed by the stretching exercises which appear later.

5. During the test, the walk should be a brisk pace and 1 mile should be covered as rapidly as possible.

6. Take your pulse rate immediately after the test. This rate should then be marked on the accompanying table that is appropriate for your age and sex.

7. Draw a vertical line through your time and a horizontal line through your heart rate. The point where the lines intersect will determine your fitness level (See Tables 6-7 to 6-16
   Rockport provides a series of 20 week walking for fitness programs that are based on the results of the walking test. These may be obtained for a nominal fee ($1.00 at this writing) by sending a request to Rockport Fitness Walking Test, 72 Howe St., Marlboro, Massachusetts, 01752.
   These charts are designed to tell you how fit you are compared to other individuals of your age and sex. For example, if your coordinates place you in the "above average" section of the chart, you are in better shape than the average person in your category.
   The charts are based on weights of 170 lbs. for men and 125 lbs. for women. If you weigh substantially more, your relative cardiovascular fitness level will be slightly overestimated. If you weigh substantially less, your relative cardiovascular fitness level will be slightly underestimated.

▎ **TABLE 6-7 20-29 year-old males relative fitness level**	▎ **TABLE 6-8 30-38 year-old males relative fitness level**

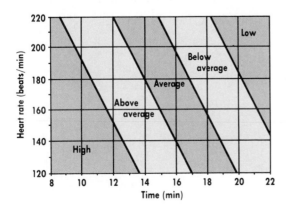

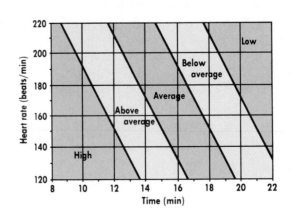

TABLE 6-9 40-49 year-old males relative fitness level

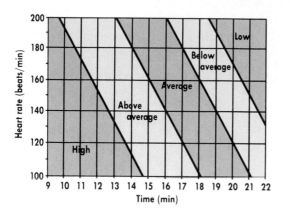

TABLE 6-10 50-59 year-old males relative fitness level

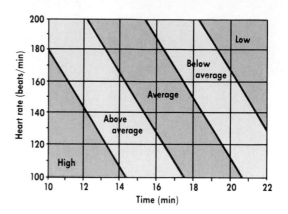

TABLE 6-11 60+ year-old males relative fitness level

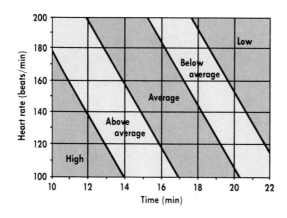

TABLE 6-12 20-29 year-old females relative fitness level

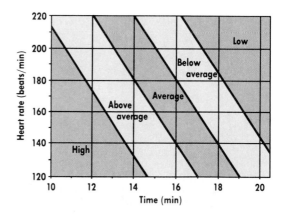

TABLE 6-13 30-39 year-old females relative fitness level

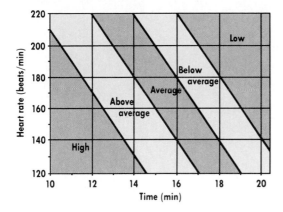

TABLE 6-14 40-49 year-old females relative fitness level

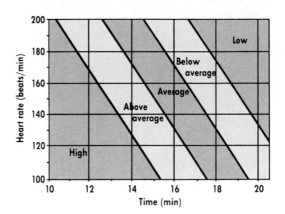

TABLE 6-15 50-59 year-old females relative fitness level

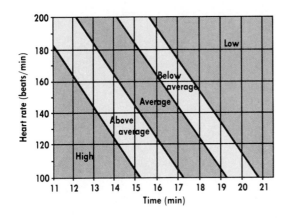

TABLE 6-16 60+ year-old females relative fitness level

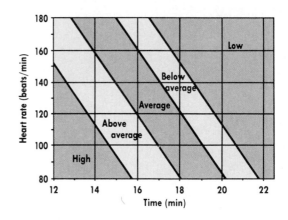

ASSESSMENT ACTIVITY   6-2

Calculating Your Target Heart Rate

Directions: Using the Karvonen Method of calculating heart rate described on p. 161, fill in the blanks below.

THR = target heart rate
MHR = maximum heart rate
RHR = resting heart rate (taken just upon waking in the morning)
TI%-training intensity

1. 220 − _____=_____
         (your age)   (your MHR)

2. THR = (MHR − RHR) × TI% + RHR

   THR = (_____ −_____) × _____+_____
         (your MHR) (your RHR)   (your desired TI%) (your RHR)

   THR = _____× _____+_____
       (your MHR − your RHR) (desired IT%) (your RHR)

   THR =_____ beats/minute

ASSESSMENT ACTIVITY   6-3

Design An Exercise Program

Directions: Design an exercise program for a 20-year old male who wishes to: (1) lose 25 lbs., (2) develop greater strength, and (3) develop cardiorespiratory endurance.

1. Suggested activities:

2. Suggested frequency of exercise:

3. Suggested intensity of exercise:

4. Suggested duration of exercise:

5. Place the activity in the weekly calendar below with the suggested amount of time devoted to each activity (place activities and time spent in minutes in the boxes below):

Sunday	Monday	Tuesday	Wednesday	Thursday	Friday	Saturday

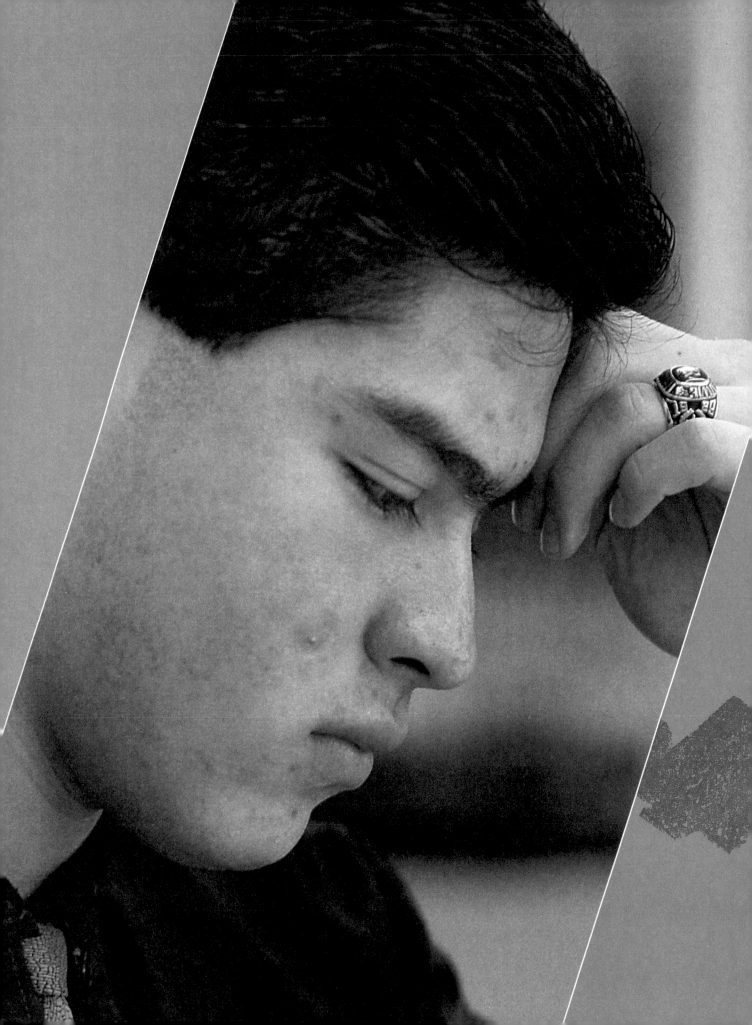

Chapter 7

Coping With and Managing Stress

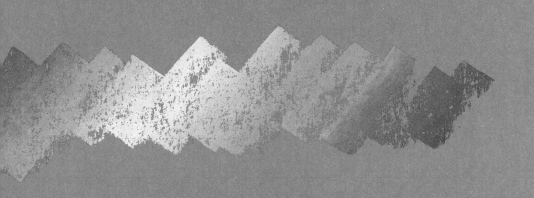

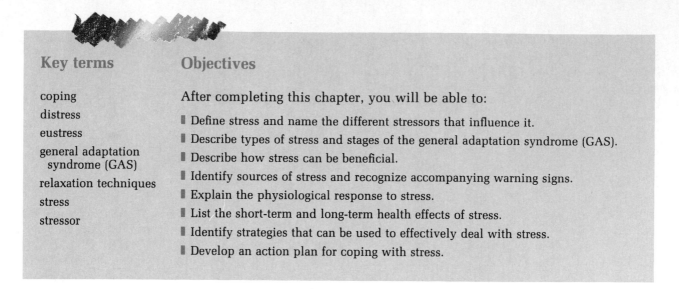

Key terms

coping

distress

eustress

general adaptation
syndrome (GAS)

relaxation techniques

stress

stressor

Objectives

After completing this chapter, you will be able to:

▌ Define stress and name the different stressors that influence it.

▌ Describe types of stress and stages of the general adaptation syndrome (GAS).

▌ Describe how stress can be beneficial.

▌ Identify sources of stress and recognize accompanying warning signs.

▌ Explain the physiological response to stress.

▌ List the short-term and long-term health effects of stress.

▌ Identify strategies that can be used to effectively deal with stress.

▌ Develop an action plan for coping with stress.

Very few topics are currently being delved into more by the media than stress. From *Reader's Digest* and *Cosmopolitan* to more serious journals, it is recognized that **stress** profoundly affects people's lives. Everyone lives with stress each day of his or her life—whether as a student, business person, parent, or athlete. Few days pass that a colleague or acquaintance does not remark negatively about the stress he or she is experiencing. This is because stress is frequently viewed as the adversary against which one must continually battle. This is a misconception. Stress is neither positive nor negative. How people deal with or react to what they perceive as stress is what determines its effect on their lives. As Dr. Bernie Siegal has stated, "It is often said that stress is one of the most destructive elements in people's daily lives, but that is only a half truth. The way we react to stress appears to be more important than the stress itself."[1] It is the *effects* of stress that can be either positive or negative. Positively used, stress can be a motivator for an improved quality of life. If viewed negatively, stress can become detrimental to health and destructive to the development of high-level wellness.

What is Stress?

Dr. Hans Selye was the first to define the term *stress* as the "nonspecific response of the body to any demands made upon it." Stress may be characterized by such diverse reactions as muscle tension, acute anxiety, increased heart rate, hypertension, shallow breathing, giddiness, and even joy. From a positive perspective, stress is a force that generates and initiates action. Using Selye's definition, it becomes apparent that stress

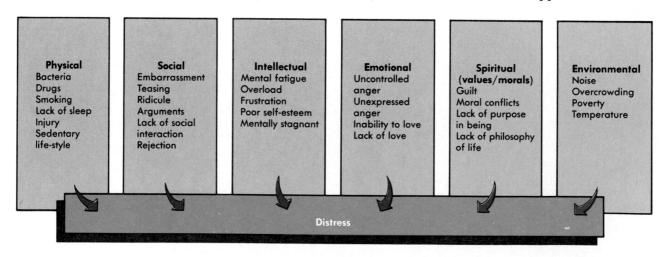

Figure 7-1 Stressors that can create distress.

can accompany pleasant or unpleasant events. Selye referred to stress judged as "good" as **eustress.** This form of stress is the force that serves to initiate emotional and psychological growth. Eustress provides the experience of pleasure, adds "specialness" to life, and fosters an attitude that tries to find positive solutions to even complex problems. Eustress can accompany a birth, graduation, getting a new car, making a new friend, accomplishing a difficult task, or succeeding in an area that has previously produced anxiety. **Distress,** on the other hand, is stress that results in negative responses. Unchecked, negative stress can interfere with the physiological and psychological functioning of the body and ultimately may result in disease or disability.[2]

Stress also provides humans with the ability to respond to challenges or dangers. Since it is both impossible and undesirable to live in an environment so totally sheltered that stress does not occur, stress cannot be avoided. It is vital to self-protection and serves as a motivator that enhances human ability.

A **stressor** is any physical, psychological, or environmental event or condition that initiates the stress response (Figure 7-1 gives some examples of typical negative stressors.) What is considered a stressor for one person may not be a stressor for another. Speaking in front of a group may be stimulating for one person and misery for another. Sky diving may be viewed as relaxing for one and terrifying for another. Some people may view taking a test as "just another event" while others experience extreme test anxiety. Fortunately, the stress response is not a genetic trait, and, since it is a response to external conditions, it is subject to personal control. It is easy to avoid sky diving if an individual has no desire to participate. Avoiding taking a test may not be so easy, but techniques and precautions can be used to lessen the effect of the stress on the person involved. For example, knowing the material thoroughly and engaging in deep breathing several minutes before a test will help dissipate anxiety.

To maximize quality of life, people *can* find positive ways of coping with stress that are effective for them.

The concept that the stress response can serve to enhance and actually increase the level of performance, be it a mental or physical, is referred to as the inverted-U, theory.[3] Whether a person is taking a test or giving a gymnastic performance, too little stress may result in a poorer effort while too much stress can inhibit effort. There appears to be an optimal level of stress that results in peak performance. Figure 7-2 depicts this concept. Exactly what is an appropriate level of stress seems to depend on the particular individual and the type of task to be accomplished. Stress can have a positive effect on an individual. Table 7-1 lists some of the potentially positive outcomes associated with stress.

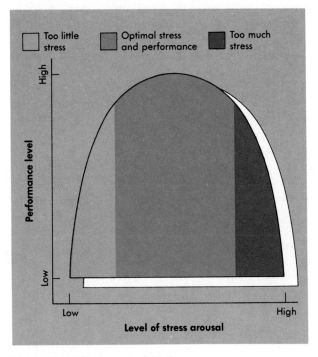

Figure 7-2 The inverted-U theory.

TABLE 7-1 Positive potential of a stress challenge

Mental	Emotional	Physical
Enhanced creativity	Sense of control	High energy level
Enhanced thinking ability	Responsiveness to environment	Increased stamina
Greater goal orientation	Improved interpersonal relationships	Flexibility of muscles and joints
Enhanced motivation	Improved morale	Freedom from stress-related disease

General Adaptation Syndrome

Our bodies are constantly attempting to maintain a physiological balance. This balance is referred to as *homeostasis*. Any event or circumstance that causes a disruption (a stressor) in the body's homeostasis requires some type of adaptive behavior. Physiologically, whether a stressor is conceived of as positive or negative, the body responds with the same three-stage process. This series of changes is known as the **general adaptation syndrome (GAS).**[4] The three phases are alarm, resistance, and exhaustion (Figure 7-3).

The *alarm* phase occurs when homeostasis is initially disrupted. The brain perceives a stressor and prepares the body to deal with it, a response sometimes referred to as the *"fight-or-flight" syndrome*. The subconscious appraisal of the stressor results in an emotional reaction. The emotional response stimulates a physical reaction that is associated with stress, such as the muscles becoming tense, the stomach tightening, the heart rate increasing, the mouth becoming dry, and/or the palms of the hands becoming sweaty.

The second stage is *resistance*. In this phase the body meets the perceived challenge through increased strength, endurance, sensory capacities, and sensory acuity. Hormonal secretions regulate the body's response to a stressor. Only after meeting and satisfying the demands of a stressful situation can the internal activities of the body return to normal. Girdano and Everly[5] state that individuals have different levels of energy storehoused to deal with stressors. In dealing with short-term stressors, only a superficial level of energy is required, allowing deeper energy levels to be protected. Superficial levels of energy are readily accessible and easily renewable. Unfortunately, all stress cannot be resolved with superficial energy levels. When long-term or deep levels of stress are experienced, the amount of energy available is limited. If sufficient stress is experienced for an extended period, loss of adaptation can result. While some scientists believe

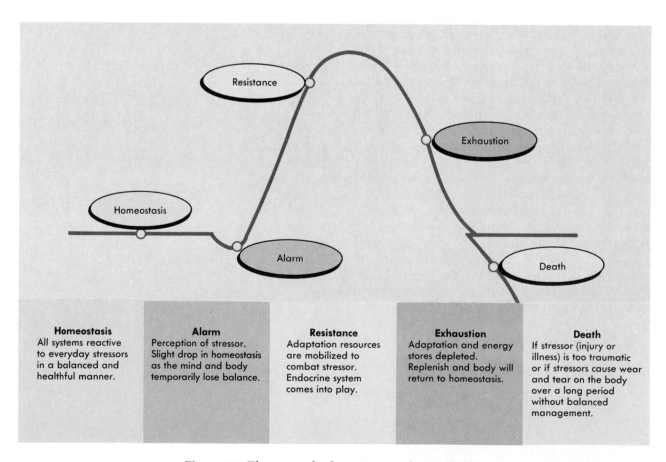

Figure 7-3 The general adaptation syndrome (GAS).

that energy stores may be genetically programmed, all people are capable of replenishing their storehouse through exercise, good nutrition, adequate sleep, and other positive lifestyle behaviors.

When chronic stressors become sufficiently long range or pervasive, the third phase, *exhaustion,* is reached. In exhaustion, energy stores have been depleted and rest must occur. While it may take anywhere from weeks to years before the effects of long-term stressors take their toll, if a person does not learn how to adequately deal with stress, exhaustion will occur. At this point, stress may affect the stomach, heart, blood pressure, muscles, and joints. Fortunately, the effects of stressors can be completely or partially reversed when adequate management techniques are initiated. The earlier these management techniques are learned and used, the fewer adverse problems will be experienced.

Sources of Stress and Warning Signs

Most stressful situations fall into one of three categories. They include (1) harm-and-loss, (2) threat, or (3) challenge.[6] Examples of *harm-and-loss situations* are the death of a loved one, loss of personal property, physical assault, physical injury, or severe loss of self-esteem. *Threat situa-* tions may be real or may be perceived as menacing and can range from being caught in traffic to being unable to understand an event. Threatening events tax a person's ability to deal with everyday life. Threat stressors are any stressors that result in anger, hostility, frustration, or depression. *Challenge situations* are those that are perceived as catalysts for either growth or pain. Often, these stressors involve major life changes and include such events as taking a new job, leaving home, graduating from college, or getting married. Challenge events are usually perceived as being good, but involve stress because they disrupt homeostasis and require considerable psychological/physical adjustment.

Being aware of the mental and physical signals associated with stress is the beginning step in learning how to manage it. Assessment activity 7-1 will aid you in identifying some of the major stressors. By continually using self-assessment to monitor for signs of stress, needless consequences of excessive stress can be avoided. The negative results of distress are shown in Table 7-2. Some indicators of excessive distress include:

1. Chronic fatigue, migraine headaches, sweating, low backaches, sleep disturbances, weakness, dizziness, diarrhea, or constipation.
2. Working or studying harder and/or longer

▌ TABLE 7-2 Negative results of distress

Mental	Physical	Emotional
Short-term effects		
Poor memory	Flushed face	Irritability
Inability to concentrate	Cold hands	Disorganization
Low creativity	Gas	Conflicts
Poor self-control	Rapid breathing	Mood swings
Low self-esteem	Shortness of breath	Chronic sleep problems
	Dry mouth	Acid stomach
		Overindulgence in alcohol, drugs, food
Long-term effects		
Bouts of depression	Hypertension	Overweight/underweight
Mild paranoia	Coronary disease	Drug abuse
Low tolerance for ambiguity	Ulcers	Excessive smoking
Forgetfulness	Migraine/tension headaches	Ineffective use of work/leisure
Inability to make decisions/quick to make decisions	Strokes	Over-reaction to mild work pressure
	Allergies	

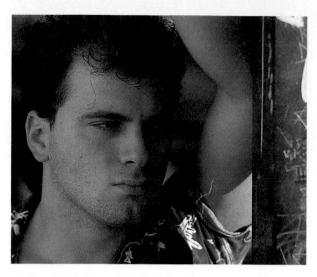

Recognizing the symptoms of excessive stress is the first step in effectively dealing with it.

but accomplishing less; an inability to concentrate; general disorientation.

3. Denying that there is a problem or troubling event.
4. Increased incidence of illness, such as colds, flu, and so on, or constant worry about illness or becoming ill; over-use of over-the-counter drugs for the purpose of self-medication.
5. Feeling depressed, irritable, anxious, apathetic, or experiencing an overwhelming urge to cry or run and hide; feelings of unreality.
6. Excessive behavior patterns, such as spending too much money, drinking, breaking the law, and addiction.
7. Accident proneness.
8. Becoming reclusive and avoiding other people.
9. Emotional tension, feeling "keyed up," being easily startled, engaging in nervous laughter, experiencing anxiety, hyperkinesia, or developing nervous tics.

Physiological Responses to Stress

Stress abounds in every aspect of life. Stress is experienced as the result of happy as well as unhappy events. However, regardless of the nature of a stressor, each time a stressful event occurs, a whole series of neurological and hormonal messages are sent throughout the body. Figure 7-4 gives a simplified version of the physiological responses to stress.

The nervous system serves as a reciprocal network that sends messages back and forth between the awareness centers of the brain and the organs and muscles of the body. Part of this system is referred to as the *limbic system*. The limbic system contains centers for emotions, memory, learning relay, and hormone production, and includes the pituitary gland, thalamus, and hypothalamus.

When a stressor is encountered, the body sends a message to the brain via the nervous system. The brain then synthesizes the message and determines if it is valid or not. If a message is not verified by the brain as being particularly threatening, the limbic system over-rides the initial response and "tells" the body to continue to function normally. If the initial response is translated as accurate, the body responds with some emotion (fear, joy, terror), and the hypothalamus begins to act.

When a stressor is perceived, the *hypothalamus* sends a hormonal message to the pituitary gland. It then releases a hormone *(ACTH)* that helps signal other glands in the endocrine system to secrete additional hormones, the primary one being *cortisol*, which provides fuel to respond with the "fight-or-flight" reaction.

Through another hormonal message the adrenal cortex increases blood pressure to facilitate the transportation of food and oxygen to the active parts of the body. Blood volume is augmented through a decrease in urine production and an increase in sodium retention, causing less fluid to be eliminated from the body. Systolic blood pressure may rise 15 to 20 mm Hg because of the presence of aldosterone.

The hypothalamus also sends a message to release the hormones *epinephrine* and *norepinephrine* that initiate a variety of physiological changes. These changes include increased heart rate, increased metabolic rate, increased oxygen consumption, increased force in the pumping of the blood from the heart, and the release of other hormones called *endorphins*, which decrease sensations of pain.

The *autonomic nervous system* is responsible for a second major set of physiological responses. In reaction to a threat, the autonomic nervous system increases heart rate, the strength of the skeletal muscles, mental activity, and basal metabolic rate; dilates the coronary arteries, pupils, bronchial tubes, and arterioles; and constricts the abdominal arteries. This same system then works to return the body to a normal, relaxed state.

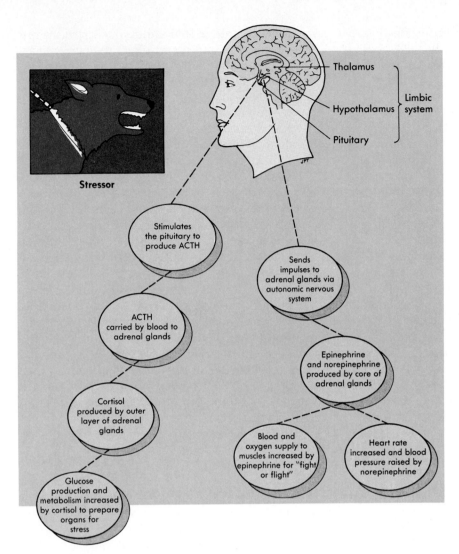

Figure 7-4 The physiological response to stress.

Health Effects of Stress

The mind and body act on each other in remarkable ways. Recent research has indicated that nerves connect the thymus and spleen directly to the hypothalamus and that white blood cells respond directly to some of the same chemicals that transmit messages from one nerve cell to another. What this means is that the immune system is in direct contact with and under at least partial control of the part of the brain that is physiologically reactive to emotions. Thus there may be a biological link between emotions and disease and even death. Mortality is three times higher in individuals with few close relationships, while people with strong support groups have additional protection against life stressors. Death rates are higher for cancer patients with pessimistic attitudes. Illness is more common among people who feel locked into strife-ridden marriages. Conversely, AIDS patients with hearty

psyches seem better able to withstand the ravages of their disease.[7]

The effects of any stressful situation take their toll on the human body. Some researchers have indicated they consider stress to be a primary enemy of overall health and a major contributor to disease. Since stress affects the immune system, the body becomes more susceptible to a multitude of ailments, from colds to cancer. Respiratory conditions such as asthma may become worse. The cardiovascular system reacts by causing the blood vessels to constrict while increasing blood volume. The net result is a rise in blood pressure that occurs over and over throughout a stress-ridden day. Multiple increases in blood pressure can eventually contribute to chronic high blood pressure. More forceful contraction of the heart elevates levels of free fatty acids, enhancing the development of clogged arteries leading to and including the heart itself. In extreme cases, sudden death can occur, especially if an individual has been experiencing high levels of uncontrolled stress for an extended period of time.

Headaches, including migraines, have long been associated with stress. Tension headaches are caused by involuntary contractions of the scalp, head, and neck muscles. Typical muscular reaction to stress is contracting or tensing. When chronic stress occurs, the body reacts by being constantly ready to respond and the muscles become *braced,* or always in a state of tension. When always braced, any more or different stress only magnifies the tension the muscles are already undergoing. Increased muscular tension manifests itself in headaches, backaches, neck aches, and other pains. The smooth muscles that control internal organs also experience bracing pains. More and more intense contractions can lead to stomachache, diarrhea, hypertension, heartburn, gastritis, diarrhea, bloating, inflammation of the pancreas, and blockage of the bile ducts.

Under the effects of stress, saliva in the mouth decreases, often making speaking awkward. Swallowing may become difficult and increases in stomach acids contribute to ulcer pain. People tend to perspire more and electrical currents are transmitted more quickly across the skin. Skin conditions such as acne, psoriasis, herpes, hives, and ecxema are exacerbated.

Stress also seems to effect the body's nutritional status and immune response to disease. Individual nutritional patterns can also influence stress management efforts. For example, eating too much or too little, eating the wrong kinds of food, and overuse of products such as caffeine or alcohol all upset homeostasis. Diets high in fat, simple carbohydrates (sugar), or processed foods place a heavy burden on various body systems, such as the cardiovascular or gastrointestinal. However, taking in too few calories can lead to breakdown of lean tissue to meet the nutritional demands of the body for normal functioning. In order to best meet the demands of stress, adequate nutrition should be maintained through a balanced and varied diet. Chapter 3 provides guidelines for developing a beneficial nutritional plan. Figure 7-5 provides some insight into the interactive nature of stress, nutritional status, and immunity.

Ultimately, no body system escapes the ef-

 Figure 7-5 Stress, nutritional status, and immunity: an interactive effect

Although the mechanism is not completely understood at this time, stress significantly effects nutritional status and, thereby, immunity. Several nutritional factors have implications for how our bodies respond to stress.*

- **Energy:** Stress can increase the body's basic caloric needs by as much as 200 %. The stress hormones increase body heat production. When this heat is released, it is not available for cell metabolism. The caloric inefficiency induced by stress accounts for the increased need for energy intake.
- **Protein:** Stress may increase the body's need for protein from 60 % to as much as 500 %. The integrity of the body's tissues, such as the skin and the tissue lining the mouth, lungs, and nose (called mucosal tissue) depend on adequate protein repair and maintenance of secretions of biochemicals that serve as protective agents. The formation of antibodies also requires protein.
- **Fats:** Dietary fatty acids influence the synthesis of a group of fatty acid derivatives called *prostaglandins.* Prostaglandins stimulate or depress other cellular and immune functions in relationship to stress.
- **Vitamins:** Vitamin A functions to maintain healthy skin and mucus membranes. Individuals who are vitamin A–deficient have fewer mucus-secreting cells and those they do have produce less mucus—thus the protection provided by the mucus lining is diminished. Vitamin C has been shown to enhance the engulfing or "eating" actions of the immune cells called *macrophages.* If vitamin C is deficient, macrophages are less mobile and less able to consume disease-causing organisms. Deficiencies of vitamins A, B_{12}, and folate can impair production of the cells that enable antibody responses. Large doses of vitamin E have been associated with suppression of B cells, which are vital to the immune response. Finally, metabolic requirements for thiamin, riboflavin, and niacin are increased in response to a stressful situation.
- **Minerals:** Deficiencies of zinc impair immune cell reproduction and responsiveness.

fects of stress. Long-term presence of certain stress-associated hormones in the brain damages receptors and cells found in the hippocampus (the hippocampus sends messages when stress is occurring). Since brain cells do not regenerate, these cells become lost forever. While it is currently unknown what kind of effect this loss will have, indications are that eventually humans become less able to respond to stress appropriately.[8] Assessment activity 7-2 provides guidelines for identifying stress style and provides suggested relaxation activities for each style.

Self-Esteem and Stress

How people feel about themselves and others and their perceptions of the stressors in their lives are all part of the psychology of stress. Ability to cope with stress often hinges on impressions of how detrimental a stressor is and how adequately resources can be mustered to deal with the situation(s). How much stress people view themselves as experiencing is also closely associated with their own sense of self-esteem. Self-esteem includes beliefs and attitudes about changes, beliefs about personal talent and skills, and the ability to deal with the changes and challenges that inevitably occur in life. Self-esteem is also the basis of self-efficacy and the locus of control. (See Chapter 1.) In fact, the single most influential factor in determining response to stress may be people's perceptions of themselves. This is because people bestow their own sense of self-efficacy, locus of control, and self-worth on themselves.

Personality and Stress

Two physicians, Friedman and Roseman,[9] have written extensively concerning personality, cardiovascular disease, and stress. These researchers have described two stress-related personality types—type A and type B. Most people are neither type exclusively but fall somewhere along a continuum between the two.

Type A personality is characterized by an urgent sense of time, impatience, competitiveness, aggressiveness, insecurity over status, and inability to relax. People with type A behavior characteristics are likely to be highly stressed. Type B people have a more laid back and unhurried approach to their lives. The type B personality does not become as upset at losing or not attaining a goal. Type Bs also tend to set more realistic goals.[10] Researchers have disagreed, however,

over whether there is a possible relationship between the stress-prone type A personality and cardiovascular disease.[11] Several studies have reported a correlation of type A behavior and cardiovascular disease, while other research literature has reported little association. There is a general feeling among researchers that being a type A personality is not a problem if there is no underlying hostility. However, regardless of whether type A individuals are more susceptible to heart disease or not, they will experience more negative effects, such as tiredness and frustration, from short-term stress. It has been suggested that some type A people are actually more resilient to stress and use their type A behaviors and traits to better resist stress. These people have been labeled "type C" and seem to channel their energies into creative endeavors without suffering the effects of high stress.

It has been generalized that "stress survivors"—people who have been found to handle stress successfully or to have successful coping abilities—have several common characteristics. Psychologist Suzanne Kobasa[12] has isolated these attributes and given a label to the type person

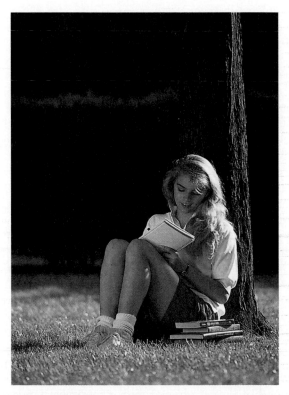

Taking control of one's life is the most important aspect of coping with stress.

who exhibits them. A *hardy personality* tends to remain healthy even under extreme stress. Characteristics of a hardy personality or *hardiness* are challenge, commitment, and control (see Assessment Activity 7-3).

Challenge is the ability to see change for what it is—not only inevitable, but an opportunity for growth and development of unique individual abilities. *Commitment* is delineated by a strong sense of inner purpose. It is necessary to *want* to succeed if success is to be achieved. Commitment is the ability to become really involved, while maintaining the discernment to know when dedication and desire are becoming harmful. *Control*, the last aspect, is exhibited by the recognition that each person has power over his or her own life and attitudes. People who have a sense of control *act* in situations rather than *react* to them. These people make their own decisions rather than let circumstances dictate those decisions for them. It is part of the attitude of making lemons into lemonade.

Coping with Stress

All events in life precipitate a reaction. How people react or respond to situations is uniquely individual. **Coping** is the term used to refer to effort(s) made to manage or deal with stress. Coping is independent of outcome—it does not mean that an individual will experience success. Coping successfully with stress may require using a variety of techniques (Figure 7-6). Since stress-related responses are based primarily on mental perceptions, developing coping strategies that achieve desirable results may need to originate with a change in attitude or outlook. If specific situations or people are perceived as disruptive, one solution is to avoid the situation or person. It is frequently possible to change job positions, to not date a particular person, or to minimize contact with a neighbor one does not like.

While there are no *easy* answers and certainly very few perfect ones to life's problems, there is always some kind of answer or solution. There may be times when dealing with a stressor reaches an impasse—where it seems as if there are no solutions, yet the tension resulting from the situation is becoming increasingly detrimental. Then it may become necessary to consider changing attitudes, goals, and/or values. When an ideology or outlook on life becomes unlivable, something must change and sometimes it needs to be the way a person thinks. This is probably

Figure 7-6 Guidelines for dealing with stress

Some guidelines for effectively dealing with potentially harmful stress are:

■ **Schedule time effectively:** Practice good time management techniques by using time wisely. This means taking time out for yourself everyday and scheduling work when you are usually at peak ability (see Assessment Activity 7-5).

■ **Set priorities:** It is necessary to know what is important to *you*. Don't attempt to work on four or five projects simultaneously. Keep efforts focused on one or two major items.

■ **Establish realistic goals:** While it is good to aim high, goals must also be achievable. Don't establish impossible expectations and then become frustrated when they are not accomplished as quickly as you would like. Write down long-range goals and then establish bench marks as checks for keeping you on track and monitoring progress. Short-term goals help you see how you are moving toward your goal and provide rewards as you advance toward success.

■ See yourself as achieving the goals: Visualize yourself as being successful. Go over in your mind what it will look and feel like to accomplish the goal.

■ Give yourself a break—Take time every day to exercise and relax.

the most difficult form of coping—when it seems the only way to cope is to change. If a long-held belief is creating stress, then it may be time to alter that belief somewhat, or even replace it with a belief or attitude or behavior that better promotes a sense of peace and personal harmony. It is frequently beneficial to seek the help of a professional counselor when attempting to resolve particularly stressful situations. Assessment Activity 7-4 provides ways to recognize some of the positive and negative behaviors that can be used to deal with stress.

Learning about and using relaxation techniques can help alleviate or even prevent detrimental effects associated with stress. Engaging in

Figure 7-7 Michelle's day—approaching stress

Event	Michelle's stress response	A better approach
7:00 AM. Late rising for first class. Stayed up late studying the night before.	Skips first class to study for exam. Misses notes from that class and cannot contact friend to see if she can use her notes. Skips breakfast.	Begin studying for a test a few days before the exam. Don't attempt to cram everything into one night. Get a good night's rest and get up early to review notes. Eat breakfast and attend first class.
Late for test.	Stays home too long and gets caught in traffic. Walks in late for the test. Doesn't have a full hour to complete the test.	Leave early to allow for traffic and parking problems. Be on time so can concentrate on test and have time to relax a few minutes.
Lunch.	Skips lunch—has a soft drink and potato chips.	Have a nutritionally balanced meal in a relaxing atmosphere. Go with friend to just chat.
Afternoon. Late for work because had to return library book.	Rushed to library. Forgot to return overdue book. Upset that had to pay fine. Had to stand in line 15 minutes at the library.	Write down when books are due and return on time. Use a daily calendar to plan activities and allot time to take care of personal business.
Evening. Watches TV until midnight. Neglects to study for test the day after tomorrow.	Too tired and "stressed out" to study so just watches TV all evening. Has a hamburger and coke for dinner.	Take a short nap after work and have a nutritious meal. Plan the evening so that some time is spent watching TV and some is spent studying. Go to bed early so can get to school on time and rested.
Next morning. Gets up late for class again.	Begins the same cycle of feeling tired and pressured and being late.	Analyze current time constraints to determine where more time needs to be alloted and how to develop a more efficient plan (see Assessment Activity 7-4).

positive self-talk and relabelling negative experiences—for example, viewing difficulties as "challenges" rather than as problems—are positive steps in reducing stress-related disorders. Eating well, taking time to enjoy life, laughing, exercising, living in the present, and "taking time to smell the flowers along the way" all serve to reduce stress. Stress can be handled effectively when individuals work on developing all their abilities to the fullest, when they develop a lifestyle that is compatible with personal values, and when they develop realistic expectations for themselves. Working toward these goals is how a wellness lifestyle is established (Figure 7-7).

The origin of successful coping is being aware of incidents and situations that are perceived as being stressful. Recognition of stressors includes awareness of how one's body responds to stress. Recognition requires continuous monitoring of the body and mind for evidence of excessive stress.

Successful coping does not "just happen." It is the outcome of real effort on the part of an individual. Assistance in successful coping may lie in the development of the quality of hardiness. Kobasa[12] has three suggestions to encourage the growth of this characteristic. One suggestion is to focus on the signals the body is sending when experiencing stress and then to think back to the event or situation that might have triggered those

...gs. Another suggestion is to recreate a re-
...event that has been stressful. After visualiz-
ing the episode, write down six ways that the
outcome could have been different—three with a
worse outcome and three with a better outcome.
It is important to recognize that things could
have been worse! At the same time, it is wise to
increase awareness of how to better handle similar situations in the future. A last suggestion is to
try something new. This can be anything a person has ever wanted to do but has never done
and can range from taking a cooking class to
changing professions. The idea is to be challenged and then to meet that challenge successfully. Trying something new and meeting the
challenge reinforces the sense of being able to
deal with life successfully.

Optimal health requires the ability to cope
with stress positively so that physical symptoms
or illness do not occur. The next section contains
techniques that should prove helpful in reducing
and coping with stress.

Relaxation Techniques

The ultimate goal in stress coping and management is to reduce the negative effects associated with stress. Different **relaxation techniques**
have proved successful and should be used based
on individual preference. A brief description of
various techniques follows:

Deep breathing. Deep breathing is the most
basic technique used for initiating a relaxation
response (a physiological change that favorably
alters body functioning), and is often the foundation for other methods. The primary benefit is
that deep breathing can be done anywhere and at
any time. It is beneficial to practice deep breathing several times a day. The methodology consists of completely filling the lungs when breathing so that the abdomen expands outward. Begin
by taking in a deep breath and then exhaling
slowly through the mouth. When inhaling think
to yourself "I am" and think "relaxed" while
slowly exhaling. A hand can be placed on the
stomach to assure that it is fully expanded. If the
stomach does not rise, the breath is not deep
enough or the abdomen is being held too tightly.
Repeat this cycle several times and then rest qui-
etly for 3 to 5 minutes.

Progressive muscle relaxation. The purpose
of progressive muscle relaxation is to create
awareness of the difference between muscular
tension and a relaxed state. Progressive muscle

relaxation is a three-step process that begins by
tensing a muscle group and noticing how the tension feels. Next, a conscious effort is made to relax the tension and experience that feeling. The
third phase consists of concentrating on the differences between the two sensations. Beginning
at either the head and working down or at the
feet and working up, all major muscle groups
should be tensed and relaxed.

Autogenics. Autogenics uses self-suggestion
to produce a relaxation response. Autogenics begins with a deep breath and a conscious effort to
relax. This technique may follow a progression
from head to feet or feet to head, as does progressive muscle relaxation, but it also uses a phrase
such as "my arm feels heavy and warm" repeated
several times before moving on to the next muscle group. Other phrases that carry a message of
calming, such as "I am completely calm and relaxed," can be used and repeated over and over.
The session can be ended by silently stating "I
am refreshed and alert." Autogenics takes practice, time, and commitment in order to achieve
the relaxation response and should be practiced
twice a day for about 10 minutes. Commercial
tapes are available that are very beneficial.

Meditation. Meditation can be approached
from a variety of perspectives. As a stress-reduction technique its purpose is to temporarily tune
out the world and invoke the "relaxation response." Meditation was first introduced to this
country on a wide scale as transcendental meditation (TM) in the 1960s. With TM, each medita-
tor is given a *mantra* (a particular word or sound
to be used while meditating). During a meditation session the person meditating concentrates
on that word or sound and attempts to eliminate
all outside distractions. The mantra is to be kept
secret to enhance attentiveness. Meditation as a
method of stress reduction uses the same pre-
cepts. Begin by taking a comfortable position on
a couch or in a chair. Several deep breaths
should be taken, slowly inhaling and exhaling.
The eyes may be shut or softly focused on an object so that the details are blurred. All thoughts
should be concentrated on a word or phrase,
such as "one" or "the Lord is my shepherd,"
"peace" or any other appropriate phrase while
continuing to breathe slowly and deeply in and
out.[13] The relaxation response can also be initiated by using the same format and then counting
breaths backward from 100 or by imagining a
white light that slowly travels throughout the
body, literally letting in light and energy while

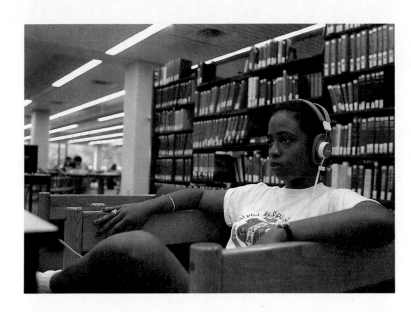

Visualization, progressive muscle relaxation, and meditation are excellent techniques to help reduce stress.

expelling tension and fear. Many commercial tapes are available that are excellent and last from 10 to 30 minutes.

Visualization. Visualization (imagery) is a form of relaxation that makes use of the imagination. Visualization begins when a person finds a comfortable position, shuts the eyes, and takes several deep breaths. Several variations of visualization can then be used. Individuals can imagine a tranquil scene, such as a beach on a sunny day or a valley with a stream or walking through a forest, and then place themselves in the scene. All the sights, sounds, smells, and feelings can be imagined that would be encountered in that situation. People suffering from a terminal illness frequently imagine scenes such as their immune system attacking or destroying or eliminating the disease or they envision themselves as healthy and disease-free with surprisingly good results. Individuals who want to make major life changes, such as losing a lot of weight or stopping smoking can envision themselves very slim or not smoking or "see" themselves in situations that create trouble for them and then plan what to do to avoid eating or smoking in that situation. A person experiencing pain from a disastrous love affair can envision his or her heart as being strong and healthy and pain-free. Visualization can also be used to improve athletic performance. Tapes are available that can assist in learning how to develop this technique.

Biofeedback. Biofeedback is based on scientific principles and is designed to enhance awareness of body functions. Sensory equipment is used to demonstrate subtle body changes such as increases or decreases in skin temperature, muscle contraction, and brain wave variations. Biofeedback enables people, through the use of the sensory equipment, to become aware of muscle tensions and then learn how to control those tensions through awareness of the sensations that are associated with relaxing. Biofeedback is to be considered an educational tool. After a few sessions, people should begin to recognize, and thereby alter, their typical bodily responses to those things that serve as stressors for them.

Music. Quiet music soothes by causing people to breathe more deeply, still turbulent emotions, reduce metabolic response, and calm the autonomic nervous system.

Humor. Laughter is a powerful stress-reducing agent. A deep laugh temporarily raises pulse rate, blood pressure, and tenses the muscles. After a good laugh, however, pulse rate and blood pressure actually go down and the muscles become more relaxed. Laughter works in two ways. Being able to laugh at a situation stimulates an appreciation for the fact that life is seldom perfect or predictable. Laughing helps keep things in perspective. Laughing also works to reinforce a positive attitude. Laughing, or even smiling, can actually alter a mood for the better.

Time management. A major contributor to stress is the pressure associated with time constraints. By effectively managing time, a great deal of stress can be eliminated. Procrastination can add to stress and undermine school work, personal relationships, and work efforts. Assessment Activity 7-5 provides a log to help manage

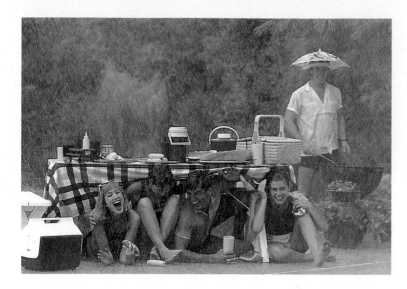

Laughter is an excellent way to reduce stress.

time more effectively. Depending on individual needs, some suggestions are:

1. Set realistic goals and priorities. These goals and priorities should be written down. Current activities should be assessed as to whether they are essential, important, or trivial. The emphasis should be placed on the first two.

2. Write down the priorities for the next day before going to sleep each night and rank order them. This provides a night to "sleep on them." They should then be approached systematically, according to need.

3. Ask for help if responsibilities become overwhelming. It is all right to say "no" when there are too many tasks to handle. Guilt over saying no only adds more stress.

4. Take a break. Every day should provide for fun, leisure, time alone, and/or relaxation. Each day is only lived once and it is important to make the most of every one.

Exercise. Since the "fight-or-flight" syndrome is there to get the body moving, exercise is a logical method of moving in response to that command. Stress is physical and causes the secretion of hormones such as epinephrine that remaining in the system in significant amounts, can create adverse effects. Physical work helps dissipate some of these effects as well as the free-floating anxiety that is a natural by-product of daily life. When a situation or person produces a particularly stressful response, exercise can be instrumental as a time to make decisions about how best to deal with it. Exercise helps clear the mind and can provide necessary "alone time" that is so difficult to find in a busy world.

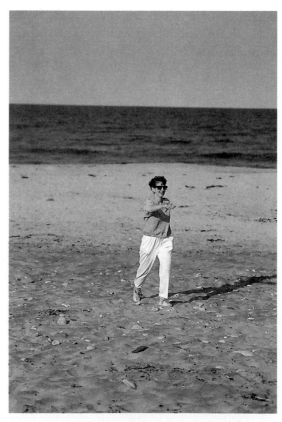

Exercise provides an effective way to cope with stress.

Summary

▌ Stress is the nonspecific response of the body to any demands made on it.

▌ Anything that creates stress is referred to as a stressor. Stressors may take the form of eustress (good) or distress (bad).

▌ The general adaptation syndrome (GAS) explains how the body responds to a stressor. The three stages are alarm, resistance, and exhaustion.

▌ The stress response can serve to enhance physical and mental performance.

▌ Whether positive or negative, each time a stressful event occurs, a whole series of neurological and hormonal messages are sent throughout the body.

▌ People's perceptions of stress are associated with self-esteem, self-efficacy, and locus of control.

▌ People who deal effectively with stress seem to exhibit hardiness in their personality. Hardiness consists of a sense of challenge (viewing stressful situations as opportunities for growth), commitment (a sense of inner purpose), and control (power over one's own life).

▌ Coping is used to refer to the effort(s) made to manage or deal with stress.

▌ There are many techniques that can help to reduce stress. They include autogenics, deep breathing, visualization, muscle relaxation, meditation, massage, biofeedback, exercise, yoga, music, and humor.

 Action plan for personal wellness

An important consideration in assuming responsibility for one's own quality of life is using information. After reading this chapter, answer the following questions and determine an action plan for enhancing your own lifestyle.

1 Based on the information presented in this chapter, along with what I know about my family's health history, the health problems/issues that I need to be most concerned about are_____

_____

_____

2 Of those health concerns listed in no. 1, the one I most need to act on is_____

_____

_____

3 Possible actions (try to be as specific as possible) that I can take to improve my level of wellness are_____

_____

_____

4 Of those actions listed in no. 3, the one that I most need to include in an action plan is_____

_____

_____

5 Factors I need to keep in mind in order to be successful in my action plan are_____

_____

_____

Review Questions

1. What is stress? What are stressors?
2. What are the stages the mind and body go through when exposed to a stressor?
3. What are some potential signals that a person is experiencing chronic stress and what are the possible effects?
4. What factors influence how an individual perceives and copes with stress?
5. Define *hardiness* and how it may help an individual effectively deal with stress.
6. What are some guidelines for handling stress positively?
7. Discuss the various stress-reduction techniques.

References

1. Siegal BS: Love, medicine and miracles, New York, 1988, Perinnial Library.
2. Selye H: Stress without distress, New York, 1975, New American Library, pp 28-29.
3. Hanson PG: The joy of stress, Kansas City, Kan, 1986, Andrews, McMeel & Parker.
4. Selye H: The stress of life, rev ed, New York, 1978, McGraw-Hill Inc.
5. Girdano D and George E Jr: Controlling stress and tension, Englewood Cliffs, NJ, 1986, Prentice Hall, p 57.
6. Folkman S: Personal control and stress and coping processes: a theoretical analysis, J Pers Soc Psychol 46:839-852, 1984.
7. Gelman D and Hager M: Body and soul, Newsweek, Nov 7, 1988, pp 88-97.
8. Greenberg J: Stress management, Dubuque, Iowa, 1987, Wm C Brown Group.
9. Friedman M and Roseman R: Type A behavior and your heart, New York, 1984, Alfred A Knopf Inc, pp 193-207.
10. Flannery RB: Toward stress-resistant persons: a stress management approach to the treatment of anxiety, Am J Prevent Med 3(1):25-30, 1987.
11. Fischman J: Type A on trial, Psychology Today 21(2):42-64, 1987.
12. Kobasa S: How much stress can you survive? American Health 5(7):64-77, 1984.
13. Benson H: The relaxation response, New York, 1985, A Berkley Book.

Annotated Readings

Gallagher W: The healing touch, American Health, Oct 1988, pp 45-53.

The writer introduces the concept of "bodywork." These are techniques that change how people can experience their own bodies and, perhaps, their minds.

Goldman D: "What's your stress style?" American Health, April 1986, pp 41-45.

Most experts agree that there is tremendous variability in the way individuals respond to stress. Consequently, it is important that a stress management program be personalized.

Maranto G: Emotions: how they affect your body, Current, Feb 1985, pp 34-41.

New research findings suggest that short bouts with stress may actually help in resisting the negative effects. The critical factor seems to be how the individual perceives a stressor rather than the actual stress itself.

Squires S: Visions to boost immunity, American Health, July 1987, pp 56-61.

The author discusses the relationship between emotional states and the immune system. The field of research is termed psychoneuroimmunology. Clinical findings indicate that imagery may serve as treatment for disease by involving the immune system.

Tierney J: The heartbeat of America, Hippocrates, Jan/Feb 1989, pp 34-36.

A humorous look at things commonly considered stressors and the way they effect blood pressure.

ASSESSMENT ACTIVITY 7-1

Stressors of Life

The stress scale below represents an adaptation of Holmes and Rahe's Life Event Scale. It has been modified to apply to college-age adults and should be considered a rough indication of stress levels and health consequences for teaching purposes.

Directions: To determine your stress score, add up the number of points corresponding to the events you have experienced in the past 12 months.

1. Death of a close family member	100	17. Increase in workload at school	✓ 37
2. Death of a close friend	73	18. Outstanding personal achievement	36
3. Divorce between parents	65	19. First quarter/semester in college	36
4. Jail term	63	20. Change in living conditions	✓ 31
5. Major personal injury or illness	63	21. Serious argument with instructor	30
6. Marriage	58	22. Lower grades than expected	✓ 29
7. Firing from a job	50	23. Change in sleeping habits	29
8. Failure of an important course	47	24. Change in social activities	29
9. Change in health of family member	45	25. Change in eating habits	28
10. Pregnancy	45	26. Chronic car trouble	26
11. Sex problems	44	27. Change in the number of family get	
12. Serious argument with close friend	40	togethers	26
13. Change in financial status	39	28. Too many missed classes	25
14. Change of major	39	29. Change of college	24
15. Trouble with parents	39	30. Dropping of more than one class	23
16. New girl or boyfriend	37	31. Minor traffic violations	20
			Total ____

Here's how to interpret your score. If your score is 300 or higher, you are at high risk for developing a health problem. If your score is between 150 and 300, you have a 50/50 chance of experiencing a serious health change within 2 years. If your score is below 150, you have a one in three chance of a serious health change. Use of effective stress reduction techniques can reduce the chances of experiencing a serious health change.

Stress Style: Body, Mind, Mixed?

Directions: Imagine yourself in a stressful situation. When you are feeling anxious, what sensations do you typically experience? Check all that apply.

_____ 1. My heart beats faster.
_____ 2. I find it difficult to concentrate because of distracting thoughts.
_____ 3. I worry too much about things that don't really matter.
_____ 4. I feel jittery.
_____ 5. I get diarrhea.
_____ 6. I imagine terrifying scenes.
_____ 7. I can't keep anxiety-provoking pictures and images out of my mind.
_____ 8. My stomach gets tense.
_____ 9. I pace up and down nervously.
_____10. I am bothered by unimportant thoughts running through my mind.
_____11. I become immobilized.
_____12. I feel I am losing out on things because I can't make decisions fast enough.
_____13. I perspire.
_____14. I can't stop thinking worrisome thoughts.

There are three basic ways of reacting to stress—primarily physical, mental, or mixed. Physical stress types feel tension in the body—jitters, butterflies, the sweats. Mental types experience stress mainly in the mind—worries and preoccupying thoughts. Mixed types react with both responses in about equal measure.

Give yourself a Mind point if you answered "yes" to each of the following questions: 2, 3, 6, 7, 10, 12, 14. Give yourself a Body point for each of these: 1, 4, 5, 8, 9, 11, 13. If you have more Mind than Body points, consider yourself a mental stress type. If you have more Body than Mind points, your stress style is physical. About the same number of each? You're a mixed reactor.

Choosing a Relaxer

Body: If stress registers mainly in your body you will need a remedy that will break up the physical tension pattern. This may be a vigorous body workout but a slow-paced, even lazy, muscle relaxer may be equally effective. Here are some suggestions to get you started:

Aerobics	Progressive relaxation
Swimming	Body scan
Biking	Rowing
Walking	Yoga
Massage	Soaking in a hot bath, sauna

Mind: If you experience stress as an invasion of worrisome thoughts, the most direct intervention is anything that will engage your mind completely and redirect it—meditation, for example. On the other hand, some people find the sheer exertion of heavy physical exercise unhooks the mind wonderfully and is very fine therapy. Suggestions:

Meditation	Autogenic suggestion
Reading	Crossword puzzles
TV, movies	Games like chess or cards
Any absorbing hobby	Vigorous exercise
Knitting, sewing, carpentry, or other handicrafts	

Mind/Body: If you are a mixed type, you may want to try a physical activity that also demands mental rigor:

Competitive sports (racquetball, tennis, squash, volleyball, etc.)
Meditation
Any combination from the Mind and Body Lists

ASSESSMENT ACTIVITY   7-3

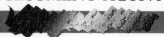

How Hardy Are You?

Directions: Below are twelve items similar to those that appear on a hardiness questionnaire. Really evaluating an individual's hardiness requires more than one quick test, but this simple exercise can be a good indication of your own "hardiness." Write down how much you agree or disagree with the following statements, using this scale:

0 = Strongly disagree
1 = Mildly disagree
2 = Mildly agree
3 = Strongly agree

_____A. Trying my best at work makes a difference.
_____B. Trusting to fate is sometimes all I can do in a relationship.
_____C. I often wake up eager to start on the day's projects.
_____D. Thinking of myself as a free person leads to great frustration and difficulty.
_____E. I would be willing to sacrifice financial security in my work if something really challenging came along.
_____F. It bothers me when I have to deviate from the routine or schedule I have set for myself.
_____G. An average citizen can have an impact on politics.
_____H. Without the right breaks, it is hard to be successful in my field.
_____I. I know why I am doing what I'm doing at work.
_____J. Getting close to people puts me at risk of being obligated to them.
_____K. Encountering new situations is an important priority in my life.
_____L. I really don't mind when I have nothing to do.

To score yourself:

These questions measure control, commitment, and challenge. For half the questions, a high score (agreement) indicates hardiness; for the other half, a low score (disagreement) does.

To get your scores on control, commitment, and challenge, first write in the number of your answer—0, 1, 2, or 3—above the letter of each question on the score sheet. Then add and subtract as shown. (To get your score on control, for example, add your answers to questions A and G; add your answers to B and H; and then subtract the second number from the first.)

Add your scores on commitment, control, and challenge together to get a score for total hardiness. A total score of **10-18 = hardy personality; 0-9 = moderate hardiness; below 0 = low hardiness.**

_____ + _____ = _____   _____ + _____ = _____   _____ + _____ = _____
(A)   (G)   (C)   (I)   (E)   (K)
                       −   −   −
_____ + _____ = _____   _____ + _____ = _____   _____ + _____ = _____
(B)   (H)   (D)   (J)   (F)   (L)
Control score = _____   Commitment = _____   Challenge score = _____
                _____ + _____ + _____ = _____
                Control   Commitment   Challenge   Total hardiness score

Paths to hardiness

Three techniques are suggested to help become happier, healthier, and hardier. They are:

Focusing: Recognize signals from the body that something is wrong. Focusing increases the sense of control over plans and puts individuals in a psychologically better position to change.

Reconstructing stressful situations: Think about a stress episode and then write down three ways the situation could have gone better and three ways it could have gone worse. Doing this helps to recognize that things could have been worse and, even more important, that there are better ways to cope.

Compensating through self-improvement: It is important to distinguish between what can be controlled and what cannot. A way to regain control is by taking on a new challenge or task to master.

ASSESSMENT ACTIVITY 7-4

Identification of Coping Styles

Directions: There are a variety of ways and methodologies to help us deal with stress. Consider each of the activities below and determine if you are currently using any of them to deal with stress.

	Often	Rarely	Not at all
Listen to music			
Go shopping with a friend			
Watch television/go to a movie			
Read a newspaper, magazine, or a book			
Sit alone in peaceful outdoors			
Write prose or poetry			
Attend athletic event, play, lecture, symphony, etc.			
Go for a walk or drive			
Exercise (swim, bike, jog)			
Get deeply involved in some other activity			
Play with a pet			
Take a nap			
Get outdoors, enjoy nature			
Write in journal			
Practice deep breathing, meditation, autogenics, muscle relaxation			
Straighten up desk or work area			
Take a bath or shower			
Do physical labor—garden, paint			
Make home repairs, refinish furniture			
Buy something—records, books			
Play a game (chess, backgammon, games, video games)			
Pray, go to church			
Discuss situations with spouse or close friend			
Others (list)			
_____			
_____			
_____			

Continued.

206   Wellness

Directions: Below is a list of negative coping behaviors. Mark them according to how much you currently use them.

	Often	Rarely	Not at all
Become aggressive			
Use negative self-talk			
Yell at spouse/kids/friends			
Drink a lot of coffee or tea			
Get drunk			
Swear			
Take a tranquilizing drug			
Avoid social contact with others			
Try to anticipate the worst possible outcome			
Think about the possibility of suicide			
Smoke tobacco			
Chew fingernails			
Overeat, undereat			
Become irritable, short tempered			
Cry excessively			
Kick something, throw something			
Drive fast in car			
Others (list)			
_____			
_____			
_____			

Scoring instructions: Count the number of positive and negative coping techniques you use.

Number of negative techniques:_____
Number of positive techniques:_____
How often do you employ negative coping strategies?
Do you use more positive than negative strategies or is it the reverse?
Do you recognize a need to change some of the techniques you are now using? If so, which ones?
What are some ways in which you can maximize your positive coping behaviors? How can you minimize your negative ones?

ASSESSMENT ACTIVITY   7-5

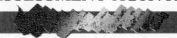

Analyzing My Use of Time

Managing your time effectively and efficiently can significantly contribute to the feelings of control you have over your life. A by-product of this sensation of control is reduced stress and tension as you are able to meet daily demands with less effort. Since the basis of change is recognizing that there needs to be a change and then determining the areas in your life that need change, a good place to begin with time management needs is by analyzing how you are currently managing your time.

Directions: Make several copies of this log and keep track of your time for a week. Include all your activities—from classess to meals to driving time to conversations with friends. At the end of the day and week, rate each hour as to how important the activities that occurred during that time were. Taking time to relax, talk to friends, and be alone are considered important to total well-being and should not be discounted.

Daily log

Time	Activities	Where	Essential, important, or trivial
6-7:00 AM			
7-8:00			
8-9:00			
9-10:00			
10-11:00			
11-12:00			
12-1:00 PM			
1-2:00			
2-3:00			
3-4:00			
4-5:00			
5-6:00			
6-7:00			
7-8:00			
8-9:00			
9-10:00			
10-11:00			
11:00 PM-6:00 AM			

Analyzing your log

1. Which activities did you find to be the most productive for you? Which were the least?
2. Where were your most productive activities performed? Your unproductive activities?
3. What time of day did you find to be the most productive for you—morning, afternoon, or evening?

   The analysis should be based on the full week's activities. You are looking for patterns of behavior that provide the best effects for you. You may find that you work best at home or in the dormitory in the afternoons or at the library in the evenings. Using this assessment, try to find the best patterns of achievement for you.

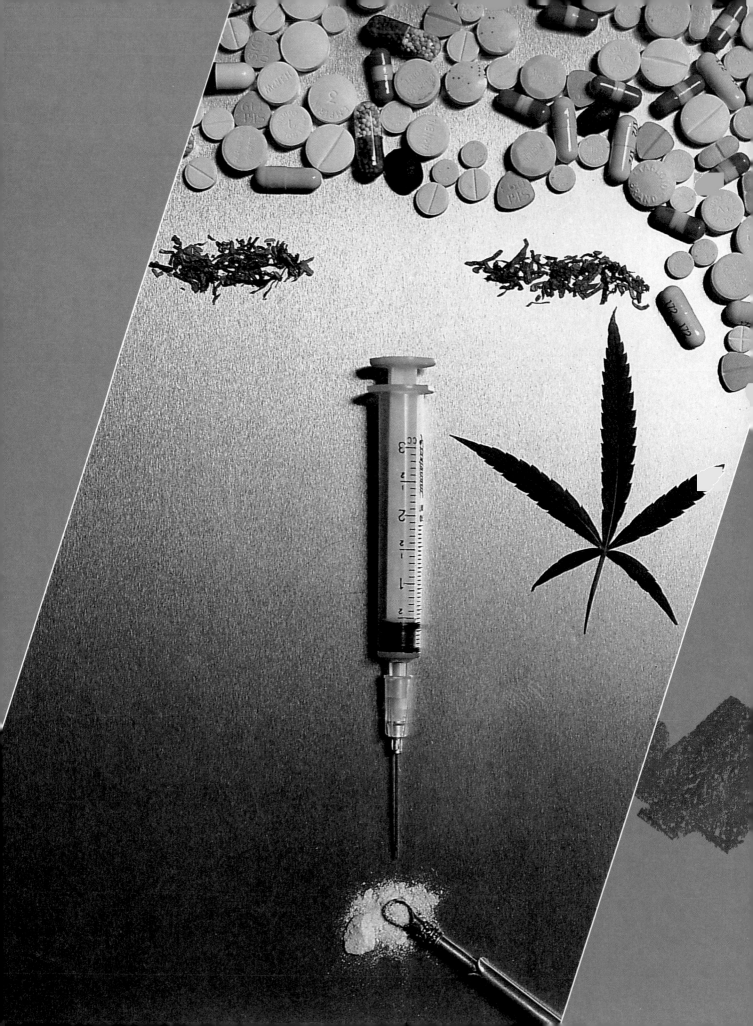

Chapter 8

Assuming Responsibility for Substance Use

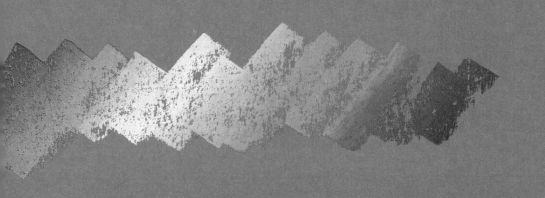

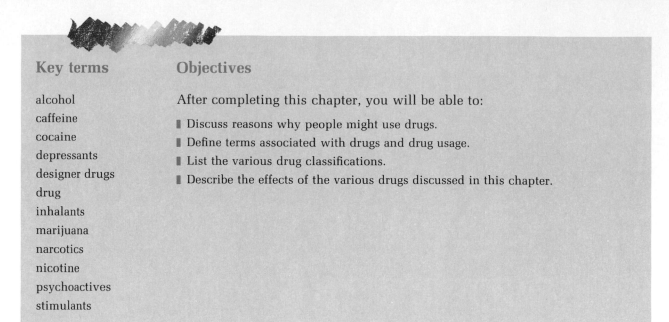

Quality of life is not necessarily concerned with doing "right" or "wrong" or being "good" or "bad." The ultimate determinant of quality of life is the decisions made by each person that affect his or her life positively or negatively. To have a high quality of life means to make intelligent choices that contribute to physical, mental, emotional, and spiritual well-being. Accurate information and recognition of the consequences of actions are necessary to make the best possible choices. The decisions individuals make are cumulative. As time goes on and aging occurs, consequences of previous actions, habits, and modes of behavior increasingly affect how the body functions. The emphasis of this book has been on personal behaviors such as exercising, weight maintenance, proper nutrition, and the prevention of cardiovascular disease. However, there are other vital areas that influence quality of life. This chapter deals with the subject of drugs. Drug use or nonuse has the potential to impact strongly on health and quality of life. For example, when a drug is used for treatment, cure, prevention, or relief of pain it is categorized as *medicine*. Many people are alive because of the therapeutic effect of drugs in preventing disease and maintaining health. It is quite clear that there are many drugs that constitute medicine but that not all drugs are used as medicines. When usage involves reasons other than medicine, even if that behavior is considered "recreational" the potential still exists for tragic consequences.

Reasons for Drug Use

A **drug** is a chemical substance that has the potential to alter the structure and functioning of a living organism. (Other terms that may be important to understanding drugs can be found in Figure 8-1.) People use drugs for a variety of reasons. Some individuals need drugs to maintain a normal life or to alleviate specific symptoms, while others indulge in drugs to alter their moods. Researchers have identified several reasons why people might use drugs.[1] They are:

1. **Recreational/social facilitation:** People frequently use drugs they feel will lessen the tension associated with social encounters. Marijuana and alcohol are particularly popular in social situations. Potential dangers in using drugs for this purpose include mental dependency on the drug and an inability to cope with social events without using the drug.

2. **Sensation-seeking:** Some people enjoy taking risks. For them, drugs fulfill the need for excitement and adventure. Others turn to drugs out of boredom or sense of inadequacy in their life. They are seeking sensations of pleasure that are artificially induced. Unfortunately, they frequently turn to increasingly dangerous drugs or to increased doses to provide equivalent or more exciting thrills.

3. **Religious/spiritual factors:** Throughout history, collectively and individually, people have used drugs in an attempt to enhance their spirituality or become more godlike. Too

Figure 8-1 Understanding drug terminology

Listed below are some terms that may be unfamiliar. These terms are useful in understanding the effects of substances.

Antagonistic: Opposing or counteracting.

Designer drugs: Illegally manufactured psychoactive drugs that are similar to controlled drugs on the FDA's schedule.

Drug abuse: The excessive and pathological use of a drug that has dangerous side effects.

Drug misuse: The use of a drug for purposes other than for what it is intended.

Effective dose: The amount that produces the desired effect.

Lethal dose: The amount capable of causing death.

Medicines: Drugs used to prevent illness or to treat symptoms of an illness.

Over-the-counter drugs (OTC): A nonprescription drug.

Physical dependence: A physiological need for a drug.

Polyabuse: The use of multiple drugs.

Potentiating: An exaggerated drug response obtained when two drugs are taken together; a much greater effect is obtained than when either drug is taken separately.

Prescription drugs: Drugs obtained only by order of a physician or dentist.

Psychoactive: Affecting mood and/or behavior.

Psychological dependence: An emotional or mental need to use a drug.

Synergistic: A combined effect that is greater than the sum of the individual effects when two or more drugs are used at the same time. The combination produces an exaggerated effect or a prolonged drug action.

Toxic dose: The amount that produces a poisonous effect.

often the drug becomes the object of worship rather than the god or spiritual essence being sought. Though many have tried, the spiritual realm has not yet been achieved through mind-altering drugs.

4. **Altered states:** Drugs are used to increase the intensity of a mood or create a state of euphoria. Some have attempted to enhance physical performance or stimulate artistic creativity.

Evidence indicates that perceptions of improvement are erroneous.

5. **Rebellion and alienation:** The use of drugs can be a deliberate act of rebellion against social values, especially the values of one's parents. Individuals who experience extreme pressures and are having difficulty coping frequently turn to drugs as an escape mechanism. This includes college-age students facing academic pressure and increased personal freedom for the first time.

6. **Peer pressure and group entry:** People who have a great desire or need to feel accepted will often use drugs to demonstrate their sameness with other members in the group. Feeling accepted, modeling behavior after someone who is admired, and attempting to create an identity or specific image are all reasons offered for engaging in drug use. Self-esteem seems to be a vital component. Individuals with high self-esteem see themselves as competent, successful, self-sufficient, accepting, outgoing, and well rounded. People with low self-esteem tend to feel isolated and unloved and lack the capacity for joy or self-fulfillment. It is in the attempt to magically overcome these sensations/perceptions that many people turn to drugs.

All the reasons why any individual uses drugs are usually not easily categorized. Most

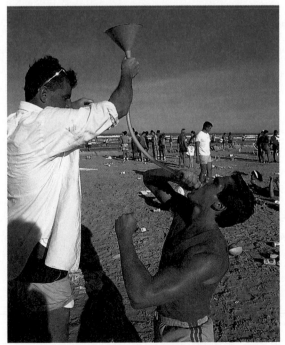

People use drugs for a variety of reasons, including rebellion, peer pressure, and sensation seeking.

TABLE 8-1 Commonly used substances

Type	Name	Appearance	How used?
Stimulants			
Amphetamines	Speed, uppers, ups, black beauties, pep pills, co-pilots, bumblebees, hearts, benzedrine, dexedrine, footballs, biphetamine	Capsules; pills; tablets	Taken orally; injected; inhaled through nasal passages
Cocaine	Coke, snow, flake, white, blow, nose candy, big C, snowbirds, lady	White crystalline powder, often diluted with other ingredients	Inhaled through nasal passages; injected; smoked
Crack cocaine	Crack, freebase rocks, rock	Light brown or beige pellets or crystalline rocks that resemble coagulated soap; often packaged in small vials	Smoked
Methamphetamines	Crank, crystal meth, crystal, methedrine, speed, ice	White powder; pills; a rock that resembles a block of paraffin	Taken orally; injected; inhaled through nasal passages
Additional stimulants	Ritalin, Cylert, Preludin, Didrex, Prestate, Voranil, Tenuate, Tepanil, Pondimin, Sandrex, Plegine, Ionamin	Pills; capsules; tablets	Taken orally; injected
Depressants			
Barbiturates	Downers, barbs, blue devils, red devils, yellow jacket, yellows, Nembutal, Secanol amytal, Tuinals	Red, yellow, blue, or red and blue capsules	Taken orally; injected
Methaqualone	Quaaludes, ludes, sopors	Tablets	Taken orally
Tranquilizers	Valium, librium, equanil, miltown, serax, Tranxene	Tablets; capsules	Taken orally
Psychoactives			
Lysergic acid diethylamide	LSD, acid, green or red, dragon, white lightning, blue heaven, sugar cubes, microdot	Brightly colored tablets; impregnated blotter paper; thin squares of gelatin; clear liquid	Taken orally; licked off paper; gelatin and liquid can be put in the eyes
Mescaline and peyote	Mesc, buttons, cactus	Hard brown discs; tablets; capsules; tablets and capsules	Discs can be swallowed, chewed, or smoked; taken orally
Phencyclidine	PCP, angel dust, loveboat, lovely, hog, killer weed	Liquid; capsules; white crystalline powder; pills	Taken orally; injected; smoked—can be sprayed on cigarettes, parsley, and marijuana
Psilocybin	Magic mushrooms, mushrooms	Fried or dried mushrooms	Chewed and swallowed
Narcotics			
Codeine	Empirin compound with codeine, Tylenol with codeine, codeine, codeine in cough medicines	Dark liquid varying in thickness; capsules; tablets	Taken orally; injected

Continued.

Type	Name	Appearance	How used?
Heroin	Smack, horse, brown sugar, junk, mud, big H, black tar	Powder, white to dark brown; tarlike substance	Injected; inhaled through nasal passages; smoked
Meperidine	Pethidine, Demerol, Mepergan	White powder; solution; tablets	Taken orally; injected
Methadone	Dolophine, Methadose, Amidone	Solution	Taken orally; injected
Morphine	Pectoral syrup, hypodermic tablets	White crystals; injectable solutions	Injected; taken orally; smoked
Opium	Paregoric, Dover's powder, Parepectolin	Dark brown chunks; powder	Smoked; eaten
Other narcotics	Percocet, Percodan, Tussionex, Fentanyl, Darvon, Talwin, Lomotil	Tablets; capsules; liquid	Taken orally; injected
Inhalants			
Amyl nitrite	Poppers, snappers	Clear or yellowish liquid in ampules	Vapors inhaled
Butyl nitrite	Rush, bolt, locker room, bullet, climax	Packaged in small bottles	Vapors inhaled
Chlorohydrocarbons	Aerosol sprays	Aerosol paint cans; containers of cleaning fluid	Vapors inhaled
Hydrocarbons	Solvents	Cans of aerosol propellants, gasoline, glue, paint thinner	Vapors inhaled
Nitrous oxide	Laughing gas, whippets	Propellant for whipped cream in aerosol spray can; small 8-g metal cylinder sold with a balloon or pipe (buzz bomb)	Vapors inhaled
Marijuana			
Hashish	Hash	Brown or black cakes or balls	Eaten; smoked
Hashish oil	Hash oil	Concentrated syrupy liquid varying in color from clear to black	Smoked—mixed with tobacco
Marijuana	Pot, grass, weed, reefer, dope, Mary Jane, sinsemilla, Acapulco gold, Thai sticks	Parsley-like substance mixed with stems that may include seeds	Eaten; smoked
Tetrahydrocannabinol	THC	Soft gelatin capsules	Taken orally; smoked
Designer drugs			
Analogs of amphetamines and methamphetamines (hallucinogens)	MDMA (ecstasy, XTC, Adam, essence), MDM, STP, PMA, 2,5-DMA, TMA, DOM, DOB	White powder; tablets; capsules	Taken orally; inhaled through nasal passages
Analogs of fentanyl (narcotic)	Synthetic heroin, China white	White powder resembling heroin	Inhaled through nasal passages; injected
Analogs of phencyclidine (hallucinogens)	PCPy, PCE, (PCP) TCP	White powder	Taken orally; injected; smoked

drug use situations involve a combination of factors. These factors vary from person to person and depend on personality, experience, perceptions of the environment, and expectations.

Drug Classification

Drugs are commonly classified according to the physiological effect they have. Based on this concept drugs are categorized as stimulants, depressants, hallucinogens, narcotics, and inhalants. There are two additional drugs that are not part of the primary grouping above but are also important. First, designer drugs are those that mimic drugs found in the previously mentioned categories. The other drug, marijuana, is difficult to classify but is usually included as a hallucinogen. Depending on the dosage, marijuana can mimic a variety of substances found in other categories.

1. **Stimulants:** Stimulants speed up the central nervous system, producing an increase in alertness and excitability.
2. **Depressants:** Also known as sedatives and tranquilizers, depressants slow down the central nervous system, causing an individual to feel relaxed.
3. **Psychoactives:** Drugs referred to as psychoactives are capable of altering feelings, moods, and/or perceptions. Marijuana is classified as a psychoactive but can exhibit effects similar to those of stimulants, depressants, and narcotics.
4. **Narcotics:** Narcotics are powerful painkillers. They also produce pleasurable feelings and induce sleep.
5. **Inhalants:** Inhalants are volatile nondrugs that cause drug-like effects if inhaled. Substances may include glue or gasoline. Some, such as nitrous oxide or amyl nitrate, may have medical uses.
6. **Designer drugs:** A drug analog that has been manufactured in an illegal laboratory and mimics a controlled substance. Designer drugs are often more powerful and less predictable than the drugs they imitate. There is a rapid increase in the number and variations of designer drugs available, making it difficult to list all the varieties.

Commonly Abused Substances

This chapter is not intended to provide a comprehensive coverage of the various classifications of drugs, but it is important to recognize the potential damage that can be done if people choose to use these substances. This text will briefly examine caffeine, alcohol, nicotine, cocaine, marijuana, and designer drugs. There are, in addition, a variety of other substances that are potentially dangerous if misused or abused. The drugs examined in Table 8-1 seem to be currently most abused.

Caffeine

Caffeine is probably the most used drug in American society. Each day millions of Americans drink, chew, or ingest caffeine in some form. **Caffeine** is a stimulant that speeds the heart rate, temporarily increases blood pressure, and disrupts sleep. It also relieves drowsiness, helps in the performance of repetitive tasks, and improves work ability. Negatively, caffeine consumption can cause insomnia, anxiety, heart arrhythmias, gastrointestinal complaints, dizziness, and headaches.

At one time caffeine consumption was thought to cause birth defects, cardiovascular disease, cancer, and fibrocystic breast disease. Current research has found no substantial association.[2,3] However, it has been recommended that pregnant and nursing women consume no more than two cups of coffee a day and that tea and caffeine-containing soft drinks should be drunk in moderation.[3] A link between caffeine and birth defects or breastfeeding problems has never been established, but it is wise to take no unnecessary risks. Further, women who suffer from premenstrual tension (PMS) would be wise to eliminate caffeine. Research has indicated that women who drink a half to four cups of caffeinated tea a day were twice as likely to suffer PMS symptoms as women who drank none at all.[3]

It is easy to consume a great deal of caffeine during the course of a day. Table 8-2 contains the amounts of caffeine found in various products. Analyzing this table, it quickly becomes apparent that several hundred milligrams can be ingested rather quickly. Becoming familiar with the amount of caffeine in a product and restricting consumption to less than 400 mg of caffeine per day seems to be an appropriate and safe way to benefit from the effects of the drug without suffering any of the negative aspects.[4]

■ TABLE 8-2 Caffeine amounts in selected products (in milligrams)

Product	Range	Average	Product	Range	Average
Coffee (5 oz)			**Prescription drugs (per dose)**		
Brewed, drip method	60-180	115	Cafergot (for migraine head-ache)	100	—
Brewed, percolator	40-170	80			
Instant	30-120	65	Darvon compound (for pain)	32.4	—
Decaffeinated, brewed	2-5	—	**Nonprescription drugs**		
Tea (5 oz)			No Doz (alertness tablets)	100	—
Brewed, major US brands	20-90	40	Vivarin (alertness tablets)	200	—
Brewed, imported brands	25-110	60	Aqua-Ban (diuretic)	100	—
Iced (12 oz)	67-76	70	Aqua-Ban Plus	200	—
Instant	25-50	30	Anacin	32	—
			Excedrin	65	—
Soft drinks (12 oz)			Midol	32.4	—
Sugar-Free Mr. PIBB	58	—	Vanquish	33	—
Mountain Dew	54	—	Duradyne	15	—
Mello Yello	52	—	Coryban-D capsules	30	—
TAB	46	—	Triaminicin tablets	30	—
Coca-Cola (classic/new)	46	—	Duradyne	15	—
Diet Coke	46	—			
Shasta Cola	44	—	**Other**		
Shasta Cherry Cola	44	—	Cocoa (5 oz)	2-20	4
Shasta Diet Cola	44	—	Chocolate milk (8 oz)	2-7	5
Mr. PIBB	40.8	—	Milk chocolate (1 oz)	1-15	6
Dr. Pepper	40.8	—	Semi-sweet chocolate (1 oz)	5-35	26
Diet Dr. Pepper	40.8	—	Chocolate-flavored syrup (1 oz)	4	—
Pepsi-Cola	38.4	—			
Big Red	38	—			
Diet Pepsi	36	—			
RC Cola	36	—			
Cherry RC	36	—			
Canada Dry Jamaica Cola	30	—			
Canada Dry Diet Cola	1.5	—			

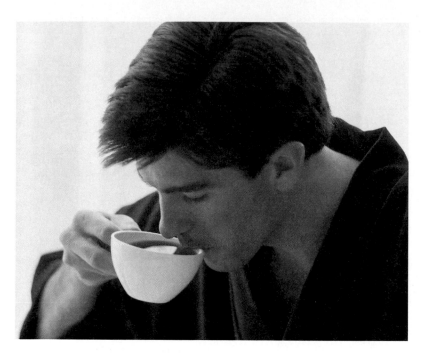

Caffeine is probably the most used drug in America.

Alcohol

The use of alcohol appears pervasive. **Alcohol** is a drug that is deemed socially acceptable by many, yet there is no other drug that causes so much physical, social, and emotional damage to individuals and families. People drink alcoholic beverages for a multitude of occasions. They drink among friends, to enhance a romantic mood, to put themselves at ease in social situations, to celebrate special occasions, when they are upset or depressed, because their role models drink, and because the advertising industry has convinced them that alcohol contributes to self-enhancement. Unfortunately, what is not mentioned is the devastation associated with alcohol. Table 8-3 contains a summary of the short-term and long-term effects of the drug. Since alcohol is one of those drugs that society has labelled appropriate and even necessary for some occasions, it may be unrealistic to expect abstinence for most people. If alcohol is to be used, the key is to use it responsibly. Figure 8-2 provides suggestions for responsible drinking.

Although there are several types of alcohol, the intoxicating agent in alcoholic drinks is *ethyl alcohol,* a colorless liquid with a sharp, burning taste. The percentage of alcohol in a beverage is measured by its *proof.* The proof is twice the percentage of alcohol. A beverage that is 40% alcohol has a proof of 80. The *blood alcohol concen-*

Figure 8-2 Responsible drinking

Following are suggestions to help each person be a responsible drinker and host.

- ❙ Drink slowly; never more than one drink per hour.
- ❙ Eat while drinking, but stay away from salty food.
- ❙ When mixing drinks, measure the amount of alcohol; never just pour.
- ❙ Serve and choose nonalcoholic drinks as an alternative.
- ❙ The host should always serve the guests or hire a bartender. It is never wise to have an open bar or serve someone who is intoxicated.
- ❙ Stop using or serving alcohol 1 hour before a party is over.
- ❙ Don't drink and drive. Have either a nondrinker drive the car or call a cab.

▮ TABLE 8-3 Short-term effects of alcohol use

Short-term or immediate effects

Blood alcohol concentration (BAC)	Effect(s)
0.00-0.05	Usually relaxed and euphoric; decreased alertness.
0.05-0.10	Exaggerated feelings and behavior; emotional instability; increased reaction time and diminished motor coordination; impaired driving; legally drunk in most states.
0.10-0.15	Lose peripheral vision; driving is extremely dangerous; unsteady when walking/standing.
0.15-0.30	Sensory perceptions significantly impaired; slurred speech; less sensitive to pain; difficult, staggering walk.
>0.30	Stupor or unconsciousness; anesthetized; death is possible at greater than 0.35.

Long-term effects

System/organ	Health risks
Breast	50% higher risk for cancer in women who drink any alcohol; 100% increase for women having three or more drinks per day.[4]
Cardiovascular	High blood pressure; irregular heartbeat; chest pain/angina; myocardial infarction; damage to coronary arteries.
General gastrointestinal	Risk of mouth, tongue, throat, esophageal, stomach, and liver cancer; pancreatitis; malnutrition; digestive impairment.
Immune	Lower resistance to infectious diseases.
Liver	Hepatitis; cirrhosis.
Pancreas	Interference with insulin production.
Small intestine	Interference with or prevention of absorption of proteins, iron, calcium, thiamine, and vitamin B_{12}.
Stomach	Bleeding from irritation; ulcers.
Muscular	Destruction of muscle fibers.
Nervous	Destruction of brain cells; interference with neurotransmitters; slowing of reaction time.
Reproductive	Impotence; decreased testosterone production; fetal alcohol syndrome; miscarriage.

tration (BAC) is the percentage of alcohol content in the blood. This percentage determines the alcohol's effect on the individual (see Table 8-3). The more quickly the alcohol is absorbed, the quicker the BAC increases.

Alcohol enters the bloodstream quickly from the stomach and even more quickly from the small intestine. In the stomach, food inhibits absorption of alcohol. Food does not affect absorption in the small intestine.[5] Other factors that effect the rate of absorption are:

1. **Rate of consumption:** How quickly the beverage is consumed.
2. **Type of beverage:** Beer and wine have substances that slow the rate of absorption. Carbonated beverages added to liquor speed absorption. This is because the carbon dioxide in carbonation allows the stomach contents to pass more rapidly to the small intestine.
3. **Body weight:** More weight means more blood and body mass, which has a diluting effect on alcohol.
4. **Tolerance to alcohol:** Some individuals just seem to remain sober while others react very quickly. One drink to a novice may have the same effect as three on someone more experienced. This is an indication that the experienced drinker's body is adapting at the cellular level to alcohol.

Alcoholism is a disease in which an individual loses control over drinking. An alcoholic is any person who suffers from the disease of alcoholism. For an alcoholic, alcohol assumes more and more importance while family, social, and/or work/school responsibilities become less important and are eventually disrupted by the desire and need for alcohol. Some alcoholics make this transition very rapidly while others are able to maintain the appearance of being only a social drinker for many years. Unfortunately, there is no way of determining in advance who will and who will not have trouble with alcohol. Alcoholism crosses all social and economic barriers and can include clergy, medical doctors, high school students, college students and their professors. Each year there is more research done that seems to link alcoholism to an inherited susceptibility or predisposition for the disease.[6] Whether the causes of alcoholism are heredity or social or a combination of these and other variables, any consumption of alcohol places an alcoholic at risk.

Treatment for alcoholism is often long term. The course of treatment is usually considered to occur in three stages: (1) detoxification—getting the alcohol eliminated from the body, (2) medical care—taking care of any health-related problems, and (3) changing long-term behavior—helping the recovering alcoholic overcome long-time drinking patterns and destructive behaviors. See Figures 8-3 and 8-4 for treatment and aftercare

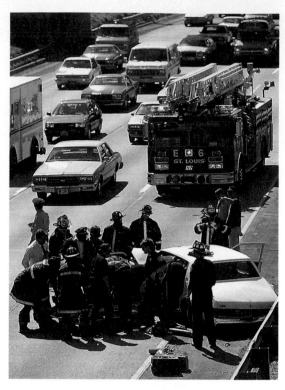

Alcohol has the potential to destroy lives socially, psychologically, and economically.

Figure 8-3 Approaches to treatment and aftercare of alcoholism

There are several approaches to providing long-term medical and psychological support to recovering alcoholics. Several current trends are listed below.

Alcoholics Anonymous (AA)

AA employs a group approach for individuals who have made a personal decision to stop drinking and want to have the support of others who have made the same decision and understand the emotions and thoughts associated with this decision. AA members view their condition as a *disease* that they are responsible for managing on a daily basis. There is a group support system as well as a buddy system to help each person through difficult times. AA also helps people with other types of drug problems or puts the individual in contact with specific groups such as Narcotics Anonymous or Cocaine Anonymous. There are also groups such as Alateen, Alatot, and Al-Anon to help the offspring and families of alcoholics.

Drug therapy

Usually part of an aftercare program, the drug Antabuse (disulfiram) is employed to create a severe reaction if alcohol is consumed. Reactions produced include headache, neck aches, nausea, vomiting, and a host of other unpleasant symptoms. Disulfiram works by blocking the enzymes that metabolize alcohol.

Group therapies

AA provides a model for many different group therapies. Another widely used approach is a behavioral model that seeks to teach coping skills. Special attention is paid to developing self-esteem and to conducting intense self-analysis to modify attitudes, emotional states, and behavior.

Figure 8-4 The twelve steps of alcoholics anonymous

1. We admitted we were powerless over alcohol—that our lives had become unmanageable.
2. Came to believe that a Power greater than ourselves could restore us to sanity.
3. Made a decision to turn our will and our lives over to the care of God *as we understood Him.*
4. Made a searching and fearless moral inventory of ourselves.
5. Admitted to God, to ourselves, and to another human being the exact nature of our wrongs.
6. Were entirely ready to have God remove all these defects of character.
7. Humbly asked Him to remove our shortcomings.
8. Made a list of all persons we had harmed and became willing to make amends to them all.
9. Made direct amends to such people wherever possible except when to do so would injure them or others.
10. Continued to take personal inventory and when we were wrong promptly admitted it.
11. Sought through prayer and meditation to improve our conscious contact with God *as we understood Him,* praying only for knowledge of His will for us and the power to carry that out.
12. Having had a spiritual awakening as the result of these steps, we tried to carry this message to alcoholics and to practice these principles in all our affairs.

Figure 8-5 Where to get help

Listed below are several telephone numbers that can be used to find information and help. In addition, there are usually local agencies that can provide information and help. For example, there are many local chapters for either Alcoholics Anonymous or Al-Anon.
National Alcohol Hotline 24-hour HelpLine: 1-800-ALCOHOL

Alcoholics Anonymous:
Contact the local chapter (listed in the phone book) or call for information throughout the United States.
[Located in New York, NY: (212) 686-1100]

Al-Anon:
Provides help for families of alcoholics. Contact the local chapter of call for information throughout the United States. [Located in New York, NY: (212) 254-7230]

BACCHUS (Boost Alcohol Consciousness Concerning the Health of University Students). [Located in Denver, CO: (303) 871-3068]

National Cocaine Hotline: 1-800-COCAINE

National Clearinghouse for Alcohol and Drug Information. [Located in Rockville, MD: (301) 468-2600]

MADD (Mothers Against Drunk Driving). [Located in Austin, TX: (817) 268-6233]

programs for recovering alcoholics and Figure 8-5 for resources.

Alcoholics remain alcoholics for life, whether or not they drink. This means recovering alcoholics must be ever careful about any products they consume, including medicines and mouthwashes, many of which contain alcohol. Currently, it is estimated that over 10 million adults and 3 million adolescents under the age of 18 are alcoholics.[6]

Tobacco Products

Tobacco products in the form of cigarettes, cigars, pipes, and various types of smokeless tobacco (snuff and chewing tobacco) all contain the drug nicotine. **Nicotine** is an addictive substance and an alkaloid poison. It affects the body by increasing heart and respiratory rates, elevating blood pressure, increasing cardiac output and oxygen consumption, and constricting the bronchi (the two main branches of the trachea that lead to the lungs). Nicotine is inhaled when smoking a tobacco product. With smokeless tobacco, nicotine is absorbed through membranes of the mouth and cheek.

Smoking is either directly or indirectly responsible for a number of conditions and diseases that are listed in Table 8-4. Some of the

TABLE 8-4 Risks of smoking[9]

Risks	Results
Coronary heart disease	It is estimated that between 169,000 and 226,000 deaths from coronary heart disease can be attributed to cigarette smoking.
Peripheral arterial disease	Smokers are two to three times more likely to suffer from abdominal aortic aneurysm than nonsmokers. Smokers have more atherosclerotic occlusions.
Lung cancer	Smoking cigarettes is the major cause of lung cancers in men and women. Rates are currently increasing faster among women than among men.
Cancer of the larynx	Laryngeal cancer in smokers is 2.0 to 27.4 times that of nonsmokers.
Oral cancers	Use of smokeless tobacco and snuff is associated with an increased risk of oral cancers. Pipes and cigars are also major risk factors. Use of alcohol seems to enhance the possibility of developing oral cancer.
Cancer of the esophagus	Smoking cigarettes, pipes, and cigars increases the risk of dying from esophageal cancer from two to nine times. Alcohol use in combination with smoking adds to that risk.
Bladder cancer	Percentage of bladder cancer attributed to smoking is estimated at 40% to 60% in males and 25% to 35% in females.
Cancer of the pancreas	Smokers have twice the risk of nonsmokers for this type of cancer.
Chronic obstructive pulmonary (lung) disease	Between 80% to 90% of more than 60,000 deaths per year from COPD are from smoking.
Peptic ulcers	Cigarette smokers develop peptic ulcers much more frequently than nonsmokers. Ulcers are also more difficult to cure in smokers.
Complications in pregnancy; illnesses in children	Smoking mothers have more stillbirths and babies with low birth weight. The hospital admission rates for pneumonia and bronchitis is 28% higher in children of smoking mothers. Asthma is more common among children of smoking mothers. Parental smoking is a risk factor associated with persistent middle-ear effusion in young children.

components of cigarette smoke are known *carcinogens* (substances that cause cancer or enable the growth of cancer cells). Nicotine, tars, and carbon monoxide are all found in cigarette smoke. The *tar* in tobacco is a black, sticky, dark fluid composed of thousands of chemicals. Many of the chemicals found in tar are cancer causing. *Carbon monoxide* is a deadly gas emitted in the exhaust of cars and in burning tobacco. The carbon monoxide level in cigarette smoke is 400 times greater than what is considered safe in industrial settings. Carbon monoxide binds to hemoglobin

more readily than oxygen interfering with the ability of blood to transport oxygen to the body, impairs the nervous system, and increases the risk of heart attacks and strokes.

Effects of smoking on the nonsmoker. *Passive smoking* is the inhalation of cigarette smoke by a nonsmoker from his or her environment. The most common form of inhaled smoke is sidestream smoke. *Sidestream smoke* is the smoke that comes from burning tobacco products and the end of the lighted tip of a cigarette between puffs[4] that is inhaled by nonsmokers when they are around people who smoke. Sidestream smoke has higher concentrations of nicotine and other carcinogenic agents than the smoke inhaled by the smoker. Many studies have shown that this passive smoking can cause cancer in nonsmokers. Nonsmokers married to smokers have a 30% greater risk of lung cancer and are more likely to experience heart attacks than nonsmoking spouses of nonsmokers.[10] There are no "safe" levels of exposure to cigarette smoke and there are no "safe" tobacco products (see Table 8-5.)

Advantages of quitting. Smoking is an extremely strong addiction. The good news is that when individuals do stop smoking, their risk of developing the listed diseases and conditions will eventually decrease to that of a nonsmoker. Although it may take several years to achieve, the effects of smoking are reversible. To quit completely, many people require the help of trained professionals. While it is difficult, the health benefits associated with quitting far outweigh the problems. For suggestions on how to stop smoking see Figure 8-6.

Cocaine

At one time **cocaine** was considered the drug of upper class America. Unfortunately, cocaine and its derivative, *crack,* have become epidemic in use. Estimates are that 25 to 30 million people have experimented with cocaine in the United States. Approximately 5 million use the drug regularly. Among young adults, 6.7% have tried crack and 40% have tried cocaine. In a recent survey of high school seniors, one in 18 admitted trying crack and 14% used cocaine in other forms.[13]

A powerful stimulant, cocaine is derived from the leaves of the South American coca shrub. Ground into a crystalline powder, the most common methods of using the drug are *snorting* it or liquefying it and then *injecting* or *freebasing* (smoking) it. When snorted, the white powder is sniffed up through the nose. The most potent, and most expensive, method of cocaine use is freebasing. The drug is usually smoked in a water pipe since this provides faster absorption into the bloodstream.

Crack is relatively easy to make and fairly inexpensive to buy. At $10 to $15 a dose, crack is the form of the drug that is most prevalent on the streets. When snorted, crack reaches the brain in about 5 minutes. When injected or smoked, it takes only a few seconds for the drug to take effect.

Figure 8-6 Smoking cessation

To quit smoking is not easy! For the person who chooses (and it is a choice) to quit, the Mayo Clinic Health Letter offers the following suggestions[11]:

1. **Set a date:** Make the date reasonably soon. Make a list of reasons why you want to quit.
2. **Start stopping before you reach the date:** Taper off on the number of cigarettes you are currently consuming. Choose a milder brand.
3. **Make your plans known:** Tell a friend, your family, and colleagues of your plans. Ask for their support.
4. **Take it one day at a time:** Get up every morning and decide not to smoke that day. Focus your attention on that one day only.
5. **Change your routine:** Avoid or change situations where you have previously smoked.
6. **Alter your surroundings:** Start new activities such as exercising or needle point.
7. **Time the urge:** Identify when your urge to smoke is the strongest. Being prepared will help you resist.
8. **Use substitutes:** Substitutes can include gum, celery, carrots, pickles, etc.
9. **Prepare a daydream:** Have a pleasant daydream ready to help fight off the desire to smoke. This can be an image of yourself without a cigarette in a situation you find highly desirable.
10. **Use relaxation techniques:** Deep breathing or progressive muscle relaxation can help.
11. **Practice positive thinking:** Tell yourself "I can make it." Remember that you *can* make it.

If you try all of the above and continue to fail, it may be beneficial for you to contact a physician for a prescription of nicorette gum. This gum contains small amounts of nicotine and helps some people overcome the nicotine addiction. Nicorette gum can be used whenever there is an urge to smoke. Initially, this may require 12 to 24 pieces a day. The use of nicorette gum can cause mouth ulcers and nausea and should not be used by pregnant or nursing women.[12]

Use of cocaine produces feelings of well-being, euphoria, and extreme exhilaration. Mental alertness seems to increase. Blood vessels become constricted, causing heart rate and blood pressure to rise. Cocaine is rapidly metabolized by the liver. Snorting cocaine results in a 5 to 15 minute "high" while the effects of crack last 20 to 30 minutes. Psychological and physical dependency on crack develops rapidly because of the brief period of stimulation. The feelings of exhilaration experienced while under the influence of the drug are quickly followed by depression.

The consequences of cocaine use on the body are extreme and highly dangerous. Cocaine use can cause headaches, exhaustion, shaking, blurred vision, nausea, impaired judgment, hyperactivity, loss of appetite, loss of sexual desire, and paranoia that can lead to violence. Snorting cocaine can destroy the septum in the nose. Freebasing may damage the liver and the lungs; fluid build-up in the lungs has resulted in death for some individuals who freebase. Cocaine can initiate strokes, bleeding in the brain, heart attacks, irregular heartbeat, and sudden death.

Women who use cocaine while pregnant have newborns that suffer withdrawal and permanent disability. Fluctuations in blood pressure in the mother can cause the baby's brain to be deprived of oxygen and the blood vessels in the baby's brain begin to break down. Essentially, the baby suffers the equivalent of a stroke. Babies born of cocaine addicts have more respiratory and kidney problems, more visual problems, lack coordination, and are developmentally retarded.[14]

Cocaine addiction is most difficult to overcome. Antidepressants seem to help reduce dependency. Tyrosine and tryptophan have also been used for treatment. These chemicals are amino acids that, when taken with an antidepressant, seem to block a cocaine high.[15]

Marijuana

Twenty years ago marijuana became a cultural phenomenon, the symbol of one generation's disregard for another. The marijuana found on the streets at that time, however, lacked the potency of current crops. Crossbreeding of more potent varieties, improved cultivation, and the part of the plant being used all contribute to increased levels of delta-9-tetrahydrocannabinol (THC), the major psychoactive drug found in marijuana. Some of the marijuana currently being grown in the United States rivals the previously stronger varieties of Mexico, Jamaica, and other areas. The THC percentage in Cannabis sativa (the Indian

hemp plant from which marijuana is derived) in U.S. grown plants can range from 2% to as high as 7%.[16] The higher the percentage of THC the more potent the drug. **Marijuana** is composed of the dried leaves and flowering tops of the cannabis plant. Hashish, which has stronger effects, is processed from the resin of the plant. The resin is either dried and pressed into cakes or sold in liquid form called hash oil. Marijuana is used more extensively than hashish in the United States.

Over 400 known chemicals constitute marijuana. More than 60 of these are cannabinoids, chemicals found only in cannabis. THC is the cannabinoid that appears most responsible for the sensations experienced by marijuana users. Cannabinoids are different from other drugs in that they are fat soluble rather than water soluble and have a decided affinity for binding to fat in the human body. This means that where other drugs might be taken in and then leave the body within relatively short periods of time, marijuana tends to attach to fatty organs such as the gonads and brain and remain there.[17] A single ingestion of THC may require up to 30 days to be eliminated from the body.

Marijuana can be eaten in baked goods such as brownies but the effects tend to be less predictable. Smoking is a more efficient and powerful technique. When inhaled, THC reaches the brain in as little as 14 seconds. Hashish is so concentrated that a single drop can equal the effects of an entire marijuana joint (cigarette). Cannabis products are difficult to classify but are considered hallucinogens.

Small doses or short-term use of marijuana creates sensations of euphoria and relaxation, often accompanied by hunger or sleepiness. Time seems to slow down and the senses appear heightened. Memory of recent events may be impaired, as well as physical coordination and perceptions. Even with small amounts of marijuana, driving ability can be detrimentally affected. Physiologically, heart rate speeds up and certain blood vessels become dilated, which may create problems for individuals with any type of heart problem. Some users experience anxiety, panic, and paranoia. In rare cases or with stronger doses, individuals may suffer from a sense of depersonalization, image distortion, and hallucinations. Chronic use seems to lead to behavioral changes in some people that may or may not be permanent. Lack of motivation or interest in activities unrelated to drug use is one result. Students have difficulty remembering when high.

Use by teenagers has been shown to lead to impairment of thinking, poor reading comprehension, and reduced verbal and mathematical skills.[4,7,16]

Some long-term effects are unknown at this time. This is partially due to the lesser potency of earlier marijuana in this country. Also, individuals vary greatly in their response to the drug. There is some indication of psychological dependence by chronic users. Increased doses are needed as tolerance develops over time. Very heavy users experience withdrawal symptoms of restlessness, irritability, tremors, nausea, vomiting, diarrhea, and sleep disturbances.[18]

Physically, marijuana appears more carcinogenic than tobacco. Known carcinogens occur in larger amounts in marijuana and when marijuana is smoked, the smoke is held in the lungs. Cannabis smoke contains more tars than tobacco smoke. Marijuana use quickly affects pulmonary function adversely and long-term use has indicated cellular changes in the lungs. People who have angina pectoris (chest pains associated with heart disease) may be significantly at risk, since more oxygen is required when using marijuana. Marijuana binds readily to hemoglobin, reducing the amount of oxygen carried to heart tissue.

Many individuals consider cannabis an aphrodisiac. Over time it actually has the opposite effect, depressing sex drive and causing impotence. Regular male users have evidenced a decrease in sperm count and reduced motility of sperm. Proportionately, more sperm appear abnormally shaped, a phenomenon associated with lessened fertility. In females, TCH blocks ovulation. Pregnant women who smoke marijuana frequently use other drugs, all of which have a detrimental effect on the fetus. Marijuana also depresses the immune system.

Therapeutic use has been and is still being explored. At this time, the most promising application seems to be as an antinausea drug for cancer chemotherapy patients.

Marijuana is a drug and an illegal one. Many people who use marijuana eventually experiment or use other, "harder" drugs, and many people engaged in other forms of drug abuse began with marijuana. As with alcohol and all other drugs, it is impossible to predict how any single person will react or who will be most adversely affected. No one starts out with the intention of having a drug become the focus of their life, but some people ultimately do allow a drug to take over and control them. Marijuana is a drug that has that potential.

Other Drugs of Concern

Drugs discussed in the following sections are ones that have been abused for many years. Unfortunately, some that had become less appealing seem to now be making a reappearance along with a dangerous new generation of illicit drugs.

Heroin. Heroin is a narcotic that is synthesized from morphine. This drug induces a strong sensation of euphoria but quickly leads to physical and psychological dependency. The physical tolerance for heroin develops rapidly. Since heroin is usually injected, addicts often share needles, which increases the risk of contracting diseases such as AIDS and hepatitis. Experts fear the younger generation may become addicted to her-

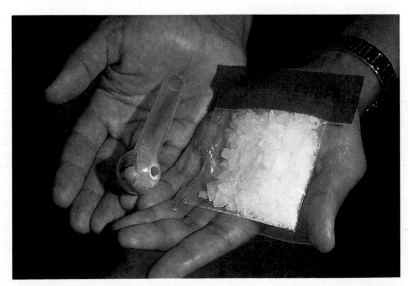

Crystal methamphetamine is more commonly know as "ice" and is extremely addictive.

oin through a substance called "moonrock"—a mixture of heroine and cocaine that can be injected, smoked, or snorted. Heroin is used in this manner to reduce the paranoia and depression that follow a cocaine high.[19]

Methamphetamine (crank). Methamphetamine is a potent stimulant that can cause uncontrollable manic behavior or paranoid thinking. The most current use of this drug is as crystal methamphetamine or "ice." While crystal methamphetamine has been touted as a safe alternative to cocaine, evidence indicates otherwise. Overdoses are often fatal and the drug is extremely addictive. In many areas of the United States, "ice" is a widespread problem.

Lysergic acid diethylamide (LSD). LSD is a hallucinogenic drug that has had a rebirth in recent years. The substance induces altered perceptions of shapes, images, time, one's own body, and sound. Tolerance to the drug develops quickly with daily use.[7] "Flashbacks" can occur in some individuals.

Phencyclidine (PCP). PCP was originally intended for use as a surgical anesthetic for humans. In actual use, however, unusual and undesirable effects on patients under its influence led to the conclusion that the drug was unsuitable for this purpose.[7] Also called "angel dust," PCP provokes a variety of unpredictable responses from users. These reactions include feelings of unreality, depersonalization, confusion, depression, anxiety, sometimes aggressive and violent behavior, acute or permanent psychosis, and coma. Users often fail to experience sensations of pain and report feeling uncoordinated in their movements. Classified as a hallucinogen, PCP

has been used as an additive to cocaine, a combination that multiplies the toxic effects of both drugs.

Designer drugs. These drugs resemble those that are controlled by the Federal Drug Administration (FDA); that is, they act like known drugs but they have a different chemical composition. Probably the two best known designer drugs that are currently being used are China white, an analog of heroin, and "ectasy." Ecstasy is an analog of the amphetamines and hallucinogens under FDA control since 1985. However, designer drugs appear so rapidly that is difficult to impossible to restrict sales. Poor quality control of these drugs can result in neurological damage or death.[19] Often, brain damage is caused with a single dose.

A Final Thought

To develop a high level of wellness each person must address the issue of his or her own drug use. Drugs prescribed as medicine can promote quality of life but unwise use severely diminishes it. There are some indications that the use of psychoactive drugs is meeting with disfavor among college students. The exception to decreasing drug use is widespread use of alcohol, which continues to be *the* most abused drug—particularly among college students. Perhaps as each person becomes more aware of the dangers associated with alcohol and drug use, a smaller percentage of college students will use them. Hopefully the general public, particularly young people of junior high and high school age, will begin to refrain from the most destructive behavioral patterns associated with drug abuse.

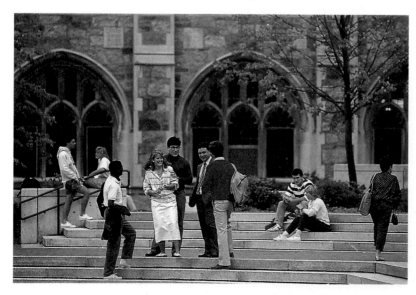

There are no safe drugs. People must choose not to use drugs.

Summary

▌ People use drugs for a variety of reasons, which include recreational/social, sensation-seeking, religious/spiritual, to achieve altered states, as a sign of rebellion and alienation, or as a result of peer pressure. Usage usually involves a combination of reasons.

▌ Drugs are commonly classified according to the physiological effect they create. The five classifications are stimulants, depressants, hallucinogens, narcotics, and inhalants.

▌ Caffeine is probably the most used drug in America. It is a stimulant that speeds heart rate, increases blood pressure, and can cause insomnia.

▌ Alcohol is a "socially acceptable" drug that is a major source of physical and emotional damage and death.

▌ The blood alcohol concentration (BAC) of ethyl alcohol is affected by the rate of consumption, the type of alcoholic beverage being consumed, the body weight of the individual drinking, and his or her tolerance to alcohol.

▌ Alcoholism is a disease in which a person loses control over drinking. It is impossible to determine who will or will not become an alcoholic. Alcoholism crosses all social, sexual, educational, and racial barriers.

▌ Nicotine is an addictive agent found in tobacco. The tars found in tobaccos are carcinogenic agents.

▌ The carbon monoxide formed when tobacco is smoked interferes with the body's ability to transport oxygen and increases the risk of heart attacks and strokes. Sidestream smoke has even higher concentrations of these agents than the smoke inhaled by a smoker.

▌ Cocaine use has become epidemic in the United States. Cocaine can be snorted, injected, or freebased (smoked).

▌ The consequences of cocaine use can range from

Continued.

Action plan for personal wellness

An important consideration in assuming responsibility for one's own quality of life is using information. After reading this chapter, answer the following questions and determine an action plan for enhancing your own lifestyle.

1 Based on the information presented in this chapter, along with what I know about my family's health history, the health problems/issues that I need to be most concerned about are:_____

_____

_____

2 Of those health concerns listed in no. 1, the one I most need to act on is:_____

_____

_____

3 The possible actions (try to be as specific as possible) that I can take to improve my level of wellness are:_____

_____

_____

4 Of those actions listed in no. 3, the one that I most need to include in an action plan is:_____

_____

_____

5 Factors I need to keep in mind in order to be successful in my action plan are:_____

_____

_____

headaches and nausea to violence and death. Cocaine addiction is difficult to overcome.

▌ The primary psychoactive ingredient in marijuana and hashish is delta-9-tetrahydrocannabinol (THC). Carcinogens can be found in more potent levels in marijuana than in tobacco. Hashish is more potent than marijuana.

▌ Short-term effects of marijuana include euphoria and perceptual impairment. Some people experience anxiety, a sense of depersonalization, and hallucinations. Long-term effects are not well documented at this time.

▌ Some drugs have been abused by society for many years. They include heroin, methamphetamine (crank), and LSD. The newest form of methamphetamine is "ice," which is smokable and more addictive, potent, and destructive than crack cocaine.

▌ Designer drugs are analogs or copycats of controlled substances and are more powerful and less predicable in the effects they create.

Review Questions

1. List reasons why people might choose to use drugs.
2. List and define the five classifications of drugs.
3. What are the positive and negative effects of caffeine on individuals?
4. What factors affect the blood alcohol concentration (BAC) of a person? How can people be responsible drinkers? What are some potential effects of long-term alcohol use?
5. Discuss the risks associated with smoking and list the steps to be used when attempting to quit.
6. Discuss why cocaine and its derivatives represent an extreme danger to anyone using the drug.
7. List and describe the effects of some of the other drugs currently being used.

References

1. Schlaadt RG and Shannon PT: Drugs of choice: current perspectives on drug use, Englewood Cliffs, NJ, 1986, Prentice Hall.
2. Mermelstein NH: Caffeine, Contemporary Nutrition 9:1-2, 1984.
3. Grounds for breaking the coffee habit, Tufts University Diet and Nutrition Letter, Feb 1990, pp 3-6.
4. Carrol CR: Drugs in modern society, ed 2, Dubuque, Iowa, 1989, Wm C Brown Group.
5. LeMonick M: Should women drink less? Time 129(6), May 1987, pp 66.
6. Biological and genetic factors in alcoholism, Research Monograph, No 9, Rockville, MD, 1983, National Institute on Alcohol Abuse and Alcoholism.
7. Ray O and Ksir C: Drugs, society, and human behavior, St Louis, 1990, Mosby–Year Book, Inc.
8. Waldinger RJ: Fundamentals of psychiatry, Washington, DC, 1986, American Psychiatric Press, Inc.
9. Felding JE: Smoking: Health effects and control, Professional Education Publication, New York, 1986, American Cancer Society.
10. The health consequences of involuntary smoking: a report of the surgeon general, Department of Health and Human Services, DHHS (CDC), Washington DC, 1986, US Government Printing Office.
11. Smoking cessation—here's how to stop, Mayo Clinic Health Letter, Aug 1987, pp 2-3.
12. Nicotine addiction, Mayo Clinic Health Letter, March 1989, p 6.
13. Hour by hour crack, Newsweek, Nov 1988, pp 64-75.
14. Morganthou T: Crack and crime, Newsweek, June 1986, p 78.
15. Wilbur R: Drugs that fight coke, American Health, Vol 6, pp 44-47, 1987.
16. Witter W and Venturelli P: Drugs and society, Boston, 1988, Jones & Bartlett Publishers Inc.
17. Mann P: Marijuana alert, New York, 1985, McGraw-Hill Inc.
18. Gerald M: Pharmacology: an introduction to drugs, Englewood Cliffs, NJ, 1981, Prentice Hall.
19. The nightmare drugs: a medical essay, Mayo Clinic Health Letter, Nov 1989 pp 1-8.

Annotated Readings

Pekkanen J: Confessions of doctors on drugs, Hippocrates, Nov/Dec 1988, pp 92-94.
Doctors, nurses, and other health professionals abuse drugs. No one knows exactly how broad the problem is, but estimates are that up to 15% of all doctors are dependent on alcohol or other mind-altering drugs.

Tierney J: The nicorette generation, Hippocrates, May/June 1989, pp 32-33.
A humorous look at the use of nicorette to break smoking addiction.

Whelan EM: To your health, Across the Board, Jan 1988, pp 49-53.
Moderate drinking may aid in prolonging life. Determining the right amount and how the statistics really apply to each person is unknown at this time.

Wolfe: Smokeless tobacco: the fatal pinch, Multinational Monitor, July/Aug 1987, pp 20-21.
This article examines the dangerous habit of using smokeless tobacco and how the advertising industry promotes smokeless tobacco as "class enjoyment."

ASSESSMENT ACTIVITY   8-1

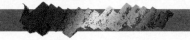

How Can You Tell If You Have a Drinking Problem?

There have been many self-tests published for people to use to determine if they are alcoholics or if they have a drinking problem. None of them should be taken as an absolute test or as providing a definite answer to that question because in most cases it is a complex, subjective judgment as to whether someone should seek help. One of the best popularly printed self-tests appeared in a "Dear Abby" column, and it is offered here as a possible guide. If these questions seem to indicate that you or a friend needs to seek help, we recommend a visit to a counselor, psychologist, or physician who is experienced in the assessment of chemical dependency.

Directions: Check all that apply:

_____

_____ 1.   Have you ever decided to stop drinking for a week or so but only lasted for a couple of days?

_____ 2.   Do you wish people would stop nagging you about your drinking?

_____ 3.   Have you ever switched from one kind of drink to another in the hope that this would keep you from getting drunk?

_____ 4.   Have you had a drink in the morning in the past year?

_____ 5.   Do you envy people who can drink without getting into trouble?

_____ 6.   Have you had problems connected with drinking during the past year?

_____ 7.   Has your drinking caused problems at home?

_____ 8.   Do you ever try to get "extra" drinks at a party because you did not get enough to drink?

_____ 9.   Do you tell yourself you can stop drinking anytime you want to, even though you keep getting drunk when you don't mean to?

_____10.   Have you missed days at work (or school) because of drinking?

_____11.   Do you have "blackouts"?

_____12.   Have you ever felt that your life would be better if you did not drink?

If you checked four or more of these, it would be a good idea to seek the guidance of a specialist in chemical dependency or to seek help directly through Alcoholics Anonymous or a similar organization. It is perfectly acceptable to go to an open AA meeting, listen to what is being said, and decide for yourself if their program would be useful to you.

ASSESSMENT ACTIVITY   8-2

Drugs in My Life

Directions: Listed below are various drugs or products that contain drugs. Estimate your involvement with each of these products.

Drug	Amount	Frequency	Expense	Reason for use
Coffee/tea (caffeine)				
Cola drinks (caffeine)				
Alcohol				
Tobacco				
Cocaine or crack				
Marijuana				
Heroin				
Methamphetamine (crank) or "ice"				
LSD				
Other				

In the last column list your motivation for use, whether it is relaxation, stimulation, to get "high," out of habit, because your friends do, or another reason. On a separate sheet of paper list the benefits you derive from use and the dangers, if any. Assess the impact of these drugs on your wellness goals. Is there a need to change any aspect of your drug use?

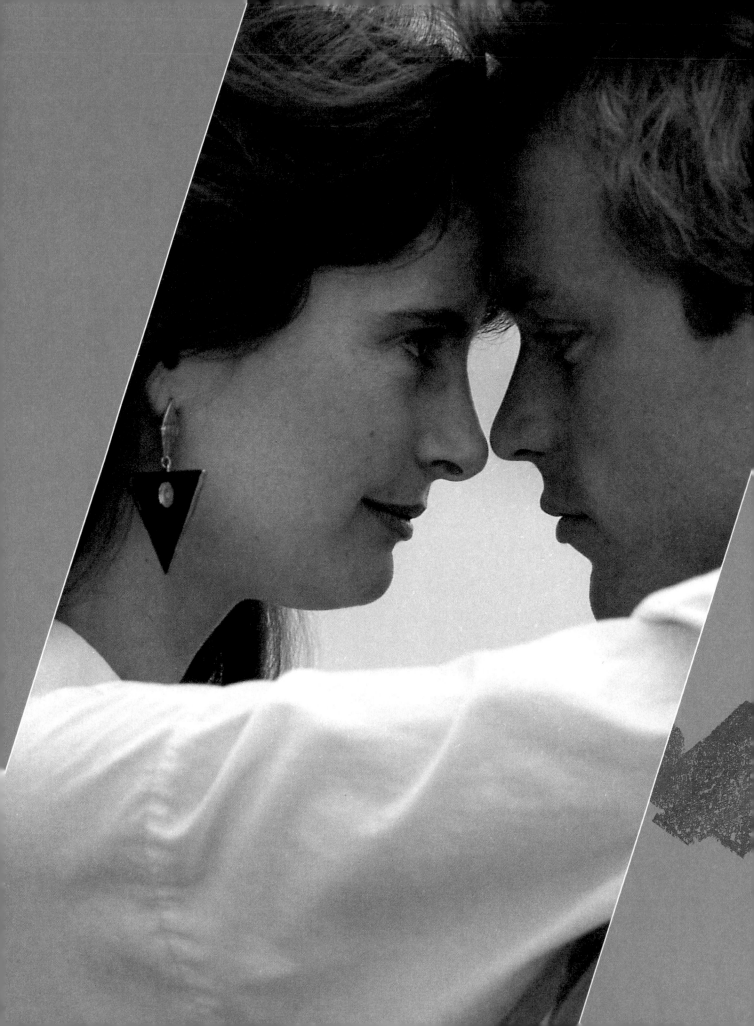

Chapter 9

Preventing
Sexually
Transmitted
Diseases

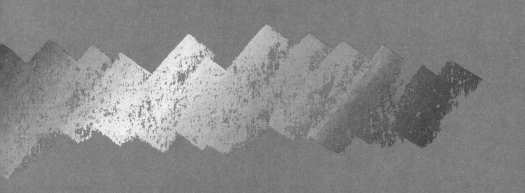

Key terms

Acquired immunode-
  ficiency syndrome
  (AIDS)

chlamydia

genital warts

gonorrhea

herpes

viral hepatitis

syphilis

sexually transmitted
  diseases (STDs)

Objectives

After completing this chapter, you will be able to:

▌ Discuss the different sexually transmitted diseases.

▌ Evaluate the risks of having multiple sexual partners.

It has been said that humans are sexual beings from womb to tomb. Sexuality is an important aspect of each of individual. Sexuality is involved in every facet of human existence, including relationships, anatomy, behaviors, thoughts, and values. Human sexuality is an area where numerous vital decisions must be made. The sexual behaviors in which each person engages is one aspect of sexuality.

There are no easy answers. Each person must come to terms with his or her own sexual behavior. If people choose to have a variety of partners, it must be realized that for each act of coitus, the sexual history of both people is brought to that union. While it may be the first experience for one, if the other partner has had intercourse with three other people, the person for whom it is the first time is essentially having sex with four other individuals. Any diseases or infections any of those four people may have is perhaps brought to this association.

Decisions concerning sexual behavior have many lifelong consequences. These choices can enhance or severely diminish an individual's feelings of well-being. Sex can be wonderful and fulfilling, but it also holds the potential for serious problems. This chapter examines some of the **sexually transmitted diseases (STDs)** that can result when people engage in behavior that puts them at risk.

Genital Warts

Warts on the genitalia, around the anus, in the vagina, and on the cervix are called **genital warts,** or *condyloma*. These warts are caused by

the *human papilloma virus (HPV)*. Experts postulate that genital warts is the third most prevalent STD, following chlamydia and gonorrhea. Between 1966 and 1981, the Centers for Disease Control reported a 459% jump in HPV patients. It is estimated that 1.2 million people become infected annually.[2] Genital warts most commonly involve people between the ages of 15 and 24.

Genital warts have a cauliflower-like appearance. In moist areas they are soft and either pink or red. On dry skin they are usually yellow-gray and hard. The warts generally appear 2 to 3 months after exposure. There are 56 distinct varieties of HPV, some of which have been specifically linked to cervical cancer[1] and cancers of the rectum, vulva, skin, and penis.[2]

Cryosurgery (freezing), electrocautery (burning), and use of the topical agent, podophyllin,

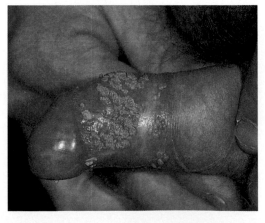

Genital warts are the results of human papilloma virus or HPV.

are all methods that have been successfully employed. Podophyllin should not be used during pregnancy or on warts in the cervical area. If the individual has had a variety of partners, the reproductive area in all partners should be checked so that treatment can be initiated if genital warts have developed.

Chlamydia

Chlamydia is the most common sexually transmitted disease in the United States with estimates of three million new cases each year.[3] The causative agent is a bacteria called *Chlamydia trachomatis.* Chlamydia is frequently found in conjunction with other STDs such as gonorrhea, herpes, and syphilis, and it may be contracted through anal or vaginal intercourse.

In men, the infection is usually manifest by inflammation of the urethra (urethritis). Infected men generally experience a burning sensation during urination and, possibly, a mild discharge. One third of all men with chronic chlamydia infection develop no symptoms.

Symptoms in women include vaginal discharge, intermittent vaginal bleeding, and ill-defined discomfort or pain on urination. Infected mothers may pass the infection to their babies during the birth process. This may result in conjunctivitis in the child or a more serious condition known as chlamydial pneumonia. Over 30,000 newborns are affected by this condition each year.[4]

When left untreated, chlamydia can lead to arthritis and damage the heart valves, blood vessels, and heart muscle itself. In men, the condition can also lead to sterility. In women, the disease can infect the uterus, fallopian tubes, and upper reproductive areas, producing a chronic condition known as *pelvic inflammatory disease (PID).* This scarring of the fallopian tubes by PID causes both sterility and increased risk of ectopic pregnancy (where the embryo is implanted outside the uterus).

Tetracycline and erythromycin are the drugs used for treatment. The drugs are taken orally for 1 to 3 weeks. It is extremely important to take the full course of medication since relapse can occur. All sexual partners should be treated or the disease can be passed back and forth.

Herpes

Herpes is caused by a virus called *herpes simplex virus (HSV).* Five different strains of the herpes virus infect human beings. The most common are herpes simplex-1 (HSV-1) and herpes simplex-2 (HSV-2). Type 1 is usually confined to nongenital areas in the form of "cold sores" or "fever blisters". It is a very common form of herpes, but it is not categorized as an STD. Type 2 generally causes lesions on and around the genital areas and is an STD. However, through either direct or indirect contact, type 1 can affect the genital area while type 2 can produce sores in the mouth. So, the common sites for type 1 and type 2 can be reversed.

Type 2 herpes appears as a single or a series of very painful blisters on the penis or inside the vagina or cervix. The blisters may also be present on the buttocks, thighs, or in the groin area. The infection usually lasts 2 to 4 weeks and then disappears but does not leave the body. The virus retreats to the nerve endings where it remains dormant for prolonged periods. Herpes can become active again without any warning; that is, the disease has the potential to be recurrent. Menstruation, stress, trauma to the skin (such as too much sunlight), lack of sleep, and poor nutrition all seem to be triggers that stimulate recurrences. Recurrences are generally less severe and of shorter duration.[5]

Men do not seem to experience any major long-term complications. Women, however, may be faced with the possibility of cancer of the cervix and infecting their newborns during the birth process. Any woman with a history of herpes should have an annual pap smear test. Physicians attending the pregnancy of a woman with a history of herpes should be informed so the clinical history can be monitored. If herpes becomes active or the physician feels the child is at risk in a vaginal birth, *cesarean section delivery* (surgical removal of the fetus through the abdominal wall) is often used to prevent the possibility of infection. Additional hazards of herpes infection are herpes encephalitis, where the virus invades the brain, and herpes keratitis, or eye infection. These two conditions are rare and can be effectively treated with antiviral drugs.

There is no cure for herpes at this time. A prescription drug, acyclovir which comes in either ointment or capsule form, is capable of helping control and treat herpes. The drug does not kill the virus, but it does seem to help shorten the duration and severity of genital herpes. The capsule form appears best suited for treatment purposes but must be taken at the first sign of a flare-up to be effective.

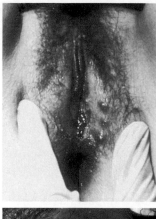

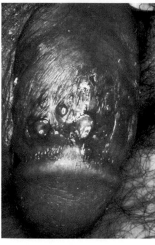

The sores associated with genital herpes are extremely painful.

Viral Hepatitis

Hepatitis is an inflammation of the liver caused by one or more viruses. There are currently four distinct known types of **viral hepatitis:** hepatitis A (once known as infectious hepatitis), hepatitis B (formerly serum hepatitis), Hepatitis C (non-A, non-B hepatitis), and the newest form called hepatitis D or delta. Hepatitis A is the least serious form and tends to be self-limiting. The spread of hepatitis A is associated with overcrowding, poor hygiene, unsanitary conditions, contamination of food and water, and direct contact with the virus, including sexual contact. Type A is a common infection in the United States with almost half the adult population having antibodies against the virus.[6] The incubation period is 2 to 6 weeks, and protection is provided if gamma globulin is administered within 10 days of exposure.

Hepatitis B was at one time spread primarily through tattoo needles, the sharing of needles by drug addicts, and transfusions of contaminated blood. It can also be spread through body secretions, including sweat, breast milk, and semen. Hepatitis B is a sexually transmitted disease that is found particularly among male homosexuals who have many sexual partners. The incubation period is 6 weeks to 6 months. A vaccine has been developed to immunize against the disease.

Hepatitis D virus cannot initiate an infection in isolation but acts together with the hepatitis B virus to create a more severe form of the disease. Hepatitis D is contracted the same way as B.

Hepatitis C is caused by one or more viruses that cannot be traced to A, B, or D. Hepatitis C is most often associated with post-transfusion patients, but there is a growing concern over possible sexual transmission.

Symptoms for all forms of viral hepatitis are similar. They include fatigue, loss of appetite, mild fever, nausea, vomiting, diarrhea, aching muscles and joints, loss of appetite, and tenderness in the upper right abdomen. A few people may have jaundiced (yellowed) skin and eyes, itching skin, darkened urine, and light-colored feces. Still others may exhibit no symptoms except those usually associated with the flu. This group does not usually seek treatment. Yet, they are still able to transmit the infection to others even though they do not have easily recognizable symptoms.

Viral hepatitis is a kind of liver injury. Most patients with hepatitis recover without serious problems. However, for some people serious scarring of the liver or even death may occur. In some cases of hepatitis B and hepatitis C, the individual with the disease becomes a chronic carrier or can develop chronic progressive hepatitis that eventually leads to liver failure.

Gonorrhea

Nearly 2 million cases of **gonorrhea** are reported each year, making it the second most prevalent STD. Gonorrhea is caused by the bacterium *Neisseria gonorrheae*, which attacks the mucus membranes of the penis, vagina, rectum, throat, and eyes. The disease is spread by vaginal, oral, and rectal contact.

Men usually know when they have gonorrhea. Even so, 20% will experience no symptoms. Symptoms appear 2 to 10 days (within an average of 3 to 5 days) after contact with the bacteria and include a thick, yellowish discharge from the penis and a painful, burning sensation on urination. These indications should cause men to seek medical treatment immediately. Untreated, gonorrhea can result in sterility.

The symptoms in women are discharge and burning on urination, but they may be so mild they are unnoticed. The bacteria can survive in the vagina and other areas of the female reproductive system for years. During this time, women are capable of infecting any sex partners as well as their fetus, if they become pregnant. Contact by the child with the bacteria during childbirth can lead to an eye infection resulting in blindness. Untreated gonorrhea can lead to pelvic inflammatory disease (PID), the leading cause of sterility in women. In both men and women, rectal and oral gonorrhea may go unnoticed. The disease can develop into a serious infection, resulting in arthritis, meningitis, skin lesions, and liver, heart, brain, and spinal cord problems.

Gonorrhea is diagnosed by obtaining a smear from the penis or cervix. Penicillin is the drug of choice for treatment. If a person is allergic to penicillin, tetracycline is usually used. It is now quite common to treat for chlamydia when gonorrhea has been diagnosed. Gonorrhea can be completely cured although there is no immunity to the disease. If a person has multiple sexual partners, it is imperative to seek medical help and advice regularly.

Syphilis

Syphilis is caused by a corkscrew-shaped bacterial spirochete called *Treponema pallidum*. Kissing, oral-genital contact, and intercourse are the most common forms of transmission. The spirochete dies quickly when exposed to air so primary entry to the body is through a break in the skin. Once in the blood stream it can set up housekeeping in a variety of organs and mimics the symptoms of many major chronic diseases. Because of this ability to mimic other diseases it is referred to as "the great imitator."

There are four stages of syphilis.

Primary syphilis. The initial sign of primary syphilis is a lesion called a *chancre* (pronounced SHANK-ER) located at the site of entry of the pathogen. The incubation period can range from 10 to 90 days with an average of 21 days before symptoms appear. The chancre can vary from the size of a pinhead to the size of a dime. Even though the chancre may look very painful, it is

not and may go unnoticed. If the lesion occurs on the labia, vagina, or rectum it can very easily be undetected. The chancre will disappear within 3 to 6 weeks.

Secondary syphilis. From 1 month to a year after the chancre disappears, the symptoms of secondary syphilis may appear. Symptoms include headaches, swollen glands, low-grade fevers, skin rash, white patches on the mucous membranes of the mouth and throat, hair loss, arthritis pain, or large sores around the mouth and genitals. These sores contain the bacteria responsible for syphilis and contact with them can spread the disease. Symptoms may be mild or severe and in rare instances no symptoms will appear at all. Even if left untreated, symptoms usually run their course, lasting anywhere from a few days to several months. The pathogen remains active in the body even with the absence of symptoms and will reappear at some later time—perhaps as long as 20 years later.

Latent syphilis. During latent syphilis there are few or no clinical signs that the disease exists even though the spirochetes are invading the various organs and systems of the body, including the brain, heart, and central nervous system. The spirochetes multiply relentlessly and begin to destroy the tissue, bones, and organs. An infected person is no longer contagious at this time.

Late syphilis. Anywhere from 10 to 20 years after the onset of latent syphilis, the disease progresses to its most devastating stage. Late syphilis can cause heart damage, central nervous damage, blindness, deafness, paralysis, and psychosis.

Penicillin is the drug of choice for treating syphilis. Individuals who are penicillin-sensitive are placed on other antibiotics. It is quite common for persons with syphilis to also have other STDs such as gonorrhea and chlamydia, thereby requiring greater doses of antibiotics.

Acquired Immunodeficiency Syndrome (AIDS)

AIDS has been recognized by the World Health Organization as a worldwide epidemic. First diagnosed in this country in New York in 1981, AIDS is found in Europe, Africa, Australia, South America, the Caribbean, Asia, and the Middle East. In many African nations there are approximately equal numbers of men and women infected, but in the United States, the vast majority of individuals with AIDS are promiscuous homosexual males, followed by bisexual men, and IV drug users. This statistic is expected to change somewhat in the future as more heterosexual individuals acquire the disease.

The virus responsible for AIDS is the *human immunodeficiency virus (HIV)*. This virus attacks the "helper" T-lymphocytes, specifically the T-4 cell, that are possibly the most critical element in the body's immune system.[7] HIV attaches to the part of the T-cell that recognizes virus infections and blocks its ability to react to them. It is thought that, over time, HIV may even multiply and destroy T-cells, leaving the body more and more defenseless against the invasion of opportunistic organisms that can lead to illness and even death.

Anyone is infected who has HIV present in their body, whether or not they exhibit symptoms. Not everyone who has been infected with the HIV virus has developed AIDS or ARC (*AIDS-related complex*) at this time. It is not known if everyone carrying the virus will develop AIDS or ARC. Many people who carry HIV are apparently healthy individuals with no indications of disease. However, even people with no obvious symptoms are fully capable of transmitting the AIDS virus to others who, in turn, may develop AIDS or ARC while the carrier remains symptomless. Once infected, a person appears capable of transmitting the virus from shortly after the time of infection until the end of his or her life. HIV apparently remains in a dormant stage for some individuals anywhere from 3 months to 6 or more years. Some people will develop chronic conditions such as fever, weight loss, diarrhea, fatigue, or swollen lymph glands. These symptoms are often referred to as the AIDS-related complex (ARC). ARC is an HIV-caused immuno-deficiency, but it is not AIDS.

AIDS seems to progress through various stages and is often associated with specific conditions such as *Kaposi's sarcoma* (an otherwise rare form of cancer) and *AIDS dementia complex* (which involves hallucinations, incoherent speech, disorientation, and memory loss). AIDS itself may include these conditions as well as the presence of opportunistic infections (ones that occur because the immune system has broken down) such as *Pneumocystis carinii pneumonia (PCP)* or *cryptoccal meningitis*.

It is not currently known why some people develop AIDS rapidly while others do not. Factors that may contribute to the advancement of the condition are weakening of the immune system through other infections, alcohol or drug abuse, poor nutrition, and stress.[8] There is no way of determining who will or will not develop AIDS. The longer the virus is in the system, the greater the chances are of acquiring AIDS. In one study spanning a 6-year period, 30% of the participants with the virus developed AIDS, 49% displayed ARC symptoms, and 21% remained free of symptoms. All of these individuals were capable of continuing to spread the disease.

There is no cure for AIDS. However, the drug AZT has been found beneficial in prolonging the lives of patients in advanced stages. AZT is quite expensive. For this reason and because AIDS is "new" with little known about the effects of different medicines on the syndrome, the drug has been previously used primarily after the onset of

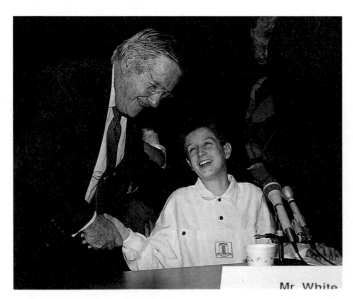

Ryan White became very active in the fight against AIDS and also in the fight to destroy the fears associated with those who have AIDS. Ryan contracted AIDS through a blood transfusion and died of complications from the disease in 1990.

the most dangerous characteristic symptoms. Earlier use of AZT may help alter or prevent the onset of some or all of these symptoms. No one has ever recovered from AIDS, however, and over 50% of those diagnosed since 1981 have died.

The number of anti-AIDS drugs is increasing. In January 1990, the Food and Drug Administration (FDA) approved a drug called *flucanazole,* an antifungal drug that is used to treat two diseases that frequently affect AIDS victims: candidiosis (thrush) and one form of meningitis. Another new drug is U-81749 which, hopefully, blocks an enzyme the AIDS virus needs to reproduce itself. U-81749 is still in the test stage, however, and is not approved for human use at this time.

AIDS is spread through intimate sexual contact, the transfusion of blood from an infected individual, and from an infected mother to her fetus during the prenatal period or birth process, or while breastfeeding. There have been no cases where AIDS or the AIDS virus have been spread through casual contact—this includes family members or friends living in close contact with infected adults or children. A *very* few health care professionals working with AIDS patients

have contracted the disease in rare situations where mishandling of blood occurred. The AIDS virus is not transmitted from toilet seats, foods or beverages, or social kissing. The virus is found in small amounts in tears and saliva, though transmission through these mediums is undocumented at this time.[9]

Anal sexual intercourse is currently the most prevalent means of spreading AIDS, whether through homosexual or heterosexual contact. This may be because this type of activity increases the likelihood of making small tears that facilitate the spread of the virus from semen to blood. Vaginal and oral sex are also considered highly dangerous. Sharing of needles among drug users or having sex with an IV drug user is placing oneself in jeopardy. Sex with a prostitute is a significant risk factor. Anyone with multiple sexual partners is at risk since there is no way of knowing with whom those partners have previously had contact. People who are not sexually active are not at risk. Individuals in a monogamous relationship where neither individual has a sexually transmitted disease or has been an IV drug user are considered safe.

Individuals who may have been or currently are at risk should consult a physician or public health department for a screening to determine if they are carrying the virus. AIDS is the most deadly of all sexually transmitted diseases, but no one has to acquire it. With education, wisdom, and reduction in behaviors known to contribute to its development and spread, AIDS can be prevented (Figure 9-1). Information on AIDS can be obtained through various sources (Figure 9-2).

Figure 9-1 Preventing the spread of AIDS[7]

AIDS can be stopped by preventing the transmission of the AIDS virus from one person to another. This means eliminating direct sexual contact with infected people and not using contaminated needles. Recommendations to reduce the possibility of becoming infected include:

- Practice abstinence or mutual monogamy.
- Always use protection (that is, latex condom and spermicide such as nonoxynol-9) if having sex with multiple partners or with persons who have multiple partners.
- Do not have unprotected sex with individuals with AIDS, those who engage in high-risk behavior, or those who have had a positive test for the AIDS virus.
- Avoid sexual activities that might cut or tear the rectum, vagina, or penis, such as anal intercourse.
- Do not have sex with prostitutes.
- Do not use IV drugs or share needles. Refrain from sex with IV drug users.

Figure 9-2 AIDS information sources

Any questions or concerns you may have about AIDS can be answered by one of the hotlines listed. They can also provide testing referral and locations of support groups. Your local health department also has valuable information.

AIDS Hotline: 1-800-342-2437
                (404) 329-1245 in Atlanta, GA

National Gay
Task Force: Crisisline 1-800-221-7044
                Hours: 3-9:00 PM Eastern Time

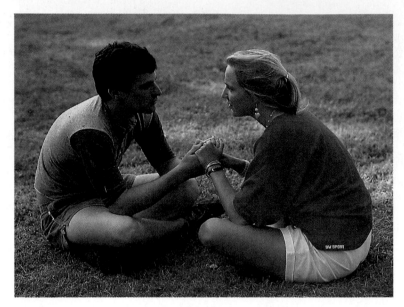

Safer sex is an individual responsibility.

Safer Sex: An Individual Responsibility

The purpose of this book is to increase awareness of how modifying lifestyles can help individuals achieve optimal wellness. Changes in dietary habits, moderate use of alcohol, avoiding use of cigarettes, and incorporation of exercise can all help prevent disease. Prevention of STDs requires similar responsibility. Sexual abstinence or a monogamous relationship are the only relatively sure ways of preventing STDs. People who choose to engage in sexual contact with more than one partner place themselves at risk. If a choice is made to have sex with someone, the tough questions concerning sexual history need to be asked. The integrity of the partner is vital. If the history is one that places either partner at high risk, contact should be considered very carefully. A condom should always be used with any new partner.

Safer sex is difficult since few people want to discuss it. Having sex should be viewed as a major decision that has the potential for lifelong consequences. While it is nice to picture a world where everyone finds that special person, falls in love, and remains with them "happily ever after," life does not always work that way. The sexual practices in which human beings engage carry varying degrees of risk and profoundly affect their futures. If a decision is made to engage in sexual intercourse, a condom should be used—a practice that can help in preventing pregnancy and the transmission of STDs. Once again, the decision for safer sexual behavior rests with each person.

Summary

▮ Genital warts, or condyloma, are caused by the human papilloma virus (HPV) and have been linked to some cancers. Cryosurgery, electrocautery, and use of a topical agent are methods of treatment.

▮ Chlamydia is a bacteria that produces the most common STD in the United States. Left untreated, it can cause arthritis, damage the heart and blood vessels, and cause sterility. Pelvic inflammatory disease (PID), resulting in ectopic pregnancies, may develop from chlamydial infection. Treatment is available.

▮ Herpes is caused by the herpes simplex virus. In humans, lesions are usually located either around the mouth or the genital area. Herpes does not go away, but remains dormant in the human body and can recur at any time. While men do not experience major long-term complications, women may develop cancer of the cervix or infect newborns during the birth process. There is no cure for herpes.

▮ Viral hepatitis is an injury to the liver. Hepatitis has several types of viruses associated with it.

▮ The second leading STD is gonorrhea. Gonorrhea can lead to sterility in males and females and PID in women. Symptoms are often unnoticed by women but can cause serious problems if left untreated. While there is no immunity to the disease, treatment is available.

▮ Syphilis is caused by a bacteria. There are four stages of syphilis, and the full effects may not be experienced for 10 to 20 years after infection occurs.

▮ AIDS is the result of the human immunodeficiency virus (HIV) that attacks the immune system. AIDS can be transmitted if an individual has symptoms or not. Deadly diseases associated with AIDS are *pneumocystis carinii* pneumonia and Kaposi's sarcoma. AIDS is only spread through intimate sexual contact, the sharing or needles, or from mother to child. There is no cure for AIDS and over 50% of the cases diagnosed since 1981 have died.

▮ The only positive way to avoid acquiring a STD is through abstinence or monogamy. Use of condoms is associated with decreased risk when a person has a number of sexual partners.

 Action plan for personal wellness

An important consideration in assuming responsibility for one's own quality of life is using information. After reading this chapter, answer the following questions and determine an action plan for enhancing your own lifestyle.

1 Based on the information presented in this chapter, along with what I know about my family's health history, the health problems/issues that I need to be most concerned about are:_____
_____
_____

2 Of those health concerns listed in no. 1, the one I most need to act on is:_____
_____
_____

3 The possible actions (try to be as specific as possible) that I can take to improve my level of wellness are: _____
_____
_____

4 Of those actions listed in no. 3, the one that I most need to include in an action plan is: _____
_____
_____

5 Factors I need to keep in mind in order to be successful in my action plan are: _____
_____
_____

Review Questions

1. How can people accept responsibility for their sexual behavior?
2. Why does chlamydia represent a serious problem?
3. Discuss why HPV is more dangerous for females than for males.
4. What are the various kinds of viral hepatitis and how are they spread?
5. List and explain the four stages of syphilis.
6. What precautions can be taken to protect against the spread of AIDS?
7. Why, if one STD is present, may it be necessary to get treatment for more than one?

References

1. Genital warts and cancer, The Health Letter 32(8):4, Oct 1988.
2. Symptoms of HPV commonly missed, The Commercial Appeal, Aug 20 1989, p 5E.
3. Chlamydia: cloak and dagger, Harvard Medical School Health Letter 13(12):7, Oct 1988.
4. *Chlamydia trachomatis* infection: Mortality and Morbidity Weekly Report 33:805-807, 1985.
5. Braude AL, Davis CE, and Fierer J, editors: Infectious diseases and medical microbiology, ed 2, Philadelphia, 1986, WB Saunders Co.
6. Crowly LV: Introduction to human disease, ed 2, Boston, 1988, Jones & Bartlett Inc.
7. Haseltine WA and Wong-Staal F: The molecular biology of the AIDS virus, Scientific American 259(4):52-64, Oct 1988.
8. Yarber WL: AIDS: what young adults should know, Reston, VA, 1987. AAHPERD.
9. The facts about AIDS, NEA Higher Education Advocate 4(13):1-14, Aug 31 1987.

Annotated Readings

Franklin D: AIDS file, Health, May/June 1990, p 17.
Based on a study of 238 gay and bisexual men, brain damage has been found in individuals with the HIV virus.

Gallup G Jr, and Gallup A: AIDS—we worry about the wrong things, American Health, June 1988, pp 50-52.
A worldwide special report that seeks information about what people know and what are the common fears concerning the AIDS epidemic.

Hall SS: Gadfly in the ointment, Hippocrates, Sept/Oct 1988, pp 76-82.
A controversial article that discuss molecular biologist, Peter Duesberg's, view that AIDS is not caused by the HIV virus. His views have generally won him the scorn of colleagues. Right or wrong, the article points out how little is actually known about the disease.

Shilts R: And the band played on: politics, people, and the AIDS epidemic, New York, 1987, St Martin's Press.
This article was written by an AIDS victim expressing his views concerning the political aspects of AIDS and the difficulties in receiving treatment.

ASSESSMENT ACTIVITY   9-1

Are You at Risk for a Sexually Transmitted Disease?

Directions: Review each of the sexual behaviors listed below. If you engage in any of the activities, assess your "personal" risk for contracting a sexually transmitted disease by checking the appropriate line.

Engage In	Activity	Risk	Precautions
_____	No sex	No risk: virtually no chance of getting an STD	No precautions necessary
_____	Sex with only one partner	Low risk: if both partners have no other sexual partners and no disease, there is almost no risk of getting an STD	Remain monogamous
_____	Sex with a variety of partners	High risk: each time there is another partner the risk increases	Choose partners carefully; use condoms and spermicides; wash after sex; do not douche; urinate after sex
_____	Your sex partner has sex with a variety of partners	High risk: the more partners the greater the risk he or she will transmit an STD to you	Be aware of symptoms (see above)
_____	Sex with someone who is or has been an IV drug user	High risk: if share needles, particularly of getting AIDS and hepatitis B	Know social and sexual history of partner (see above)
_____	Oral sex	No risk for Activity (1); little risk for Activity (2); high risk for Activities (3), (4), and 5	Know your partner; do not engage in oral sex if history is not known

After reviewing the different categories of activities, are there areas of concern for you?_____

Making a Decision

The decision to have sexual intercourse is a major one. There are many factors that affect this decision and many factors that will be affected by it. People engage in sexual activity for a variety of reasons often unrelated to love and often without regard to the consequences of that behavior.

Directions: Listed below are several factors that can influence or not influence your decision to engage in sexual activity. Rank each of these factors as to how they affect your behavior both now and when in a situation where you have to make this decision. This is an activity for your eyes only and is not one to be handed in so answer as truthfully as possible.

Factor	Not Important	Slightly Important	Important	Very Important	Extremely Important
Risk of AIDS					
Risk of other STD					
Risk of pregnancy					
Sexual history of partner					
Partner not an IV drug user					
Biological gratification (physical sensations)					
Need for money					
Desire to be accepted by partner/ cultural group					
Dissipation of stress or to get mind off other problems					
Intense need to feel loved/cared for					
Sign of commitment in a relationship					
Expression of love for partner					
Monogamous relationship					
Desire for a variety of partners					
Evidence of desirability					
Proof of sexual prowess					

In examining your responses, consider asking your potential partner to also take this assessment as a basis for a discussion on the advisability of engaging in sexual intercourse at this time with this person. As you assess your responses, note the factors that are important to you in making this decision.

What are the most important factors?_____

Does the person you are considering have sex with have any factors that you consider to be negative? What are they?_____

How important are these factors to you?_____

How severe are the potential consequences of you or your partner's ideas and/or actions?_____

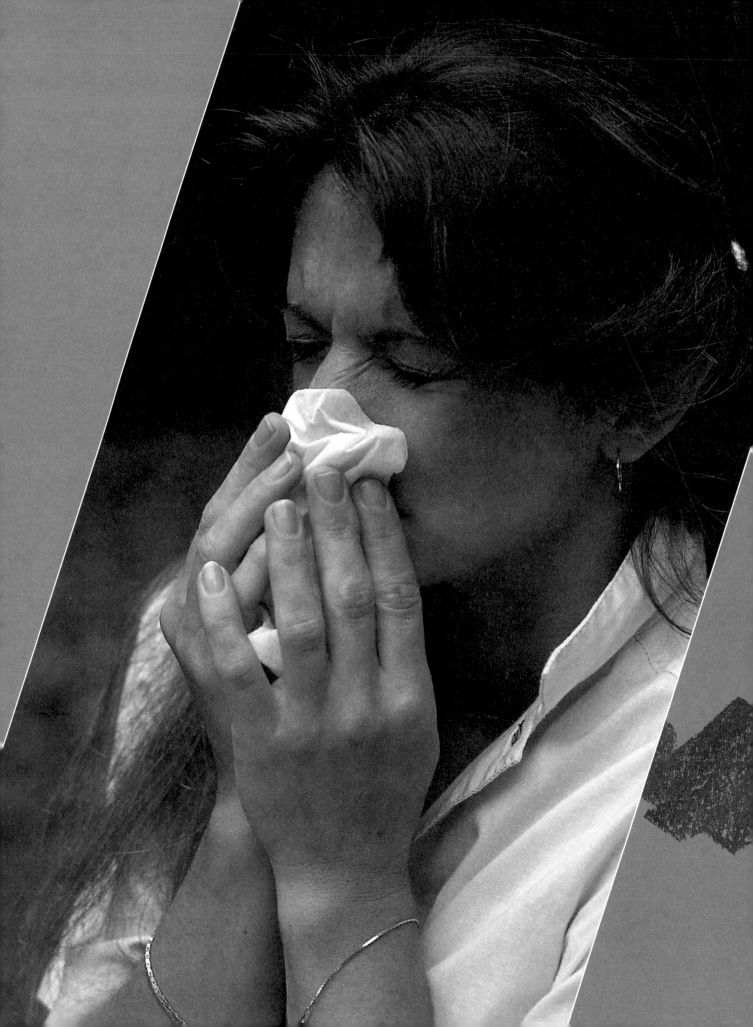

Chapter 10

Impact of Lifestyle on Common Conditions

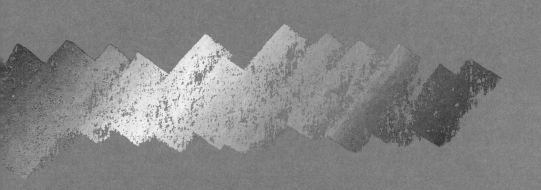

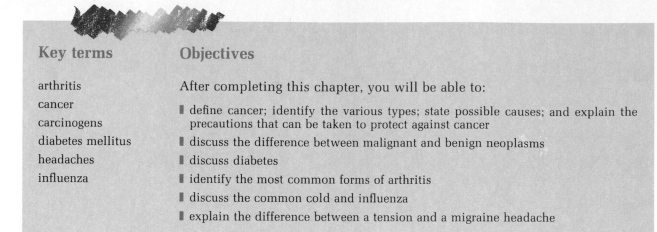

This chapter will focus on conditions that are detrimentally affected by lifestyle. If precautions are taken against the onset of these diseases, the impact of them on the body may be lessened or even avoided. While it is not possible to cover every condition that is affected by lifestyle, those that are found frequently and where lifestyle has the greatest impact are discussed. The diseases/conditions include cancer, diabetes, the common cold, headaches, and influenza. The effects of a positive lifestyle are primary in all of these, including the importance of early detection for optimal treatment.

Cancer

With the possible exception of AIDS, there is probably no disease that strikes more fear in peo-

ple than cancer. The term **cancer** refers to a group of diseases characterized by uncontrolled, disorderly cell growth. Although it strikes more frequently with advancing age, cancer causes the death of more children than any other disease. There are over 100 different kinds of cancers. Three out of ten Americans will develop the disease. While one out of every five people with cancer will die from it, it is important to remember that diagnosis of cancer does not have to mean a death sentence. The American Cancer Society estimates there are over 5 million Americans alive today who have a history of cancer. Three million of these are considered cured because they have survived for 5 years or more with no further symptoms of the disease.[1] It is possible to reduce the chances of developing cancer by assuming control of the things you do ev-

---

▮ **TABLE 10-1 Type of cancer and most common sites**

Type of cancer	Most common site	How spread
Carcinoma	Tissues covering body surfaces and lining the body cavities. Sites include the breast, lungs, intestines, skin, stomach, uterus, and testes.	Lymphatic and circulatory system
Sarcoma	The connective system. Sites include bones, muscle, and other connective tissue.	Circulatory system
Lymphomas	Develop in the lymphatic system, the infectious regions of the neck, armpits, groin, and chest. Hodgkin's disease is an example.	Lymph system
Leukemia	The blood-forming areas, bone marrow and spleen particularly. Characterized by abnormal increase in the number of white blood cells.	Circulatory system

ery day (see Figure 10-1).

Cell growth is controlled by DNA (deoxyribonucleic acid) and RNA (ribonucleic acid) in the nucleus of each cell in the body. If the nuclei lose the ability to regulate and control this growth, cellular metabolism and reproduction is disrupted and a mutant cell is produced that has a variation in form, quality, and function from the original. When a mass of these cells develop, it is called a neoplasm. A neoplasm, also called a tumor, may be either *malignant* (cancerous) or *benign* (noncancerous). A malignant neoplasm is the most dangerous and can become life-threatening quickly if not treated rapidly. Cancer cells have the ability to crowd out normal cells, invade surrounding tissue, and move through the lymphatic or circulatory system to infiltrate other areas of the body. The process by which cancerous cells spread from the original location to another location is called *metastasis*. This ability of cancerous cells to metastasize makes early detection critical. Benign tumors, on the other hand, are enclosed by a membrane that prevents them from invading other tissue. A benign tumor is not life threatening unless it is in an area that interferes with normal functioning. Table 10-1 contains types of cancer and where they are most often found.

Causes of Cancer

The causes of cancer are not understood. Correlations have been found linking cancer to everything from genetic factors to exposure to the sun's radiation. It is well established that there are many **carcinogens** (cancer causing agents) that trigger development of cancer. (Table 10-2

TABLE 10-2 Substances proven to be carcinogenic

Substance	Site of cancer
Aflatoxins	Liver
Alcohol	Liver, larynx, throat, esophagus, breast
Alkylating agents	Bladder, hematopoietic tissue
Anabolic steroids	Liver
Aromatic amines	Bladder
Arsenic	Skin and lung
Asbestos	Lung
Benzene	Bone marrow
Beryllium	Prostate
Bis(chloroethyl) ether	Bronchus
Bis(chloroethyl)sulfide	Respiratory tract
Cadmium	Prostrate
Chlornaphazine	Bladder
Chrome ores	Lung
Chloramphenicol, melphalan	Bone marrow
Coke (a type of coal)	Bronchus, lung
Diethylstilbestrol	Vagina
Immunosuppressive drugs	Lymphoid tissue
Nickel ores	Lung and nasal sinuses
Nitrates, nitrites, and nitrosamines	Stomach, liver, bladder, kidney
Oral contraceptives	Liver
Phenacetin (acetophenetidin)	Kidney
Radiation	Blood-forming areas
Soots, tars, and oils	Skin and lungs
Tobacco	Lungs, mouth, pharnynx, larynx, esophagus, bladder
Ultraviolet light	Skin
Vinyl chloride	Liver
Wood dust	Nasal sinuses
Wood and leather dust	Respiratory tract

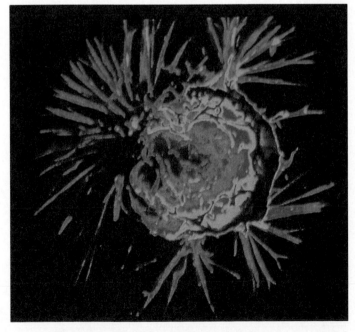

Cancer cells are distinctively different from normal cells in shape and size.

contains a list of substances known to be carcinogenic.) Although controversial, some scientists believe there is a genetic predisposition or connection for development of cancer.[2] Determining if cancer has been inherited, is a result of lifestyle, or is caused by environmental influences or some combination of these factors has not yet occurred. There is an increased probability for certain types of cancer to appear within families. If a woman's mother or sister has had breast cancer, she is at greater risk for developing this disease. It is also known that some cancers are sex related. A great majority of breast cancers occur in women. At one time men far exceeded women in lung cancer rates. However, until the 1960s smoking was not as common for women as for men.

Much research appears to link psychological states with the prevalence of disease in individuals. It has been postulated that people with positive, involved attitudes and who view life's twists and turns as opportunities for personal growth seem to have fewer diseases and recover from them more often. Individuals who feel lonely and depressed and lack appropriate social support have been shown to be more cancer-prone than their mentally healthy counterparts. However, a 1989 study from the National Institute on Aging found no relationship between attitude and development of cancer in 6403 individuals. While depression is not desirable, it is not necessarily a precursor to cancer.[2]

Although some of these concepts are controversial, it is generally accepted that substances

Figure 10-1 Five things to do and not do to prevent cancer

What to do

1. Eat more cabbage-type vegetables. Eat more broccoli, cauliflower and brussels sprouts. All cabbages and kale are examples. These vegetables protect against cancers of the colon, rectum, stomach and lung.
2. Add more high-fiber foods. Eat more peaches, strawberries, potatoes, spinach, tomatoes, wheat and bran cereals, rice, popcorn, and whole-wheat bread. Fiber protects against cancer of the colon.
3. Choose foods with Vitamin A. Eat more carrots, peaches, apricots, squash, and broccoli. Fresh foods are the best source. They are far better than vitamin pills. Vitamin A protects against cancers of the esophagus, larynx, and lung.
4. Choose foods with Vitamin C from grapefruit, cantaloupe, oranges, strawberries, red peppers, green peppers, broccoli, and tomatoes. These will help you fight against cancers of the esophagus and stomach.
5. Practice weight control. Plan to exercise and eat foods low in calories. A good exercise for most people is walking. Obese people have a high chance of getting cancers of the uterus, gallbladder, breast, and colon. Check with your doctor before you start an exercise program or a special diet.

Points to keep in mind: Not all of the DOs and DON'Ts are equal. Smoking is the most harmful risk. People who smoke and drink have an even greater cancer risk.

What to avoid

1. Trim fat from your diet. Eat lean meat, fish, low-fat dairy products. Cut extra fat off meats and skin poultry before cooking. Avoid pastry and candies. A high-fat diet raises the chance of getting cancer of the breast, colon, and prostrate. Calories loaded with fat cause weight gain.
2. Avoid salty foods. Stay away from nitrite-cured and smoked foods. Bacon, ham, hot dogs, and salt-cured fish are examples. People who eat these foods have a greater chance of getting cancers of the esophagus and stomach.
3. Stop smoking cigarettes. Smoking is the main cause of lung cancer. It causes three out of ten cancers. Pregnant women who smoke harm their babies. Parents who smoke at home cause breathing and allergy problems for kids. Chewing tobacco can cause cancers of the mouth and throat. Pick a day to quit and call the American Cancer Society for help.
4. Go easy on alcohol. If you drink a lot, you may get cancer of the liver. It is worse to smoke and drink. This increases the chances of getting cancers of the mouth, throat, larynx, and esophagus.
5. Avoid too much sun. It sun causes skin cancer and other damage to skin. Use a sunscreen. Wear long sleeves and a hat between 11 AM and 3 PM. Do not use indoor sunlamps, tanning parlors, or pills. Be alert for changes in a mole or sore that does not heal. If these occur, go to a doctor.

such as tobacco, tobacco smoke, alcohol, asbestos, herbicides, and pesticides are carcinogens. The National Academy of Sciences indicated in 1982 that diet was a factor in 60% of cancers in women and 40% in men. (Chapter 5 provides guidelines for cancer prevention as related to diet—also see Figure 10-1.) One of the major carcinogens may be radiation from the sun. People who, by nature of their occupation or for cosmetic purposes, have spent hours in the sun acquiring a tan have an increased risk for skin cancers (see Figure 10-2). Finally, as mentioned in

the previous chapter, the herpes viruses have been connected with cancer of the cervix. Viruses may be involved in the development of some forms of leukemia, Hodgkin's disease, and Burkett's lymphoma. The exact role of viruses in causing cancer is not known but it has been suggested that they provide an opportunistic environment for cancer development. Other researchers have suggested that it is a combination of factors, of which the virus may play a part, rather than the virus itself that causes a cancer.

Cancer Sites

The American Cancer Society reports each year on the incidence and number of deaths from cancer for a variety of sites (Figure 10-3). For both sexes the cancer that kills most often is lung cancer. For over 50 years breast cancer was the major cause of cancer deaths in women. An increase in lung cancer for women is directly attributed to the rise in the number of women smokers.

The breasts are still the most prevalent site for females and the prostate is the leading cancer site for males. In 1989 it was estimated that 103,000

Figure 10-2 Skin cancer—the case against too much sun

Every year more than 400,00 Americans are diagnosed with skin cancer. Fortunately this type cancer is the easiest to detect and most forms can be treated successfully. The most important risk factor for skin cancer is excessive exposure to the sun. The types of skin cancer are:

▌ **Basal cell carcinoma:** This type of skin cancer is the most common of the three types of skin cancer. Basal cell carcinoma grows slowly and usually does not spread to other areas of the body.

▌ **Squamous cell carcinoma:** This is the second most frequent type. Like basal cell cancer, squamous cell rarely spreads to distant organs but it does grow faster than the basal cell kind.

▌ **Malignant melanoma:** A much less common form of skin cancer, melanoma can be very dangerous if not detected and treated early. Every year about 22,000 people develop melanoma and approximately 5500 die from it. No one is immune, although darker skinned individuals who seldom sunburn are at less risk. Melanoma has a strong tendency to spread to other areas of the body. Melanoma may appear suddenly without warning or it may begin near a mole or other dark spot in the skin. Some birthmarks or congenital moles carry an increased risk and should be observed closely for changes. Excessive exposure to the sun increases the risk, especially for individuals who have been severely sunburned in their teens or twenties.

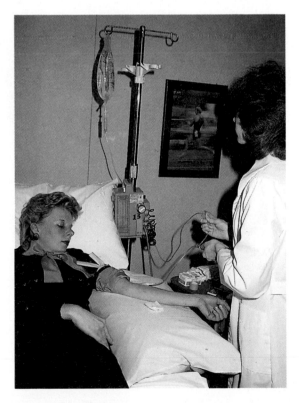

Treatment for cancer includes the use of chemotherapy.

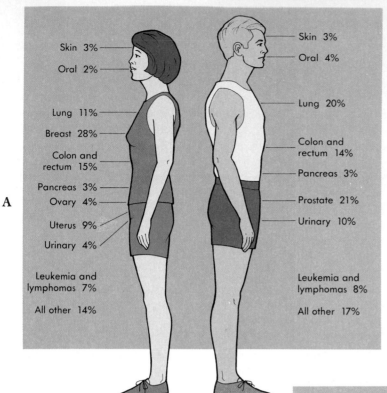

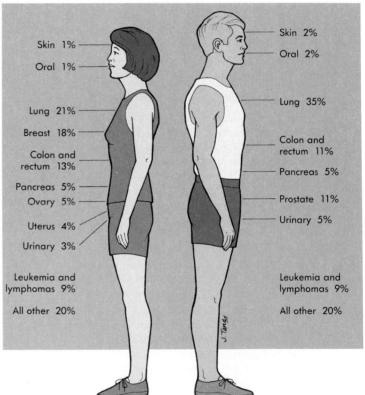

Figure 10-3 Cancer incidence (A) and death (B) by site and sex—1989 estimates

new cases of prostate cancer would be reported. For any cancer, early detection is imperative. Figures 10-4, 10-5, and 10-6 provide suggestions for check-ups for prevention and early detection

Treatment

Treatment of cancer is constantly undergoing change. Cancer is often treated surgically. A sur-geon removes the malignant tissue plus some additional normal tissue. Today, the tendency is to remove less surrounding normal tissue and combine surgery with *chemotherapy* and/or *radiotherapy*. Radiotherapy is the use of radiation to either destroy cancer cells or destroy their reproductive mechanism so they cannot replicate. This treatment can cause unpleasant side effects such as diarrhea, itching, and difficulty of swallowing. When cancer has spread throughout the body, chemotherapy is used. Chemotherapy is the use of drugs and hormones to treat such cancers as acute leukemia and testicular cancer. There are about 50 anticancer drugs in use.

The latest technique for treating cancer is *immunotherapy*. This process involves stimulating the body's immune system to help destroy malignant growths. Interferon and interleukin-2 (proteins produced by the body to protect against viral invasions of healthy cells) are being researched in this capacity. Interferon is used for treatment of a rare blood cancer called *hairy cell leukemia*. Interleukin-2 is under study in the treatment of kidney cancer and melanoma.[1]

Figure 10-4 Cancer-related checkup guidelines

Listed below are the guidelines for healthy people for early cancer detection. These are guidelines not rules. They apply only if none of the seven warning signs are present. The seven warning signs are:

C hange in bowel or bladder habits
A sore throat that doesn't heal
U nusual bleeding or discharge
T hickening or lump in breast or elsewhere
 I ndigestion or difficulty in swallowing
O bvious change in wart or moles
N agging cough or hoarseness

Checkups for healthy people:

▎A cancer-related checkup that includes the thyroids, testes, prostate, mouth, ovaries, skin, and lymph nodes
    Every 3 to 4 years for people age 20 to 40
    Every year for people age 40 and over
▎Breast
    Examination by a physician every 3 to 4 years for people age 20 to 40
    Self-examination every month regardless of age
    Baseline mammogram for people age 35 to 39, every 2 for people up to age 50 and annually after 50
▎Uterus
    Pelvic exam every 3 years for people age 20 to 40
    Annual pelvic exam after age 40
▎Cervix
    Minimum of once every 3 years after two negative tests 2 years in a row for people age 20 to 40
    Pap test following same guidelines as for cervical exam if under 20 and sexually active
    Unless at high risk because of family history, multiple sex partners, or early age of first intercourse, for people age 40 and over same guidelines as for cervical exam
▎Testes
    Self-examination every month for people age 20 and over
▎Colon and Rectal
    Digital rectal examination every year for people of both sexes age 40 and over
    Stool blood test annually for people of both sexes age 50 and over
    Proctology exam every 3 to 5 years after two negative annual examinations for people age 50 and over

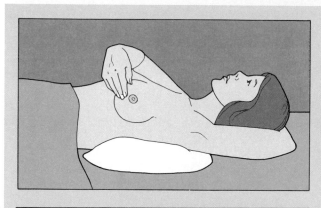

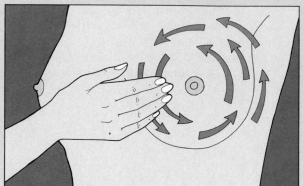

Figure 10-5 Breast self-examination

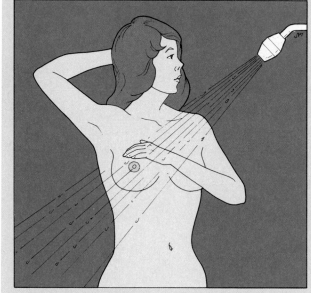

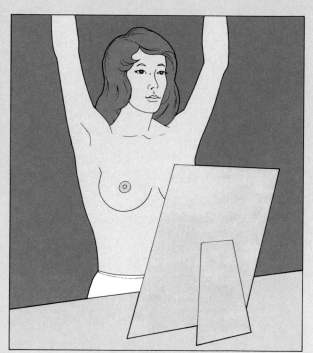

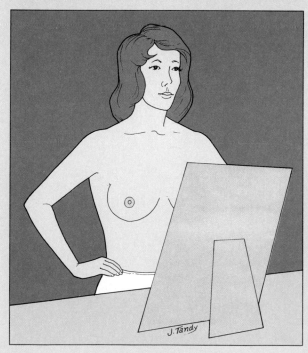

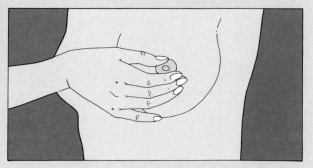

J. Tandy

Figure 10-5 Breast self-examination—cont'd

1 Lying in bed, place a pillow under one shoulder to elevate and flatten breast. Examine each breast using the opposite hand, first with arm under head and again with arm at side.
2 Make small rotary motions with flat pads (not tips) of fingers.
3 Palpate breasts in concentric circles from rim inward toward nipple. Feel for knots, lumps, thickenings indentations, or swellings. Be sure to include armpit.
4 In shower, wet, soapy skin makes it easier to feel lumps. Keep one hand overhead and examine each breast with opposite hand.
5 In front of a large mirror, stand arms relaxed at sides. Examine breasts for swelling, dimpling, bulges, retractions, irritations, sores, or changes in mole or nipple color, texture, or orientation. Repeat with arms extended, and again with arms clasped behind head.

6 Repeat inspection in step 5 while contracting chest muscles: first clasp hands in front of forehead, squeezing palms together, then place palms flat on sides of hips pressing downward. This highlights bulges, indentations, etc. which may signal growth of tumors.
7 Bend forward from hips, resting hands on knees or two chair backs. Use mirror to examine breasts for normal irregularities and abnormal variances; both are pronounced in this position.
8 Squeeze nipples to inspect for secretions/discharge.
9 Report any suspicious findings to your doctor without delay.
10 Supplement your self-examination with a breast exam by your doctor as part of a regular physical exam and cancer checkup.

Figure 10-6 Testicular self-examination

Cancer of the testes-the male reproductive glands-is one of the most common cancers in men 15 to 34 years of age. It accounts for 12% of cancer deaths in this group. The best hope for early detection of testicular cancer is a simple three minute monthly self-examination. The best time is after a warm bath or shower when the scrotal skin is most relaxed.

Roll each testicle gently between the thumb and fingers of both hands. If you find any hard lumps or nodules, see your doctor promptly. They may not be malignant, but only a doctor can make the diagnosis.

Following a thorough physical examination, your doctor may perform X-ray studies for the most accurate diagnosis.

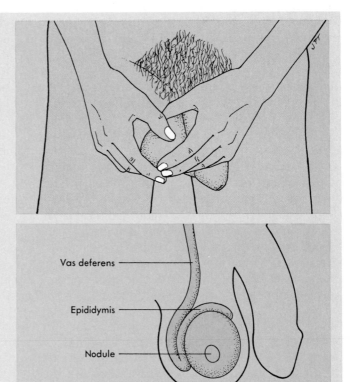

Diabetes Mellitus

Diabetes mellitus is a metabolic disorder involving the *pancreas*. The pancreas fails to produce an *enzyme* called insulin. (An enzyme is a complex protein capable of inducing changes in other substances without undergoing changes themselves.) A lack of insulin results in an inability to store or use *glucose*, the blood sugar the body uses as its primary energy source. As a result, diabetics cannot use the energy they consume and high glucose levels build up in the blood and urine, a condition known as *hyperglycemia.* Large amounts of sugar in urine require additional water so the sugar can be diluted for elimination. The increased need by the body for water leads to a depletion of the body water stores, causing excessive thirst and frequent urination. When the body becomes unable to completely break glucose down as a source of energy, fat must be used. Fat is metabolized differently than glucose and its breakdown is incomplete when glucose is not available. Incomplete metabolism causes an excess amount of chemicals called ketone bodies to build up in body. The buildup of ketones is used to perform the functions that glucose would perform under normal conditions (supplying energy), but the excess amounts of ketone bodies disrupt the body's chemical balance, altering the blood's chemistry, and making it more acidic. Acidic conditions in the body are extremely hazardous to health.

Diabetes can be a serious disorder. Symptoms include excessive thirst, increased urination, hunger, a tendency to tire easily, wounds that heal slowly, blurred vision, and frequent skin, vaginal, or urinary tract infections. Dehydration and build-up of ketones can result in *ketoacidosis* (the accumulation of ketones) and can cause nausea, vomiting, abdominal pain, lethargy, and drowsiness. This often leads to severe sickness, coma, and even death. Of equal significance is that prolonged periods of elevated glucose levels disrupt normal enzyme and membrane functions. Chronic complications that may result include eye disease, kidney disorders, painful nerve and muscle symptoms, and decreased circulation. Diabetes is a leading cause of foot or leg amputations. Diabetes can also produce impotence in males, chronic diarrhea, and increased risk of heart disease and heart attacks in both sexes. Of the 10 to 11 million people with diabetes in the United States, nearly 4 million are unaware they have it. By the time individuals realize they have this condition, they may have already suffered severe consequences.[4]

While there are varying degrees of diabetes, it is generally divided into two diagnostic categories. Type I diabetes is insulin-dependent diabetes. Initial onset of type I diabetes occurs most commonly in children and young adults, although it may develop at any age. Symptoms may be quite sudden and sometimes progress rapidly, requiring quick intervention in order not to be fatal. Type I diabetics produce little or no insulin and require insulin injections to function. Before insulin was discovered, the average life span for a type I diabetic was 2 years after diagnosis. Properly treated, these people can now live almost as long as the general population.

Type II diabetes is found primarily in individuals over the age of 40. Type II diabetics have either developed a resistance to insulin activity or experience insufficient insulin action. Their bodies are usually capable of producing adequate amounts of insulin—something a type I diabetic cannot do. The difficulty in type II diabetes is that body cells become resistant to insulin at the receptor sites (the place where insulin attaches to the cell). Type II diabetes is linked so strongly to obesity that it can be considered a symptom.[5] Eighty per cent of all type II diabetics are overweight at the time of diagnosis. The chance of developing type II diabetes doubles with every 20% of excess weight.[6] Primarily, and often the only, treatment necessary for type II diabetics is weight loss, although some individuals will still require medication or injections of insulin to help control the condition.

The causes of diabetes are not known. It has long been thought that type I diabetes was genetically linked, but this may not be as strong a connection as originally believed. There seem to be a number of factors, including viral infections, chemical injury, or other environmental components, associated with the development of diabetes. The predominant factor with type II diabetes is obesity.

There is no cure for diabetes. Many individuals with type II diabetes can control the disease through weight loss, exercise, and adequate nutrition. It is estimated that 50% to 85% of all complications of diabetes are preventable or treatable, but diagnosis and proper treatment are necessary. Negligence of diabetes and its complications may result in early death.

Arthritis

Arthritis is an inflammatory disease of the joints. There are over 100 varieties of arthritis including gout, ankylosing spendylitis, systemic lupus erythemotosis, osteoarthritis, and rheumatoid arthritis. Osteoarthritis and rheumatoid arthritis are found most often. Both result in pain and deformed joints.

Osteoarthritis is the most common form of arthritis. It is characterized by deterioration of the articular cartilage that covers the gliding surfaces of the bones in certain joints. The cartilage develops small cracks, leading to erosion of the cartilage and causing localized inflammation and painful motion.[7] The deterioration associated with osteoarthritis seems to be related to the wear and tear of daily living, age, and injury. Other factors may include heredity, diet, abnormal use of joints (for example, throwing a curve ball year after year), or an impaired blood supply to affected joints. Disability most often afflicts the weight-bearing joints of the ankles, knees, hips, and spine. Treatment for osteoarthritis includes aspirin and cortisone drugs to relieve pain. Sometimes mild exercise, heat, cold, or a combination of heat and cold application accompanied by massage are used as treatment. Exercise is used for therapeutic purposes to help maintain range-of-motion and to strengthen the muscles that can help alleviate joint problems. Exercise is usually prescribed by a physical therapist. Occasionally, surgery is employed to replace joints or repair tendons and ligaments.

Rheumatoid arthritis is found three times more often among women than men. Onset of rheumatoid arthritis is usually between the ages of 20 and 50. While the exact causes are unknown, it is theorized that this form of arthritis is an *autoimmune disease* (one in which there is an immune response against the cells of a person's body). Symptoms of rheumatoid arthritis include joint swelling, redness, stiffness, pain, muscle atrophy, joint deformity, and limited mobility. The condition is unpredictable since it can suddenly flare up and just as suddenly go into remission. Many times emotional stress is associated with an attack. The frequently disease results in disability. Treatment for rheumatoid arthritis is the same as for osteoarthritis. Emphasis is placed on relieving the pain and improving mobility.

The Common Cold

There are over 110 viruses, known as rhinoviruses, that can cause the *common cold*. An individual may develop a temporary immunity to one or two viruses and still be infected by another one. Any time people are together, viruses causing the common cold are present. Colds can be contracted by shaking hands, sneezing, or breathing. Evidence indicates that hand-to-hand contact is the main way a cold is spread. As infected individuals blow or touch their noses, the virus is transferred to their hands. When an uninfected person touches the infected person's hands, the virus is again transferred to the uninfected individual. Touching the face with hands that carry the virus leads directly to developing a cold. Frequent hand washing may prevent the spread of the virus.

The signs and symptoms of a cold are readily recognizable. They include a feeling of listlessness, general aches and pains, watery eyes, and

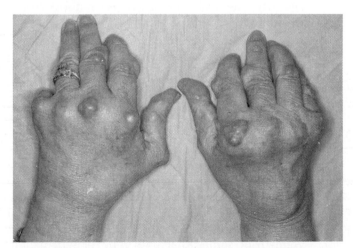

Rheumatoid arthritis can be very painful and disfiguring.

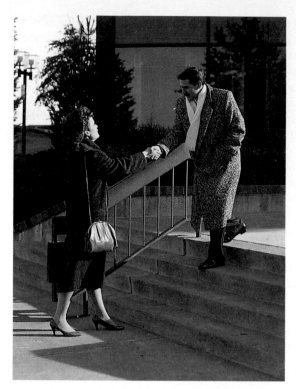

The common cold is spread most often by hand-to-hand contact.

runny nasal passages. As the cold progresses, the nasal membranes swell, resulting in a stuffy nose. Infections affecting the throat can lead to sore throats and coughing. These symptoms tend to last 7 to 10 days. As an old axiom points out, if a cold is treated it will go away in 7 days and left alone, it will last a week.

Antibiotics are of no help in curing the common cold since they only affect bacterial infections. Over-the-counter nasal sprays may offer temporary relief, but should be avoided since they can create additional swelling in the nasal passages when the effects of the spray wear off (known as a rebound effect). Nasal sprays can also become habit forming if used for prolonged periods. Research is being conducted with interferon to prevent colds.[8] Interferon is a protein manufactured by the immune system after a virus has invaded an organism. It prevents the spread of a virus to cells adjacent to infected cells.[8] It is being used by people to whom a cold poses significant danger, such as patients receiving chemotherapy for cancer, the elderly, and transplant patients. Interferon has not been approved for sale at this time. The best advice for treating a

cold is still to take aspirin (or ibuprofen or acetaminophen), drink plenty of liquid, eat a nutritious diet, and get plenty of rest.

While cough syrups may offer temporary relief, many physicians question the effectiveness of these products. Cough syrups fall into two groups: suppressants and expectorants. Suppressants turn off the brain's cough center while an expectorant supposedly loosens phlegm. It is particularly important for people suffering from emphysema or other chronic lung condition to avoid using suppressants.

Influenza

Influenza, or "flu," is also caused by a virus. There are three primary strains of the influenza virus: A, B, and C. Most influenza develops from the A and B strains. These strains have the capacity to change genetically, reappearing in an altered form every few years. Symptoms of all types of flu are similar and include chills, fever, weakness, headache, sore throat, dry cough, nausea, vomiting, and muscular aches and pains. All symptoms may not be present and the severity varies greatly from person to person. Treatment for flu is the same as for the common cold. Aspirin should not be taken by children or teenagers since the potentially fatal Reye's syndrome can develop.

Vaccines are available that can prevent a particular type of influenza. Current recommendations are that priority should be given to children and adults with chronic cardiovascular and lung disorders, residents of nursing homes, medical personnel who may transmit the virus to high risk patients, everyone over 65, and anyone with conditions such as diabetes, kidney disease, hereditary anemias, and impaired natural immunity.[9]

Headaches

One of the conditions causing great discomfort to people is the headache. Some **headaches** may be the result of injury or brain disease, but most are caused by distress, tension, and anxiety. *Tension headaches* are the most common. Caused by involuntary contractions of the scalp, head, and neck muscles, tension headaches may be precipitated by anxiety, stress, or allergic reactions. Tension headaches can often be relieved by massaging the scalp and muscles in the neck. Aspirin or some other pain reliever will usually alleviate a tension headache.

Migraine headaches are characterized by throbbing pain that can last for hours or even days. Nausea and vomiting occasionally occur. Migraines seem to be initiated by stress and range from mild to severe. The exact cause of migraines is unknown, but it is thought they originate with spasms in the arteries near the surface of the brain.[10] People who experience migraines may have advance warning symptoms, such as dizziness, sensitivity to flashing lights, the appearance of a blind spot, or an indescribable feeling that a head ache is coming. Techniques such as deep breathing, progressive relaxation, biofeedback, meditation, and visualization seem to help relieve the pain associated with migraines.

People who have symptoms and know a migraine is coming may be able to avoid it by taking medications that contain ergot alkaloids. Beta blockers (used to treat angina) may also be helpful.

Cluster headaches are similar to migraines but are characterized by intense pain in the nostril and either the right or left eye. The eye and nose water and the skin over the throbbing area may become red. The person suffering from cluster headaches may experience pain for weeks or even months. Each headache usually lasts 2 to 3 hours. Individuals may be symptom free for weeks or months. There is some association of cluster headaches with stress, overwork, or emotional trauma.[11]

Summary

▌ Cancer is a group of diseases characterized by uncontrolled, disorderly cell growth.

▌ When the DNA and/or RNA in the nucleus of each cell lose the ability to regulate and control cellular metabolism, mutant cells develop. A mass of mutant cells is a neoplasm and may be either malignant or benign.

▌ The process by which cancerous cells spread from their original location to another location is called metastasis.

▌ Carcinogens are agents that trigger the development of cancer. The tendency to develop cancer has been linked to genetics, stress, and psychological outlook, as well as carcinogens.

▌ The cancer site that has the highest incident of death in males and females is the lungs. This is followed by the prostate for males and breasts for women.

▌ Cancer may be treated surgically, often in combination with chemotherapy and radiotherapy. A relatively new technique involves immunotherapy.

▌ Diabetes is a metabolic disorder where the pancreas either fails to produce sufficient insulin, resulting in a lack of glucose, or the receptor sites become less sensitive. This inability can lead to a number of conditions, including ketoacidosis that may result in death.

▌ Hyperglycemia is a condition where large amounts of sugar build up in the blood.

▌ There are two major categories of diabetes. Type I usually occurs early in life and requires insulin injections. Type II is found mainly in obese individuals over 40. Most type II diabetics can control their condition without insulin injections.

▌ Arthritis is an inflammatory disease of the joints. The most common form of arthritis is osteoarthritis, which is characterized by deterioration of the cartilage covering the surfaces of the bones in certain joints.

▌ It is believed that rheumatoid arthritis is a disease of the immune system that results in joint swelling, pain, deformity, and decreased mobility.

▌ The common cold is caused by rhinoviruses, of which there are over 110 varieties. Antibiotics do not cure colds.

▌ Influenza is caused by only three strains of virus, but these agents have the ability to change and reappear is different forms from year to year. Since influenza can range widely in severity, certain high risk groups are encouraged to have an annual flu vaccine.

▌ Headaches are divided into three categories—tension, cluster, and migraine. People who experience migraines can use techniques such as deep breathing and meditation to alleviate or prevent onset of a headache.

Action plan for personal wellness

An important consideration in assuming responsibility for the individual's own quality of life is using information. After reading this chapter, answer the following questions and determine an action plan for enhancing your own lifestyle.

1 Based on the information presented in this chapter, along with what I know about my family's health history, the health problems or issues that I need to be most concerned about are:_____
_____
_____

2 Of those health concerns listed in number 1, the one I most need to act on is:_____
_____
_____

3 Possible actions that I can take to improve my level of wellness are (try to be as specific as possible):_____
_____
_____

4 Of the actions listed in number 3, the one that I most need to include in an action plan is:_____
_____
_____

5 Factors I need to keep in mind to be successful in my action plan are:_____
_____
_____

Review Questions

1. Describe the process by which cancer cells develop. What characteristics differentiate cancer cells from other cells?

2. List and explain the factors that possibly contribute to development of cancer. What are the leading types and sites for cancer in males and females?

3. Explain how type I and type II diabetes differ and describe the symptoms of each? What can happen when these symptoms are ignored? What are some of the factors that contribute to type II diabetes?

4. What is arthritis? Explain the differences in the two most common forms of the condition, their causes, and the preferred methods of treatment.

5. What causes colds? What are some of the methods being used to treat colds?

6. Influenza viruses act somewhat differently than the viruses that cause colds. How many are there and how do they differ from cold viruses? Why should children not be given aspirin when suffering from influenza?

7. Explain the difference between tension headaches and migraine headaches. How do the causes, symptoms, and treatments differ?

References

1. American Cancer Society: Cancer Facts and Figures-1989, Atlanta, Ga, 1989, The Society, p. 3.
2. Is There a Cancer Personality?: The Johns Hopkins Medical Letter, Health After 50 2:1, Mar 1990.
3. Krontirus TG: The emergency genetics of human cancer, New England J of Med 309(4):404, 1983.
4. Payne W and Hahn D: Understanding your health, 1989, St. Louis, Times Mirror/Mosby College Publishing.
5. Diabetes Mellitus, CareFast, 1:3, May 1989, p. 3.
6. Hamrick M, Anspaugh D, and Ezell G: Health, Columbus, Ohio: Charles E. Merrill, 1986, p. 665.
7. Osteoarthritis: Daly City, Calif, 1988, Krames Communications, Patient Information Library.
8. Interferon-Can it Prevent the Common Cold?: Mayo Clinic Health Letter 5:6, 1987.
9. This is a Good Time to Get Your Flu Shot: Mayo Clinic Health Letter 4:8, 1986.
10. Headaches: Harvard Medical School Health Letter 12:5-7, 1987.
11. Taber's Cyclopedic Medical Dictionary, Philadelphia, Pa, 1986, FA Davis Co.

Annotated Readings

Boly W: Cancer, Inc., Hippocrates, January/February 1989, pp. 38-48.
A group of rebel scientists are selling innovative treatments for cancer. If a person is willing to pay the extreme costs of the treatments they can be a guinea pig. It is expensive, but it just might work!

Rados B: And here's help-Modern pharmacy's answers to chicken soup, FDA Consumer, November 1988, pp. 7-13.
The FDA reviewed nonprescription (over the counter) cough and cold remedies and reported that the discomfort associated with colds can be eased.

Roach M: How I blew my summer vacation, In Health, January/February 1990, pp. 72-80.
Describes the author's visit to a common cold unit in England. She discovers many of the myths concerning the common cold, and her lack of immunity to the Coronavirus.

Yulsman T: Sweet news on the sugar disease, American Health, April 1987, pp. 57-59.
Emphasizes the government report that clearly indicates that if there is a history of diabetes in a family, the offspring in that family should maintain proper weight, and exercise regularly to maintain a healthy lifestyle and prevent diabetes.

Cancer Awareness Inventory

This inventory was developed to help with early detection and treatment of cancer. It is a collection of the common symptoms for various cancer sites. If you have symptoms, check with your physician. The chances are that you will not have cancer but these symptoms do suggest a potential problem with your health. It is always wise to be safe and consult your physician when you are assuming self-responsibility for your health.

Directions: For each cancer site check any of the symptoms you experience.

Are you experiencing . . .	Do you have symptoms?

Bladder

1. Blood in urine? _____
2. Unusual change in bladder habits? _____
3. Discomfort in urination? _____
4. Change in flow in urination? _____
5. An urge to urinate more frequently? _____

Bone

1. Pain in the bone or joint? _____
2. Swelling in the bone or joint? _____
3. Unusual warmth in the bone or joint? _____
4. Protruding veins along the bone or joint? _____

Breast

1. Thickening or lump in the breast? _____
2. Lump under the arm? _____
3. Thickening or reddening of the skin of the breast? _____
4. Puckering or dimpling of the skin of the breast? _____
5. Nipple discharge? _____
6. Inverted nipple, if nipple was previously erect? _____
7. Persistent pain and tenderness of the breast? _____
8. Unusual changes in the nipple and areolae? _____
9. Benign breast lumps? _____

Colon/Rectum

1. Continuous constipation or diarrhea? _____
2. Rectal bleeding? _____
3. Change in bowel habit? _____
4. An increase in intestinal gas? _____
5. Abdominal discomfort? _____

Lung

1. An unusual cough? _____
2. Shortness of breath? _____
3. Sputum streaked with blood? _____
4. Chest pain? _____
5. Recurring attacks of pneumonia or bronchitis? _____

Lymphomas

1. Painless enlargement of a lymph node or cluster of lymph nodes? _____
2. Profuse sweating and fever? _____
3. Weight loss? _____
4. Unexplained weakness? _____
5. Unusual itching? _____

Oral

1. A sore in the mouth that does not heal?
2. Lump or thickening that bleeds easily?   _____
3. Difficulty in chewing or swallowing food?   _____
4. The sensation of something in the throat?   _____
5. Restricted movement of the tongue or jaw?   _____
6. Poor oral hygiene?   _____

Prostate

1. Weak or interrupted flow or urine?   _____
2. Inability to urinate or difficulty in starting urination?   _____
3. A need to urinate frequently, especially at night?   _____
4. Blood in urine?   _____
5. Urine flow that is not easily stopped?   _____
6. Painful or burning urination?   _____
7. Continuing pain in lower back, pelvis, or upper thighs?   _____

Skin

1. Obvious change in wart or mole?   _____
2. Unusual skin condition?   _____
3. Chronic swelling, redness, or warmth of the skin?   _____
4. Unexplained itching?   _____
5. Overexposure to the ultraviolet rays of the sun?   _____

Testicular

1. An enlargement and change in the consistency of the testes?   _____
2. A dull ache in the lower abdomen and groin?   _____
3. Sensation of dragging and heaviness?   _____
4. Difficulty with ejaculation?   _____

Thyroid

1. A lump or mass in the neck?   _____
2. Persistent hoarseness?   _____
3. Difficulty in swallowing?   _____
4. Overexposure to head and neck X-ray treatments?   _____

Uterine/cervical (women only)

1. Irregular bleeding?   _____
2. Unusual vaginal discharge?   _____
3. Positive Pap smear, Class 2 to 5, some signs of abnormality? _____
4. Recurring herpes simplex virus?   _____
5. Fibroid tumors of the uterus?   _____

Application

   Any statement you have checked should be carefully evaluated. Chances are that you do not have cancer, but only a physician can determine the problem. If the symptom appears severe (for example, blood in the stool) see a physician immediately. However, pain in a joint may be observed for a short period to see if there is improvement. Never wait longer than 2 weeks to see a physician if the symptom persists for that long.

1. How many symptoms have I checked?_____

2. How serious do these symptoms seem?_____

3. Should I see a physician now or wait?_____

ASSESSMENT ACTIVITY

10-2

Are You at Risk for Diabetes?

Directions: Check the appropriate column in response to the questions below to assess your probability of having diabetes. The more questions that are answered with a *yes*, the higher the probability you have of being diabetic.

	Yes	No
1. Is there a history of diabetes in your family?	_____	_____
2. Do you tire quickly or seem to always be fatigued?	_____	_____
3. Do you urinate frequently?	_____	_____
4. Are you constantly thirsty?	_____	_____
5. Is your vision blurry?	_____	_____
6. Have you suddenly lost weight?	_____	_____
7. Are you overweight?	_____	_____
8. Do you eat excessively?	_____	_____
9. Do wounds heal slowly?	_____	_____
10. Is your skin frequently itchy?	_____	_____

Taken alone, any *yes* answer does not necessarily indicate you are a diabetic. However, if you have answered *yes* more than five times, consult your physician for a urine test.

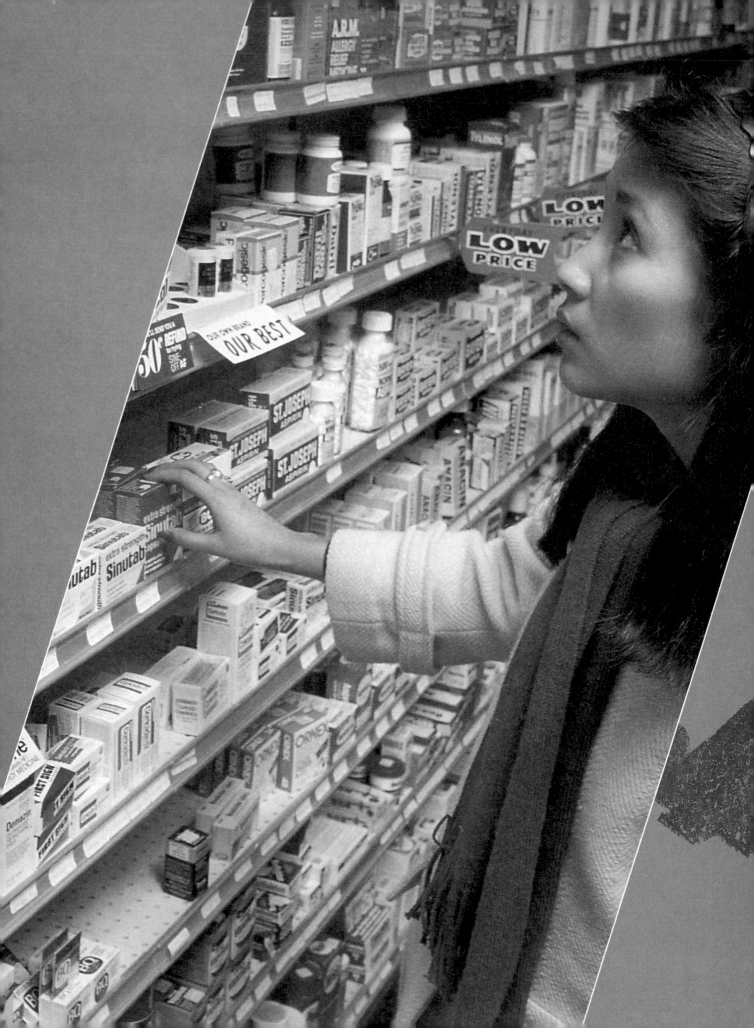

Chapter 11

Self-Responsibility in the Health-Care Market

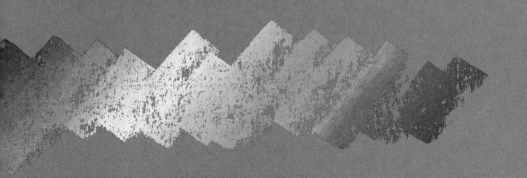

Key terms	Objectives

Key terms

contraindications

deceptive advertising

diagnostic laboratory tests

health maintenance organization (HMO)

immunization

implied consent

informed consent

primary-care physician

reliability

selective health examinations

validity

Objectives

After completing this chapter, you will be able to:

▮ Explain how to evaluate the accuracy and validity of health information

▮ Discuss criteria to consider in determining when, where, and how to choose health care

▮ Describe the functions and purposes of the three major components of a physical examination

Traditionally, Americans have adopted a rather passive attitude toward their use of health care. Whether it's taking medicine, purchasing health-care products, undergoing surgery, or having a diagnostic test administered, the general attitude was simply to follow orders. Fortunately, this attitude is changing. People are beginning to view themselves as active participants in their health care. They are asking questions, placing demands on *health care providers* (people and/or facilities which provide health care services), getting second opinions, and sometimes even refusing treatments. People now seem to realize that they must assume more responsibility for safeguarding their health. With this responsibility, however, comes the awesome challenge of knowing what people can and should do for themselves. The purpose of this chapter, therefore, is to lay the groundwork for becoming an informed, active participant in the health-care marketplace.

Understanding Health Information

The first, and perhaps most difficult, challenge for each of us is to make sense out of what is commonly called the health information explosion. So much is written about health by so many people that it is virtually impossible to keep abreast of all the new information. Many popular magazines regularly print health articles; newspapers often devote entire sections to medicine;

the publications of health newsletters abound; television programs feature numerous health stories; and a plethora of scientific health-related studes are published daily. Interest in health information appears to have reached an all-time high.

The availability of so much health information does not occur without its drawbacks. The major drawback is that so much of the information is confusing, sometimes even contradictory. Even medical experts have trouble separating fact from fiction. It is not unusual to see some new finding headlined one day and completely refuted the next. It is increasingly difficult to know what or whom to believe. For some people the ubiquity of refutations and contradictions leads to an attitude sometimes referred to as *health fatalism*, which maintains that nothing can be believed. People with a fatalistic view disregard health information because they believe that new findings will inevitably disagree with facts previously accepted as true.

Several examples illustrate this point. Cyclamate at one time was considered a safe sugar substitute. In 1969, however, an experiment seemed to show that rats in which cyclamate pellets had been surgically implanted were more likely to develop tumors. A health *hysteria cycle* followed. The cycle began with press releases suggesting that an artificial food ingredient was poisonous. These charges were based on data that could not be replicated but they still created a fear that forced the chemical off the market. After 17 years of research in which the National Cancer Institute fed a group of monkeys enough cyclamate to sweeten 150 cans of soda per animal per week, cyclamate was proven to be safe. Rather than developing tumors, the monkeys flourished. Research proved that cyclamate is safe. The cycle ends when cyclamates return to the shelves of U.S. stores—years after it has been legally sold in other countries.

Cholesterol is another good example. Few, if any, risk factors related to heart disease has received so much publicity. At one time the evidence was so convincing that many people formed a simple cause-effect relationship between cholesterol and atherosclerosis. Later studies, however, proved that some people with high blood cholesterol didn't have atherosclerosis. Conversely, some people with low blood cholesterol had advanced cases of atherosclerosis. The hysteria surrounding cholesterol finally gave way to the discovery of the high-density and low-density lipoprotein theory of heart disease.

What is the point of these examples? It would be a serious mistake to conclude that since the initial claims about cyclamates and cholesterol weren't completely and entirely true that all health information cannot be trusted. Such a conclusion would reflect a fatalistic attitude, which is not conducive to a healthy perspective towards life. Perhaps a more appropriate approach would be to adopt a skeptical and suspicious attitude, especially toward health claims which appear to be extreme and sensational. Remember that the First Amendment to the U.S. Constitution, which guarantees freedom of the press, also guarantees Americans the right to publish health distortions. Just because something is printed doesn't make it true. Publishers are not obligated to prove that their claims about health are true. It is just as important to discriminate in your search for valid and reliable information as it is to shop for products and services.

Guidelines for Evaluating Health Information

Application of the guidelines which follow should help facilitate a discriminating search for correct health information.

Avoid Jumping to Conclusions

Most health misinformation is actually based on facts, not lies. The problem is that facts get exaggerated and sometimes lead people to wrong conclusions. This happens many times because much health literature is based on research involving statistical *relationships* or associations between two or more events. Relationships are helpful clues to health but they can not and do not establish *cause and effect* relationships. The mistake many people make is to read and/or hear about a new health finding and erroneously conclude that one event causes the other (in other words, cause and effect).

A good example is provided by Vickery in the popular newsletter *Taking Care*. "The first physicians who investigated malaria concluded that it was caused by damp, stale air because it was more likely to occur in low-lying, swampy areas. It was several hundred years before it was demonstrated that it was a malaria parasite caused by mosquitoes which caused malaria. Malaria, mosquitoes, and bad air are all associated with each other, but these associations do not prove that any one factor caused any of the others."[1]

One of the areas most commonly abused by reference to cause and effect relationships is cancer. Hardly a week passes without someone suggesting that something will cause or cure cancer based on an association they have discovered in the medical literature. The association may appear significant, but the suggestion of cause and effect is usually wishful thinking.

It is important to remember that relationships are based on statistical procedures. While these relationships may provide a basis for better understanding health concerns, they usually fall short of supporting many of the sweeping generalizations and conclusions that make headlines in the media.

Beware of Oversimplifications

In our desire to make sense out of the complex world of health and medicine, there is a tendency to oversimplify the truth. Potato chips are a good example. Potato chips have long been reputed as a junk food. Since it is a common item in vending machines and because it is a popular snack food, common logic would suggest that they are a worthless food. To do so, however, would be misleading. Actually, the quick cooking process of potato chips preserves its nutrients better than mashed, boiled, or baked potatoes. The truth is that ounce per ounce, potato chips provide more nutrients than other forms of potatoes. Be careful, however, in oversimplifying this fact and forming the generalization that this is the preferred way to eat potatoes. Because potato chips are cooked in oil, they are high in fat and

■ **TABLE 11-1 Health newsletters: reliable sources of information on general health topics**

Title of newsletter	Published	Address
Consumer Reports Health Letter	Monthly	Consumers Union 256 Washington St. Mount Vernon, NY 10553
Harvard Medical School Health Letter	Monthly	79 Garden St. Cambridge, MA 02138
The Health Letter	2 issues/Monthly	P.O. Box 19622 Irvine, CA 92713
The Johns Hopkins Medical Letter	Monthly	P.O. Box 420235 Palm Coast, FL 32142-0235
Mayo Clinic Health Letter	Monthly	200 First Street SW Rochester, MN 55905
Taking Care	Monthly	The Center for Corporate Health Promotion 1850 Centennial Park Drive Reston, Virginia 22091
University of California, Berkeley Wellness Letter	Monthly	Health Letter Associates P.O. Box 412 Prince Street Station New York, NY 10012-0007

Subscription rates vary according to newsletter; approximate range is $20 to $25 per year.

loaded with calories, and not recommended for people trying to lose weight. The truth, therefore, is not so simple. By being aware that the truth is not simple for most health issues, the tendency to oversimplify and overgeneralize health information can be thwarted.

Health Discoveries Take Time

Discovery means excitement and headlines, and the media uses this to market its products.

But a cardinal rule of science is that it must be possible to replicate findings. Health information based on a dramatic discovery is not usually worth your time unless it is confirmed in several follow-up studies or experiments.

Criteria of Valid, Reliable Health Information

If information is to be trusted, it should be valid and reliable and based on scientifically controlled studies. In health research, **validity** re-

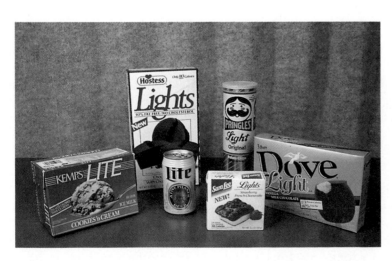

Legally meaningless and unregulated words are used to promote products.

fers to truthfulness. If a study is designed and conducted properly, its findings are likely to be valid. However, if a study has flaws, its findings and conclusions are not necessarily valid. A good example relates to vitamin E and aging. Some time ago it was found that adding vitamin E to human cells in the laboratory stimulated cell division and growth. This was used to support the erroneous conclusion that vitamin E would delay the aging process. This was not a valid conclusion because this simple laboratory experiment cannot possibly explain something as complex as aging.

Reliability is another key criterion for evaluating health information and refers to the extent that health claims can be consistently verified. If a claim is reliable, it can be demonstrated to occur consistently in study after study; that is, it can pass the test of time. Any health claim worth considering will be based on several studies or experiments.

Health information also must stand the rigors of scientifically controlled, *double-blind* studies. The classic study includes at least two groups in which one is an *experimental* group and receives some form of experimental treatment, and the other is a *control* group and receives no treatment. The double-blind feature of a study means that neither the researcher nor the subjects knows who is receiving an experimental treatment. If a researcher wanted to prove, for example, that a particular brand of soap prevents athlete's foot it would be necessary to form two groups. One would use the experimental soap and the other would use a *placebo* or soap substitute. Researchers administering the soap treatment wouldn't know which soap they were using, nor would the subjects in the experimental and control groups. Therefore, if the experimental group has significantly fewer cases of athletes foot, it is possible to attribute the results to the treatment.

The experimental-control, double-blind requirement of scientific research is a difficult standard to pass. When evaluating new health claims, it is a good idea to inquire about the nature and design of the study behind the claims.

Another consideration of a scientifically controlled study is characteristics of the study population. Scientific studies require random sampling of subjects which represent the racial, religious, gender, and cultural characteristics of the population at large. It is a mistake to place much confidence in so-called medical break-throughs that are based on a small number of *homogenous*, or similar, subjects.

Sources of Information

Valid and reliable health information comes from respected journals, magazines, and newsletters. Such publications have health or medical editors and subject their articles to peer review and criticism by other scientists. A partial listing of reliable sources of health information published in newsletters that contain no advertisements is presented in Table 11-1.

Be on guard for information that appears to be motivated by commercial interests. Watch for claims based on anecdotes, case studies, testimonials, and personal observations. Chances are good that they reflect personal bias or serve a hidden agenda.

Deceptive Advertising

Health claims in advertising have increased as Americans have become more health conscious. While many claims are accurate, the Federal Trade Commission's Bureau of Consumer Protection, which regulates advertisements, cautions consumers to be on guard against deceptive advertising. **Deceptive advertising** misleads consumers to their detriment; overstates the quality of a product; or exaggerates the performance of a product.[2] Deception is particularly common in the area of nutrition, where advertisements play on the appeal of certain catchwords and phrases.

While food and nutrition per se are beyond the scope of this chapter (see Chapter 3 for in-depth discussion on nutrition), it is useful to analyze the subtle and sometimes blatantly deceptive words which the food industry uses to mislead consumers. If deception in food labels can be discerned, it may be possible to develop a discriminating eye for valid, reliable health information in other areas of health care.

Legally meaningless and unregulated words which are flaunted include "natural," "wholesome," "organic," "health food," "lite," "low-calorie," and "high energy." Government surveys indicate that 63% of people believe "natural" foods are more nutritious than other foods, and 47% are willing to pay a 10% premium for "natural" fare.[3] So it's not surprising that labels highlight "natural" whenever possible. That's why one lemonade manufacturer proclaims "100% Natural Lemon Flavor" on a chemical concoction in

Figure 11-1 Deceptive words on health product labels

The meaning of terms on labels are not always apparent. Here are some legal definitions for terms you are likely to see on labels. Note that these definitions (which represent the most important ones) may change in the future as labeling laws change.

Diet or dietetic: Usually the product contains no more than 40 kilocalories per serving (also called low-calorie), or has at least one-third fewer kilocalories than the regular product (also called reduced-calorie).

Imitation: The product does not follow the usual recipe for that type of product. For instance, more water may have been added to margarines to make it lower in kilocalories. Note that such products may also be lower in nutrients, such as protein, vitamins, or minerals.

Natural: This term is usually meaningless. It simply states that the product occurs in nature. When applied to meats, it means the meat contains no added artificial flavors, colors, preservatives, or synthetic ingredients.

Sugar-free: The product cannot contain sucrose (table sugar), honey, fruit juice, molasses, or other simple sugars.

Light (lite): There are no laws concerning the use of this term with beer or other foods. It may or may not be lower in kilocalories than the standard product (read the label).

Low-calorie: The product contains no more than 40 kilocalories per serving and no more than 0.4 kcalories per gram.

Sodium-free: The product contains less than 5 milligrams of sodium per serving.

Very-low-sodium: The product contains no more than 35 milligrams of sodium per serving.

Low-sodium: The product contains no more than 140 milligrams of sodium per serving.

Reduced sodium: The product contains 75% less sodium than the product it replaces.

No artificial flavors: The product contains no flavors other than those from naturally occurring products.

No artificial coloring: The product contains only colors from naturally occurring products, such as beet juice, grape skin, or carrot oil.

May contain one or more of the following: The product can contain any of the ingredients listed after this phrase. Usually the ingredient(s) will be the one(s) found to be least expensive at the time of production.

No cholesterol: The product contains no cholesterol.

Cholesterol-free: The product contains less than 2 milligrams of cholesterol per serving.

Low-fat: Milk described as such can contain 0.5% to 2% milk fat. Low-fat meat can contain no more than 10% fat by weight.

New: The product is either brand new or has been substantially changed within the last 6 months.

Organic: This term has no legal meaning as far as the U.S. federal law is concerned.

Wheat: The product contains wheat but not necessarily whole wheat. The label will say whole wheat if the product uses only whole-wheat flour.

Enriched: The vitamins thiamin, riboflavin, and niacin and the mineral iron have been added to the product to replace (and in some cases augment) that lost in processing.

Fortified: Vitamins and/or minerals that were not originally present have been added to the product. There are other fine points to labeling laws.

which everything but the flavor is artificial. "Natural," along with the terms "organic," and "health food" have not been defined by the federal government and are considered inherently deceptive. For this reason some states have enacted legislation which places limits on the use of ambiguous health terms. For example, some states now have guidelines for what can be called "organic."

Even terms which have been regulated may be misleading. (See Figure 11-1) Many people think "light" means fewer calories. Before 1986, "light" could mean anything—less potato chips, less air, less package. Now it must be less in something related to nutrition—calories, sodium, fat, etc. Still, it can be deceptive. For example, there is no particular nutritional difference between one brand's extra "light" pancake mix and those regular mixtures sitting next to it on supermarket shelves. When asked what light stands for a company spokesperson said it means the pancakes have a "thinner, flatter" texture.[4] In another example the extra light olive oil made by one company provides the same number of calories as its regular brand. In this case the extra light means that the oil has a milder taste.

The Food and Drug Administration (FDA), which oversees the labeling of food products other than meat and poultry, has not developed a legal definition of "lite" and "light." The only time "light" has a well-defined meaning is when it appears on meat and poultry products which are regulated by the U.S. Department of Agriculture (USDA). The USDA requires that meat and poultry labeled "light" must be at least 25% lower in fat, sodium, or calories than similar versions and that the label must state where the reduction lies.

Seeking Health Care

Answers to the following questions provide clues to the use of health-care services, providers, and products:

1. When should we seek health care?
2. What can we expect from a stay in the hospital?
3. How can we select a health-care professional?

When to Seek Health Care

Many people tend to fall into two groups regarding health care: those who seek health care for every ache and pain and those who go to the opposite extreme and avoid health care unless under the duress of extreme pain. Both groups fail to make wise use of the health-care establishment. Those in the first group fail to understand that too much health care can be ineffective or even harmful. They also fail to recognize the powerful recuperative powers of the body. It is estimated that 80% of patients who seek medical care are unaffected by treatment, 10% get better, and 9% experience an *iatrogenic* condition in which they get worse because of the medical treatment. Those in the latter group fail to recognize the value of early diagnosis and detection of disease. The challenge for each of us is to try to learn the difference between both extremes.

Perhaps the best way to find a balance between too much and too little health care is to establish a physician-patient relationship with a general practitioner. The general practitioner may be a *family practice physician* or an *internist* who specializes in internal medicine.

It is important to visit your doctor while in good health. Not only does this permit your doctor to serve as a facilitator of wellness, but it also provides a benchmark for interpreting symptoms when they occur.

A second important way to balance health care is to trust your instincts. Nobody knows when something is wrong with your body better than you do. Health as well as illness is an individual matter and subject to a wide variation in interpretation. If you are attuned to your body, it is helpful to remember that you are your own best expert for recognizing signs and symptoms of illness.

There are several signs and symptoms that warrant medical attention without question. Internal bleeding, such as blood in urine, bowel movement, sputum, vomit, or from any of the body's openings, require immediate attention. Abdominal pain, especially when it is associated with nausea, may indicate a wide range of problems from appendicitis to pelvic inflammatory disease and require the diagnostic expertise of a physician. A stiff neck when accompanied by a

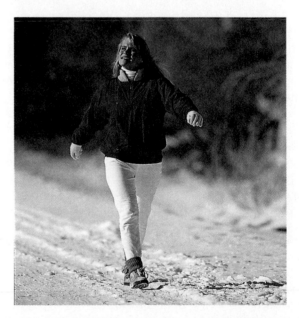

You are the best judge when it comes to recognizing the signs and symptoms of illness in your body.

fever may suggest meningitis and justifies immediate medical intervention. Of course, injuries, many first aid emergencies, and severe disabling symptoms require prompt medical care.

There is debate as to when medical care is called for in the case of fever. An elevated temperature may be a sign that the body's immune system is responding to an infection and working to destroy *pathogens* or disease-producing organisms. On the other hand, if left untreated for an extended time, a fever may cause harm to sensitive tissues in the body, such as connective tissue found in joints and tissues in the valves of the heart.

Normal body temperature is 98.6° F but varies with exercise, rest, climate, and gender. Fever means a reading over 99° F. It is not usually necessary for an adult to seek medical care for a fever. Home treatment in the form of aspirin, acetaminophen, and sponge baths will usually lower fever. You should consult your physician if fever remains above 102° F despite your actions, or, in the case of a low-grade fever (99° to 100° F) if there is no improvement in 72 hours. Consult a physician if fever lasts more than 5 days, regardless of improvement. Symptoms such as sore throat, ear pain, diarrhea, urinary problems, or skin rash may be the cause of the fever and should be treated as such. Fever in young children should be discussed with a physician.

Choosing a Hospital

A hospital is driven by the goal of saving lives. It may range in size and service from a small unit which provides general care and low-risk treatments to large, specialized centers offering dramatic and experimental therapies. You may be limited in your choice of a hospital by factors beyond your control, including insurance coverage, your physician's hospital affiliation, and type of care available.

In selecting a hospital it is important to remember that you are not shopping for a hotel with all of its perks. Hospitals are life-saving places that have already benefitted almost all of us or surely will help sometime in the future. At the risk of stirring feelings of paranoia, it is important to know that they also can be dangerous places. Well known hospital hazards are unnecessary operations, unexpected drug reactions, harmful or even fatal blunders, and hospital-borne infections. Boston University researchers recently reported on a five-month study of an unnamed hospital in which 290 (36%) of 815 patients became ill and 15 died as a result of complications and mishaps at a teaching hospital. This was significantly worse than a similar study 20 years earlier when 20% suffered some ill effect as a result of an adverse reaction to a drug, test, or treatment.[5]

The greatest risk that the hospital presents is infection. "Some 40 million Americans enter hospitals every year, and about two million of them get infections that sometimes are fatal. The Centers for Disease Control estimates that 80,000 to 100,000 patients die each year as a direct or indirect result of hospital-incurred infection. At least a third of these infections are preventable."[6]

What can lay people do to ensure proper and safe care while in the hospital? Consider the following guidelines:

▌ If you have a choice of hospitals, inquire about their accreditation status. Hospitals are subject to inspection to make sure they are in compliance with federal standards. Policies implemented in 1989 require the release of information upon request to state health departments regarding a hospital's mortality rate, its accreditation status, and its major deficiencies.[7]

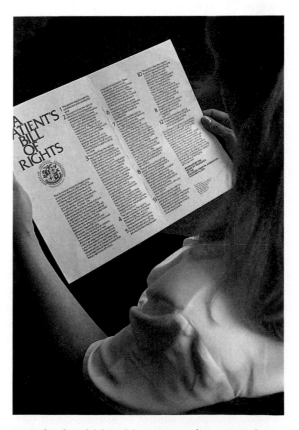

Hospitals should be able to provide you with an information booklet for a Patient's Bill of Rights.

- Before checking into a hospital, decide on your accomodations. Do you want to pay extra for a single room? Do you want a non-smoker for a roommate? Do you need a special diet? Do you need a place to store refrigerated medicine? If someone will be staying with you, will they need a cot? Try to avoid going in on a weekend when little will be done. When you get to your room, speak up immediately if it's unacceptable.
- Be familiar with your rights as a patient. Hospitals should provide an information booklet that includes a Patients' Bill of Rights. If not, ask for it. The booklet will inform you that you have the right to considerate and respectful care; information about tests, drugs, procedures; dignity; courtesy; respect; and the opportunity to make decisions, including when to leave the hospital.
- Make informed decisions. Before authorizing any procedure, patients must be informed about their medical condition, treatment options, expected risks, prognosis of the condition and the name of the person in charge of treatment. This is called **informed consent.** The only times hospitals are not required to obtain informed consent are cases involving life-threatening emergencies, unconscious patients when no relatives are present, and/or compliance with the law or a court order such as examination of sexually transmitted diseases. If you're asked to sign a consent form, read it first. If you want more information, ask before signing. If you're skeptical, you have the right to postpone the procedure and discuss it with your doctor.
- Authorization of a medical procedure may be given nonverbally, such as an appearance at a doctor's office for treatment, cooperation during the administration of tests, or failure to object when consent can be easily refused. This is called **implied consent.**
- Weigh the risks of drug therapy, X-ray examinations, and lab tests with their expected benefits. When tests or treatments are ordered, ask about their purpose. Ask about the possible actions if a test finds something wrong. If none of the actions are acceptable to you, why be subjected to the test? Also, ask about their possible risks. For example, the injection or ingestion of X-ray dyes makes body structures more visible and greatly facilitates a physician's ability

to make a correct diagnosis. However, they can cause an allergic reaction which ranges from a skin rash to circulatory collapse and death. Finally, inquire about prescribed drugs. Taking medication can be tricky. Studies suggest that almost one patient in five will suffer an adverse drug reaction.[8] Avoid taking drugs, including pain and sleeping medication, unless you feel confident of their benefits and are aware of their hazards.
- Know who is in charge of your care. Make sure you know what doctor is responsible. Record his or her office number and when you can expect a visit. If your doctor is turning you over to someone else, know who it is. If your doctor is not available and you don't know what's happening, ask for the nurse in charge of your case.
- Stay active within the limits of your medical problem. Many body functions begin to suffer from just a few days' inactivity. Moving about, walking, bending, and contracting muscles help clear body fluids, reduce the risk of infections (especially in the lungs), and help to cope with the stress of hospital procedures which add to the depression and malaise of hospitalization.
- Be alert. Throughout your stay keep asking questions until you know all you need to know. According to some experts, "the biggest improvement in health care in the last 15 years has not been technological advances. It's been patients asking questions. The more questions, the fewer mistakes, and the more power patients have in the doctor-patient relationship."[5]

Selecting a Health-Care Professional

Choosing a physician for your general health care is an important and necessary duty. In the interest of brevity, only physicians are discussed here. This information, however, applies to the selection of all health-care practitioners. You must select one who will listen carefully to your problems and diagnose them accurately. At the same time, it is just as important to find a physician who can move you through the modern medical maze that technology has made more and more complicated (see Table 11-2).

For most people good health care means having a **primary-care physician,** the professional who assists you as you assume responsibility for your overall health and directs you when special-

TABLE 11-2 Health care specialists

Name of specialist	Field of specialty
Medical specialists:	
Allergist	Allergic conditions
Anesthesiologist	Administration of anesthesia (for example, surgery)
Cardiologist	Coronary artery disease; heart disease
Dermatologist	Skin conditions
Endocrinologist	Diseases of the endocrine system
Epidemiologist	Investigates the cause and source of disease outbreaks
Family practice physician	General care physician
Gastroenterologist	Stomach, intestines, digestive system
Geriatrician	Diseases and conditions of the aged
Gynecologist	Female reproductive system
Hematologist	Study of blood
Immunologist	Diseases of the immune system
Internist	Treatment of diseases in adults
Neonatologist	Newborn infants
Nephrologist	Kidney disease
Neurologist	Nervous system
Neurosurgeon	Surgery of the brain and nervous system
Obstetrician	Pregnancy, labor, childbirth
Oncologist	Cancer, tumors
Ophthalmologist	Eyes
Orthopedist	Skeletal system
Otolaryngologist	Head, neck, ears, nose, throat
Otologist	Ears
Pathologist	Study of tissues and the essential nature of disease
Pediatrician	Childhood diseases and conditions
Plastic surgeon	Use of material to rebuild tissues
Primary care physician	General health and medical care
Proctologist	Disorders of the rectum and anus
Psychiatrist	Mental illnesses
Radiologist	Use of X-rays
Rheumatologist	Diseases of connective tissues, joints, muscles, tendons, etc.
Rhinologist	Nose
Surgeon	Treats diseases by surgery
Urologist	Urinary tract of males and females and reproductive organs of males
Dental specialists:	
Dentist	General care of teeth and oral cavity
Endodontist	Diseases of tooth below gum line (performs root canal therapy)
Orthodontist	Teeth alignment, malocclusion
Pedodontist	Dental care of children
Periodontist	Diseases of supporting structures
Prosthodontist	Construction of artificial appliances for the mouth
Other specialists:	
Chiropractor	Emphasizes the use of manipulation and adjustment of body structures to treat disease
Naturopathic physician	Emphasizes lifestyle and dietary therapies in the prevention and treatment of diseases
Optometrist	Examines and tests eyes for visual defects
Osteopath	Emphasis on structural integrity of the body; uses manipulation along with medical therapies
Podiatrist	Care and treatment of the foot
Psychologist	Study of human behavior

ized care is necessary. Because the primary-care physician will see you first with your health problem, he or she should be familiar with your complete medical history, as well as your home, work, and other environments. One of the best reasons to see a primary-care physician, even in the absence of medical complaints, is to make it possible for him or her to know you as an individual, not just a collection of symptoms (Figure 11-2). A physician can better understand you in periods of sickness if he or she also sees you during periods of wellness.

For adults, primary-care physicians are usually *family practitioners*, once called *general practitioners*, and *internists*, specialists in internal medicine. *Pediatricians* often serve as primary-care physicians for children. *Obstetricians* and *gynecologists*, who specialize in pregnancy, childbirth, and diseases of the female reproductive system often serve as primary-care physicians to female patients. In some places general surgeons may offer primary care in addition to the surgery they perform. Some *osteopathic* physicians also practice family medicine. A doctor of osteopathy (DO) emphasizes manipulation of the body to treat symptoms.

If you want a female physician, you will have a better chance to find one in the near future. Currently, only 13% of doctors are women. However, the numbers are growing. One third of medical students are now women.[9]

There are several sources of information for obtaining the names of physicians in your area.

▎ Local and state medical societies can identify doctors by specialty and tell you a doctor's basic credentials. Make sure you check on the doctor's hospital affiliation. Also, make sure the hospital is accredited. An-

other sign of standing is the type of societies in which the doctor has membership. The qualifications of a surgeon, for example, are enhanced by a fellowship in the American College of Surgeons (abbreviated as FACS after the surgeon's name). An internist fellowship in the American College of Physicians is abbreviated FACP. Membership in academies indicates a physician's special interest.

▎ All physicians board certified in the United States are listed in the American Medical Directory published by the American Medical Association and is available in larger libraries.

▎ The American Board of Medical Specialists (ABMS) publishes the Compendium of Certified Medical Specialties which lists physicians by name, specialty, and location.

▎ Ask several pharmacists to recommend names. Narrowing the list can be facilitated if you can pin down a couple of specialists who are willing to pick their favorite.

▎ Hospitals can give you names of staff physicians who also practice in the community.

▎ Local medical schools, if available, can identify faculty members who also practice privately.

▎ Many colleges and universities have health centers which keep a list of physicians for student referral.

▎ Friends may have recommendations, but allow for the possibility that your opinion of the doctor may be different.

Once you've identified a leading candidate, make an appointment. Check with the office staff about office hours, availability of emergency care at night or weekends, backup doctors, procedures

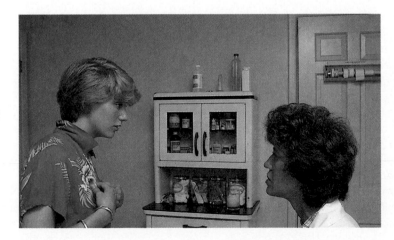

A correct diagnosis is most dependent on what a patient tells her doctor.

▉ TABLE 11-3 Communicating with health care professionals

Term

Here are some words, abbreviations, suffixes, and prefixes that are often used in health and medical care.

a	(Prefix) Without
Abberation	Different from normal action
Acute	A condition that occurs suddenly
Adult	Developed fully
Affinity	Attraction
Algia	(Suffix) Pain in
Arrest	Stopping, restraining
Asymptomatic	Without symptoms
Bowel	Intestine
Cardiac	Relating to the heart
CAT	(Abbreviation) Computerized assisted X-ray
CCU	(Abbreviation) Coronary Care Unit
Chronic	A condition that occurs for a long time
Coma	Complete loss of consciousness
Congenital	Existing at or before birth
Contraindication	A reason for not prescribing a drug, procedure, or treatment
Coronary	Relating to the heart
Degenerative	Deterioration of a part of the body
Diagnosis	Determination of a disease
Dilation	Stretching, increase in size
Distention	Widening or enlargement
Dose	Amount of medication to be given at one time
Dysfunction	Impairment of function
Edema	Swelling from accumulation of fluid
EKG, ECG	(Abbreviation) Electrocardiogram
Embolus	Blood clot floating free in the bloodstream
Endemic	Disease prevalent in a particular area
ER	(Abbreviation) Emergency room
Etiology	Refers to the cause of a disease
Extra	(Prefix) Outside of
Gastr	(Prefix) Stomach
GP	(Abbreviation) General practitioner
Hem	(Prefix) Blood
Hemorrhage	Bleeding

when you call for advice, hospital affiliation, and payment and insurance procedures. Don't wait until you have a medical crisis to look for a doctor. Schedule your first visit while in good health. Once you have seen your doctor, reflect on his or her actions. Did he or she seem to be listening to you? Were your questions answered? Was a medical history taken? Were you informed of possible side effects of drugs or tests? Was respect shown for your need of privacy? Was he or she open to the suggestion of a second opinion? Answers to these questions make it possible to determine if your doctor seems to be the kind of person you could trust with your confidence as well as your life.

Patient-physician communication. Most doctors aren't disinterested in you, but they are busy—so busy that many patients complain that their doctor can't or won't listen to them. This is a problem because, according to the American Society of Internal Medicine, 70% of correct diagnoses depend on what you tell your doctor. But be prepared to talk fast! In a recent study[10] of 74 visits to seven doctors, researchers found that only 16 patients were allowed to explain the problem fully. In 70% of the visits doctors interrupted their patients before they completed their first statement. Usually the interruption occured within 18 seconds. It was not surprising, therefore, that when the American Medical Associa-

▋ TABLE 11-3 Communicating with health care professionals—cont'd

Term	
Hyper	(Prefix) Excessive
Hypo	(Prefix) Insufficient
Indication	Condition that leads to a prescribed drug, procedure, or treatment
ICU	(Abbreviation) Intensive Care Unit
Innate	Hereditary, congenital
Innocuous	Harmless
Insidious	Refers to a disease that doesn't show early symptoms of its advent
Ism	(Suffix) Condition, theory, method
Itis	(Suffix) Inflammation
IV	(Abbreviation) Intravenous (within a vein)
Jaundiced	Yellow
Malady	Illness
Malaise	Uneasiness
MD	(Abbreviation) Medical doctor
MI	(Abbreviation) Myocardial infarction
Myo	(Prefix) Muscle
Opothy	(Suffix) Cause unknown
Pernicious	Severe, fatal
Primary	Principal, most important
Prognosis	Medical outlook of a disease
Pulmo	(Prefix) Lung
Renal	Kidney
Sign	Something tangible that can be observed
Stenosis	Constricted, decreasing in size
Symptom	Intangible evidence of a disease
Symptomatic	Relating to symptoms
Syndrome	Set of symptoms that occur together for unknown causes
Systemic	Affecting all systems of the body
Thrombus	Solid blood clot
TIA	(Abbreviation) Transient ischemic attack
TPR	(Abbreviation) Temperature, pulse, respiration
Trauma	Injury from external force
Tumor	Growth

tion conducted a study on public attitudes towards physicians, 37% of those surveyed did not believe doctors take a genuine interest in their patients. Only 45% believed doctors usually explain things well to their patients.[11] Fortunately, medical schools are beginning to emphasize communication skills. More physicians seem to realize that good medicine means establishing good rapport with patients. Of course, it's a two-way street. Patients can do much to facilitate the development of a physician-patient partnership which includes good communication. Understanding the meaning of commonly used medical words, abbreviations, suffixes, and prefixes can enhance this communication (Table 11-3). Here are some tips:

▋ When you see your physician about a problem, state the most important problem first. Doctors tend to believe that the first thing a patient says is most important.

▋ Be as specific as possible. If you have a headache, where does it hurt? How long does it last? How often does it occur?

▋ Know your family history. Since many illnesses may run in families, you may be at higher risk for certain diseases. Prior to your first visit, do some homework. Contact your parents and close relatives to learn of their health problems, especially heart disease, cancer, stroke, arthritis, diabetes, alcoholism, and tuberculosis.

▋ List medications and treatments you are receiving, including over-the-counter drugs. Also be prepared to identify any allergies and drug reactions.

- Ask questions. You might even bring a written list of questions. Try to make them brief and specific. Ask about anything that is unclear and repeat the answers in your own words.
- Before leaving the doctor's office make certain you know the diagnosis or how to follow the recommended treatment. If drugs are prescribed, inquire about the possible **contraindications** (reason for not using a drug), side effects, and the possible substitution of generics.

Second opinions. In medicine, as in any other area of decision-making, two heads are often better than one. This is expecially true for conditions involving elective surgery, chronic pain, and recurring illnesses. In many situations, a second opinion is appropriate and peace of mind is a sufficient reason for seeking it. A recent editorial in the *Harvard Medical School Health Letter* provides some helpful advice to the question, "When is a second opinion needed?" "As a general rule, patients should seek a second opinion whenever they are uncomfortable with the explanations offered by a physician, are not happy with the progress of recovery, question the proposed course of action, or simply feel the need for verification."[12] In some cases, such as elective surgery, your health insurer may require a second or third opinion before authorizing payment for certain treatments. (See Figure 11-2 for advice on getting a second opinion.)

If you decide to ask for a second opinion, common courtesy would dictate that you discuss it with your physician. Your physician may suggest bringing in a consultant who will assess your situation and discuss it with you and your physician. You can also ask your physician for the name of someone to see separately.

A physician may feel that a second opinion is a waste of time or money. Regardless, your wish for more information should be respected. Reputable physicians do not feel threatened by another opinion; to the contrary, they may welcome another perspective on a difficult case. If your physician expresses displeasure for or resists your wish to have a second opinion, it may be time to consider looking for another doctor.

Assessing Your Health

There is a plethora of tests, procedures, gadgets, and machines for assessing various aspects of health and wellness. They range from the hands-on physical examination to the use of sophisticated diagnostic tests. There is some debate, however, as to when and how often they are to be administered or how effective they are.

The Physical Examination

Until recently the annual physical examination was considered one of the sacred cows of medicine. It was viewed as a normal and necessary part of health care. Now, there is considerable debate among medical experts as to who needs a physical examination, how often it is needed, and what it should include.

A report[13] of recently published medical studies concluded that many of the routine procedures doctors use in a physical examination on healthy adults are virtually useless. Much of the touching, probing, thumping, and listening serves little purpose except to reassure patients, the report asserted. Of course this conclusion is controversial and many professional groups hold stubbornly to the view that the routine physical is necessary.

While many physicians are reluctant to elimi-

Figure 11-2 How to get a second opinion

If you are considering elective surgery and want a second opinion, here are sources for referral:

- Ask your primary-care physician for the names of two or three experts in the field.
- Call a medical center or hospital and ask to talk to the chief of surgery for a surgical opinion or to the chief of medicine for a nonsurgical question.
- Call the county medical society.
- Call the Second Surgical Opinion Hotline (800-638-6833) for medical organizations that provide referrals on surgical questions.
- Call Health Benefits Research Corporation, which offers a Second Opinion Hotline (800-522-0036, 800-631-1220 in New York) and referral service. Consultation with a board-certified specialist is available for a fee.

nate the annual physical, the emphasis today is in the use of **selective health examinations,** that is, the practice of using specific tests for specific problems. The assumption is that tests are more useful if they are matched to specific complaints. This is juxtaposed to the practice of using a shotgun approach in which a battery of tests are administered in the absence of signs or symptoms.

Criticisms of the comprehensive annual physical examination for a healthy adult are not meant to undermine the doctor-patient relationship. They simply cast doubt about the efficacy of the physical. However, this does not nullify the value of regular visits to the doctor. To the contrary, seeing a physician for a limited exam at regular intervals can be good preventive medicine.

How Often is a Physical Examination Needed?

The American Medical Association advises healthy adults to get a checkup every 5 years until age 40, then one every 1 to 3 years.[14] Yearly physicals are advisable for children under 6 and adults over 60, even if they don't have symptoms.[15]

Regardless of age, individuals with a family history of heart disease, strokes, high blood pressure, cancer, and diabetes can benefit by periodic checkups, even if they are in good health. The same is true for individuals whose health habits or occupation put them at higher than normal risk for chronic diseases and disabling conditions. Even in these cases, good judgement and discretion should rule the choice of tests to be included in the physical examination.

Components of a Physical Examination

The three basic tools for completing a physical examination are medical history, hands-on examination, and diagnostic/laboratory tests.

A *medical history* is probably the most important part of the physical examination, especially during the first visit with your physician. It includes a history of habits, lifestyle, family history, and symptoms. Many physicians use *health risk appraisals,* detailed questionnaires which provide information about health habits.

This is one area of the physical examination for which a patient can prepare. By following the guidelines for communicating with your physician presented earlier in this chapter, patients can help their physician obtain an accurate health profile. This is important because a diagnosis can be made 80-90% of the time with only a thorough history and hands-on exam.[16]

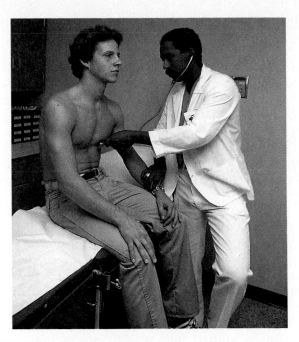

The stethoscope is just one of many instruments that physicians use to detect potential problems.

The *hands-on* exam is the second part of the physical examination. It consists of examination by touching, looking, and listening.

Physicians can feel or palpate for enlarged glands, growths, and tumors with procedures like the breast exam, pelvic exam, rectal exam, and hernia exam. Thumping the back and chest lets the physician know if any fluid has built up in or around the lungs. Tapping a knee for reflexes may reveal nervous system damage. A stethoscope is the physician's basic listening device and is used to listen to the heart, lungs, abdomen, and glands located near the surface of the skin. Possible problems that can be detected with the stethoscope range from a heart murmur to such conditions as poor circulation, lung infection, intestinal blockage, and possibly even an overactive thyroid gland.

Physicians have access to a number of instruments to visually inspect for signs of trouble. An *ophthalmoscope* is used to view the brain by looking into the eye. The first sign of some brain diseases is an unhealthy-looking optic nerve. Leakage in the blood vessels of the eye may be signs of diabetes or hypertension. An *otoscope* is used to inspect the ear, particularly the tympanic membrane. The *proctoscope* and *sigmoidoscope* are used to examine the rectum and colon. And the *laryngoscope* and *bronchoscope* provide a look at the larynx and bronchial tubes.

The last part of the physical exam includes **diagnostic laboratory tests** which may vary from a simple urinalysis to invasive dye tests. The effectiveness of these tests receives mixed reviews. On the plus side, tests conducted for specific symptoms may be invaluable in pinpointing disabling conditions. They may be just as valuable for what they don't reveal as they are for what they do reveal. This can be reassuring to the patient and physician.

On the negative side, there appears to be a test glut in which many physicians rely too heavily on lab tests. Also, patients often demand or acquiesce to more tests than necessary, sometimes more than is good for them. A recent report[16] suggests that at least 25% of all medical tests contribute little to health. For example, when researchers at the University of California, San Francisco studied 2000 patients hospitalized for surgery, they found that 60% of the blood tests routinely ordered were unnecessary. Only one in about 450 revealed abnormalities, and they were ignored because they either were not noticed or were dismissed as not significant. The researchers concluded that if a thorough history turns up no hint of a medical problem, routine testing is a waste. According to one physician quoted in a popular magazine, "indiscriminately ordering a battery of tests in the hope that something will turn up is the desperate move of an insecure examiner.[17]

Thus, when you go for a physical exam you can help determine which tests you are willing to be subjected to by asking the right questions.

▪ What do you expect to find? Start by asking why you need the test. How will it help facilitate a diagnosis? Ask about alternatives. Then ask about the disadvantage of waiting and not testing. Sometimes the best test is the test of time. Agreeing to a test because it is routine procedure is not a satisfactory explanation.

▪ What risks are associated with the test? No test is risk-free; therefore, it is important to compare potential benefits and risks.

One problem with tests is that they are not 100% accurate. For example, the accuracy of such common tests as community screening for cholesterol levels has been the subject of considerable debate.[18] An inaccurate result can lead to a wrong diagnosis. A *false positive* may occur in which a test incorrectly reveals an abnormality

and consequently provokes needless anxiety. The concomitant self-fulfilling prophesy causes some people to begin feeling and even acting sick. Conversely, normal results do not necessarily indicate good health. *False negatives* may occur in which test results indicate normality even though a person is sick. These results may lead to a false sense of health and may delay much needed treatment at critical stages of a disease.

Statistically, test results are accurate for about 95% of the population. Thus 5% of patients can be expected to have a false positive or false negative on any given lab test. Other factors which may cause test errors include certain medications, exercise, stress, eating, time of day, and mistakes in handling or processing specimens.

Another problem with tests is that they may be associated with physical risks. Some of the more common risks are infection, bleeding, damage to vital structures, and reactions to anesthetics, drugs, and dye-contrast materials. A California study[16] of 303 patients found that as many as 14% who had invasive diagnostic procedures develop one or more complications.

▪ What are the options after the test? If a test is positive, then what? If none of the options is plausible to you, why have the test administered? If it is impossible to treat a disease that a test reveals, the test is not justified. The diagnosis of treatable diseases, on the other hand, usually justifies the test.

▪ Asking your physician about the value of a test need not be perceived as a time of confrontation. Instead, it should be viewed as a time for communication, for questions and answers. If approached with sincerity and courtesy, discussions about the physical exam in general and lab tests in particular can serve as a basis for forming an active partnership with your physician in making decisions about your health care.

Common Diagnostic Lab Tests

Now, more than ever before, Americans are having diagnostic tests performed (see Figure 11-3). Depending on your health status, sex, age, symptoms, or risk for a disease, some of the more common tests listed may be recommended when you go in for a checkup.

Multiple blood screening tests check for high blood sugar which indicate diabetes; blood urea nitrogen, an indicator of kidney function; calcium, for signs of an overactive parathyroid gland; and blood count, a screen for anemia.

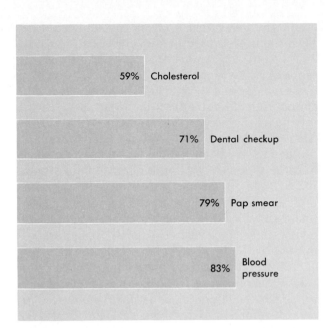

Figure 11-3 Percentage of adults having four common diagnostic tests.

Blood cholesterol screening is recommended for everyone over 20. According to the National Heart, Lung and Blood Institute, 25% of the population have cholesterol levels in the high range (240 mg/dl or above). If cholesterol is high, retesting is recommended. If it is still high, it is important to check *high-density lipoproteins* (HDL), *low-density lipoproteins* (LDL), and triglyceride levels. An LDL level of less than 130 mg/dl is desirable; an HDL reading below 35 mg/dl is considered a major risk factor for cardiovascular disease; and a desirable triglyceride level is usually 30 to 150 mg/dl.[19] (See Chapter Five for a more thorough discussion of cholesterol.)

Hemoccult tests are used to detect hidden blood in the bowel movement. If the test is positive, it may indicate signs of an early cancer of the colon. If this happens, don't jump to a conclusion. There are many causes for blood in the stool. However, see your physician for further testing. Individuals over 50 years of age should either test themselves (home screening kits are available in most pharmacies) or have their stools tested for blood every year.[20]

Pulse rate may be an indicator of a health problem. It is easy to measure pulse rate by counting the wrist or carotid pulse for a minute. A normal resting heart rate is between 60 and 80 beats a minute. Resting heart rates above 80 per minute put a person in a higher risk category for

heart attacks and sudden death.[20] The high heart rate itself doesn't increase the risk. It is just an indicator of basic problems such as cigarette smoking, too much caffeine, stress, anxiety, hyperthyroidism, and most commonly, a poor level of physical fitness.

Slow heart rates are normally found in physically fit individuals; in these cases, it is a sign of good health. But very slow rates, below 50 per minute, can occur in people who are not fit and who have a possible heart problem. These individuals, of course, should seek medical advice.

Blood pressure measurements should be monitored on a regular basis, especially for individuals who have had a previously high reading or who have a family history of hypertension (high blood pressure). Inexpensive, accurate, home blood pressure kits can be purchased at most drug stores. Ask your pharmacist for a recommendation. Individuals who have measurements higher than 140 over 85 should keep a home record of their blood pressure and present them to their physician during periodic checkups.

Mammography, an X-ray examination of the breast, detects early signs of breast cancer. The

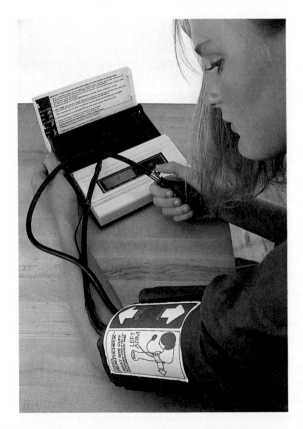

A growing number of tests and instruments are available for self-assessment.

American Cancer Society advises women to have a mammogram every one to two years between 40 and 49, and annually after age 50. High risk women may be advised to have mammograms more often and at an earlier age.[15]

A *pap smear* is used to detect cancer of the cervix. The American Cancer Society recommends an annual Pap test starting at age 18 or when sexual activity begins, whichever comes first. Pap smears should not be done during the menstrual period. The test is more accurate during the first half of the cycle if oral contraceptives are taken. Mid-cycle is preferred in most other menstruating women. Regardless of when the test is done, the technician reading the smear must know if you're taking oral contraceptives or estrogen replacement therapy, as well as when your last menstrual period began. Only with this information can the smear be accurately interpreted.[21]

Tonometry is used to detect elevated pressure in the eye, an indicator of glaucoma. It is a painless test and should be employed every two to three years past age forty or annually if family history suggests a higher risk.

Electrocardiograms (EKG) are used to detect irregularities of the heart. While there is some debate about its use as a routine screening procedure for *asymptomatic* (without symptoms) low risk individuals, an EKG reading by age 35 provides a benchmark for subsequent comparisons. Chest pain, hypertension, or symptoms of cardiovascular disease justify earlier EKG's.

Chest X-ray examinations are valuable diagnostic tools for people with chest symptoms, respiratory diseases, or heart problems. For people without such symptoms, their routine use is questionable. Several groups of experts, including those associated with the Food and Drug Administration, recommend discontinuation of chest X-rays in most cases. Still, if you go to a hospital or in many cases your doctor's office, you can anticipate a chest X-ray more out of the need to comply with business policy than for its diagnostic potential. You will want to avoid a chest X-ray if there is any possibility of being pregnant.

Immunizations for Adults

Many people are under the illusion that **immunizations** (administration of a preparation or vaccine, usually in the form of injections, for providing immunity or preventing a disease) are for only children. Consequently, many thousands of

adults die every year of diseases they would not have acquired if they had received standard vaccines. Consider some startling statistics recently reported in two health publications[22,23]: 91% of tetanus cases and 87% of hepatitis B cases in this country affect adults over the age of 20. Half the rubella cases are among adults. While deaths from measles, rubella, mumps, tetanus, and diptheria have been reduced to about 12 a year, most of these are among older people—a complete reversal of 30 years ago. Also, 40,000 people die a year from pneumococcal infections; influenza viruses kill 20,000 more. Of the 300,000 people who contract hepatitis B, 10,000 are admitted to a hospital and about 5000 die.

Adult immunization is recommended to prevent or ameliorate seven diseases. They include influenza, pneumonia, hepatitis B, measles, rubella (German measles), tetanus, and diptheria. Table 11-4 provides immunization information for each of these diseases.

Paying for Health Care

The cost of health care in the United States is expensive and fast becoming more so. A large majority of Americans would not be able to afford the cost of medicines, physicians' fees, or hospitalization without some form of health insurance. Decisions regarding the type of insurance policy purchased influence to a major extent where you go for health care, who provides the health care, and what medical procedures can be performed. The three basic health insurance plans to choose from include a private, fee-for-service plan; a prepaid group plan; and government-financed public plan.

Private, Fee-For-Service Insurance Plan

Until recently this was the principal form of health insurance coverage. In this plan an individual pays a monthly premium, usually through an employer, which entitles him or her to seek health care on a fee-for-service basis. Upon incurring medical costs, the patient files a claim to have a portion of these costs paid by the insurance company.

Prepaid Group Insurance

In this type of insurance, health care is provided by a group of physicians organized into what is referred to as a **health maintenance organization (HMO).** HMOs provide an advantage in that they cover most, in some groups all, of an in-

■   **TABLE 11-4 Immunization schedule for adults**

Immunization	Who	Shots	Precautions	Side effects
Tetanus and diphtheria	All adults	3 in initial series; boosters every 10 years	Pregnancy, previous reactions	Reddening of the skin, joint pain
Measles	All adults	One; no boosters	Pregnancy, allergy to eggs, reactions to antibiotics	Occasional fever and mild rashes
Rubella (German measles)	All adults, especially women of child-bearing age	One; no boosters	Same as for measles. Women should avoid conception within three months of vaccination.	Joint pain
Mumps	All adults, especially males	One; no boosters	Same as for rubella	Allergic reactions and swelling of the salivary glands
Pneumonia and flu	All adults over 65 and chronically ill adults	One for pneumonia with revaccination every 6 years for some people; flu shots yearly	Pregnancy	Mild pain or redness
Hepatitis B	Adults at risk because of job, travel, or exposure to infected people	Three; no boosters	None	Some soreness

dividual's medical expenses. For an annual fee, usually paid through payroll deductions by an employer, and often a small deductible, HMOs can provide a full range of medical services. Instead of paying on a fee-for-service basis, your premium is used as a prepayment for any health care service. For most people, this makes health care less expensive than private insurance over a long period of coverage. The major disadvantage of HMO's is that you are restricted to seeing those physicians who are included in a particular group.

Government Insurance

In this type of plan the government at the federal, state, or local level pays for the health care costs of elgible participants. Two prominent examples of this plan are Medicare and Medicaid. Medicare is financed by social security taxes and is designed to provide health care for individuals 65 years old and over; the blind; the severly disabled; and those requiring certain treatments such as kidney dialysis. Medicaid is subsidized by federal and state taxes. It provides limited health care, generally for individuals who are elgible for benefits and assistance from two programs: Aid to Families with Dependent Children and Supplementary Security Income.

Summary

■ Health information that can be trusted is based on scientifically controlled studies that yield consistent results over time.

■ Signs and symptoms that warrant immediate medical attention are signs of internal bleeding, abdominal pain associated with nausea, a stiff neck accompanied by fever, and serious first aid emergencies and injuries.

■ People can help to ensure proper and safe care while in a hospital by checking on the hospital's accreditation status, deciding on accomodations prior to admission, knowing their rights as a patient, discussing treatments and procedures with their physician, asking questions, and staying active.

■ Good health care means establishing a doctor-patient relationship while in good health.

■ When telling a physician about a problem, good communication is enhanced by presenting the most important problem first, being as specific as possible, being familiar with your family medical history, knowing the names of medicines you are taking, and by asking questions.

■ The three major components of a physical examination are medical history, hands-on examination, and diagnostic laboratory tests.

■ The seven diseases for which adults need to maintain immunination are influenza, pneumonia, hepatitis B, measles, rubella, tetanus, and diptheria.

■ The three basic options for paying for health care include private, fee-for-service insurance; prepaid group insurance; and government insurance.

 ## Action plan for personal wellness

An important consideration in assuming responsibility for the individual's own quality of life is using information. After reading this chapter, answer the following questions and determine an action plan for enhancing your own lifestyle.

1 Based on the information presented in this chapter and what I know about my family's health history, the issues related to the health care market that I need to be most concerned about are:

_____

_____

_____

2 Of the health care issues listed in no. 1, the one I most need to act on is: _____

3 The possible actions that I can take to improve my ability to understand health information and to make better use of the health care market are (try to be as specific as possible): _____

_____

4 Of the actions listed in no. 3, the one that I most need to include in an action plan is: _____

_____

5 Factors I need to keep in mind to be successful in my action plan are: _____

_____

_____

Review Questions

1. How do the concepts of "health fatalism" and "health hysteria cycle" present a negative influence on the understanding of health information?
2. What criteria must a research study satisfy before its claims can be trusted?
3. What are some techniques and strategies that manufacturers and producers of health products use to mislead and/or deceive the public?
4. Why is it important to see a physician while in good health?
5. What can lay people do while in a hospital to ensure that they receive safe and proper care?
6. What is the major role and function of a primary-care physician?
7. List four sources of information for identifying physicians and specialists in your geographical area.
8. Identify four techniques that will facilitate communication between patient and physician.
9. Discuss the purpose and potential value and risks of the three major components of a physical examination.
10. Compare and contrast the three basic plans of health insurance.

References

1. Vickery D: Viewpoint—understanding health information, Taking Care 8(January):7, 1986.
2. Nutrition claims in advertising, H.E.—Xtra 14(3):6, 1989.
3. Eisenberg A and Murkoff H: How to read a food label, American Health 3(July/August):52, 1984.
4. The meaning of light remains vague, Tufts University Diet and Nutrition Letter 6(9):1, 1988.
5. Cohn V: How to survive the hospital, American Health 7(March):99, 108, 1987.
6. United Press International: Hospitals infect patients; threat grows, CDC says, Commercial Appeal 146(311):C3, 1985.
7. Mayer D: Accreditation panel to release hospital information to health care financing administration, Medical Benefits 6(11):12, 1989.
8. Vickery D: The terrible I's: the hidden hazards of hospitalization, Taking Care 7(9):5, 1985.
9. Kiplinger Washington Editors: Shopping for a new doctor, Changing Times 40(6):51, 1986.
10. Shell E: How to talk to your doctor in 18 seconds, American Health 6(1):82, 1987.
11. Gibbs N: Sick and tired, Time 134(5):49, 1989.
12. Second opinions, Harvard Medical School Health Letter 14(4):1, 1989.
13. Browne M: Analysis discovers wasted motion in routine physical examinations, The Commercial Appeal 150(43):C3, 1989.
14. Oppenheim M: The 'big 4' tests you really need, American Health 3(September):80, 1984.
15. Carey B: Do you need a physical, In Health (March/April):80-82, 1990.
16. Sobel D: When not to take medical tests, American Health, 5(9):59, 54, 1986.
17. Blau N: The test glut, Health 17(1):36, 1985.
18. Moore T: The cholesterol myth, The Atlantic Monthly 264(3):37-70, 1989.
19. Kolata G: Cholesterol tests: 9 tips—what your blood will tell, American Health 7(1):42, 1988.
20. Lamb L: Do it yourself medical testing, The Health Letter 29(12):3, 2, 1987.
21. Annual pap smears, Consumer Reports Health Letter 1(2):15, 1989.
22. Norton C: Not just for kids, Hippocrates 3(5):75, 1989.
23. Shots for grownups, Harvard Medical School Health Letter 13(10):1, 1988.

Annotated Readings

1. Bennett W, Goldfinger S and Johnson G: Your good health, Cambridge, Massachusetts, 1987, Harvard University Press.
   Published by the editors of the Harvard Medical School Health Letter, this book presents information and advice on a variety of health topics.
2. Kunz J: The American Medical Association family medical guide, New York, 1982, Random House Publishers.
   An encyclopedia of health information that serves as a useful reference. Includes 99 symptom charts for making a self-diagnosis; also includes 68 full-color visual aids for making self diagnosis.
3. ABC's of the human body, Pleasantville, NY, 1987, The Readers Digest Association.
   Full-color presentation on the systems of the body with many health tips and advice. Contains a comprehensive index.
4. Editors of Consumer Reports books: The new medicine show, Mount Vernon, NY, 1989, Consumers Union of the United States.
   Practical guide to some everyday health problems and health products including but not limited to pain relievers, cold remedies, indigestion and antacids, constipation and diarrhea medicines, diet and nutrition aids, skin and hair care, teeth and gums, and generic and brand-name drugs.
5. Sobel D and Ferguson T: The people's book of medical tests, New York, 1985, Summit Publishers.
   Presents information on 200 medical procedures including purpose of tests, how tests are performed, how long tests take, risks, and costs.

ASSESSMENT ACTIVITY

11-1

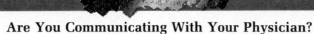

Are You Communicating With Your Physician?

Directions: Using the scale below, circle the appropriate number for each question. Total your responses and find your score at the bottom of the activity.

When I go to my physician for a health problem,	Almost always	Very frequently	Frequently	Occas- ionally	Never
1. I plan ahead of time how I'm going to describe my problem.	5	4	3	2	1
2. I describe my most important problem first.	5	4	3	2	1
3. I check with my immediate family to determine if my problem runs in the family	5	4	3	2	1
4. I take a list of medications, over-the-counter drugs, and treatments I am receiving.	5	4	3	2	1
5. Before the visit, I prepare a written list of questions to ask.	5	4	3	2	1
6. I ask about anything that is unclear to me.	5	4	3	2	1
7. I repeat in my own words the physician's answers to my questions.	5	4	3	2	1
8. I understand the doctor's diagnosis of my problem.	5	4	3	2	1
9. I make sure I know the benefits and risks of prescribed treatments.	5	4	3	2	1
10. I know if and when to return for a follow-up visit.	5	4	3	2	1

Scoring: 46−50 = Excellent communication (you're getting the most from your visit.)
41−45 = Good, better than most.
36−40 = Average, but who wants to be average?
31−35 = Fair, reevaluate your communication style.
Less than 30 = Poor, are you really trying?

ASSESSMENT ACTIVITY   11-2

Are Your Immunizations Working for You?

Directions: For each of the adult immunizations listed below indicate the dates of your initial immunization and most recent booster shot. Check the immunization schedule in Table 3-4 and determine if your immunizations are current. If it is, write "yes" in the last column. If it is *not*, write "no" in the last column. A "no" means that you need to discuss your immunizations with your health care provider.

Immunization	Dates of Initial shot	Booster shot	Yes/No
Tetanus and Diphtheria			
Measles			
Rubella			
Mumps			
Pneumonia			
Influenza			
Hepatitis B			

ASSESSMENT ACTIVITY   11-3

Assessing Results of Diagnostic Tests

Directions: Use this assessment to record the dates and results of commonly administered diagnostic medical tests. The blank spaces at the bottom can be used to list additional tests. Refer to information in this chapter to review the purposes of these tests.

Diagnostic test	Date	Results
Blood sugar		
Blood urea nitrogen		
Calcium		
Blood count		
Cholesterol		
High density lipoprotein		
Low density lipoprotein		
Triglyceride		
Hemoccult		
Pulse rate		
Blood pressure		
Mammography[*]		
Pap Smear[*]		
Prostate[†]		
Tonometry		
Electrocardiogram		
Chest X-ray		
Dental check-up		

[*]Women   [†]Men

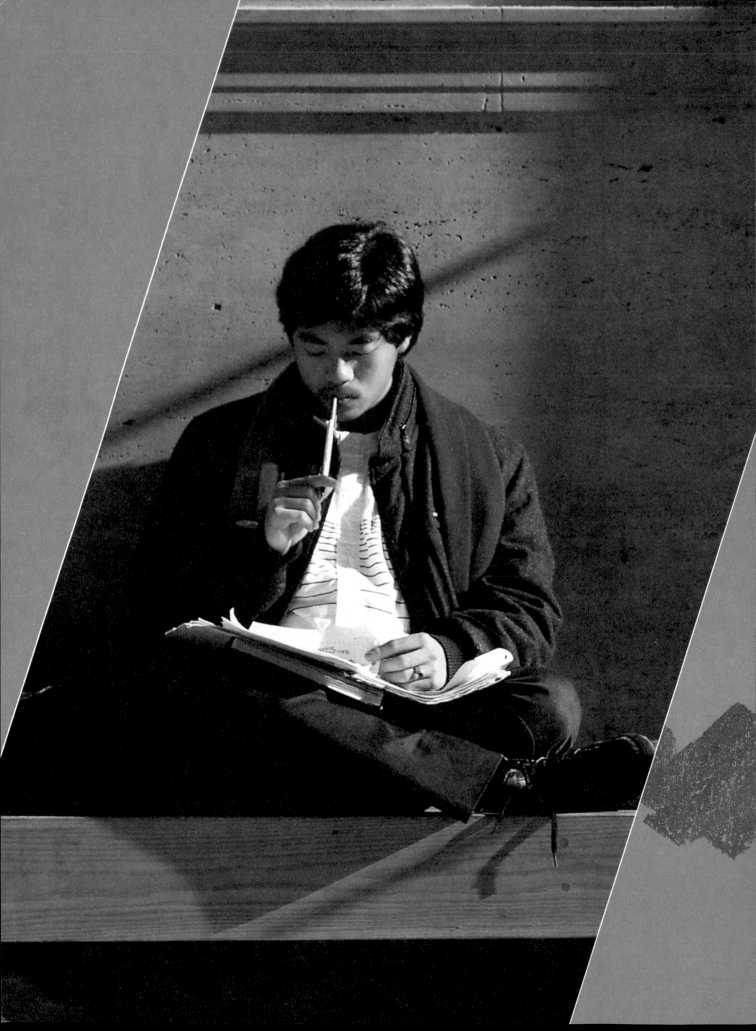

Chapter 12

Developing an Action Plan for Lifetime Wellness

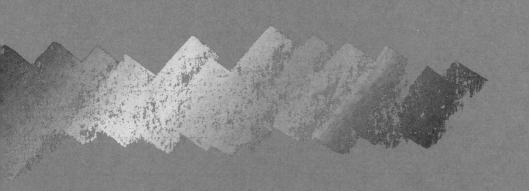

This chapter is for you. Throughout the term, you have been reading about topics that specifically relate to quality of life. Your health and state of wellness encompass every aspect of living, whether physical, social, psychological, emotional, spiritual, or environmental. The more you take charge of each of the components affecting your life, the greater the chances are that you will live a healthy and fulfilling life.

In this chapter, you are asked to bring together all the knowledge and information you have acquired this term to form a comprehensive picture of where you are in relationship to where you would like to be from a wellness perspective. Consider all the assessment activities you have completed this term, including the Action Plans for Personal Wellness. These should provide you with insight into the areas you might want to consider for change. Next, you need to analyze your health history. Assessment Activity 12-1 is designed for this. Using this health history in combination with the previous assessments you have completed, your next task will be to formulate an action plan for changing at least one of those behaviors that are detrimental or ineffective in attaining high level wellness to ones that are more conducive to personal development. Some experts have suggested that the easiest starting point is an exercise or aerobic program. However, where you decide to make changes is a personal decision. Along with the assessment activities and action plans, this chapter contains forms and exercises that will help you accomplish this task. Further, it is strongly suggested that Appendix A, the Lifestyle Assessment Inventory, be retaken to isolate changes and the current status of your lifestyle.

The purpose of the following assessment is to increase your awareness of your present medical condition and your medical history. If your lipid profile is somewhat elevated, this may be an area

in your life that needs attention and change. Recognizing a family history of breast cancer should contribute to your desire to not engage in behaviors that have a strong correlation to breast cancer. While there are many things you cannot control in your life, there are also many things you can. All the information that can be gathered about yourself from a medical perspective contributes to your decision-making ability when it comes to lifestyle and behavioral change.

Assessing Your Personal Wellness

In Chapter 1, Figure 1-2 is labeled *The dimensions of wellness*. Using this figure, the information you have gathered during the term, and Assessment Activities 12-2 and 12-3, you will now assess your current level of functioning based on the wellness model. For your convenience, the definitions of each component are restated below:

▌ **Spiritual:** The belief in some force that serves to unite human beings. This might include nature, science, or a higher power and includes a person's morals, values, and ethics. Everyone has their perception of spirituality. It is this component that provides meaning and direction in life and enables each person to grow, learn, and meet new challenges. Optimal spirituality is our ability to discover, articulate, and act on our own basic purpose in life.[4]

▌ **Social:** The ability to interact successfully with the people and the environment of which each person is a part. It is developing and maintaining intimacy with specific others as well as respect and tolerance for those with differing opinions and beliefs.

▌ **Emotional:** The ability to control stress and to express emotions appropriately and comfortably. Emotional health is being able to recognize and accept one's feelings and express them appropriately as well as not allowing ourselves to be defeated by setbacks and failures.

▌ **Intellectual:** The ability to learn and effectively use information for personal, family, and career development. Intellectual wellness indicates the striving for continued growth and the ability to learn to deal effectively with new challenges.

▌ **Physical:** The ability to carry out daily tasks, develop cardiovascular fitness, use adequate nutrition, and invest in positive lifestyle habits.

Writing a Contract for Lifestyle Change

Before writing a wellness contract(s), several steps should be considered. Some of these need to be formulated prior to writing the contract and some will be worked on while the change is occurring. Some steps are ongoing. See Assessment Activity 12-4.

1. **Identify your goal.** The purpose of the previous assessment has been to help you identify your personal goal. Knowing what you want is the first step in any action.

2. **Record your present behavioral pattern.** When you want to change a current behavior, it is a good idea to record your current pattern of the behavior. Recording can help increase your awareness of when, and probably why, you engage in this behavior. This can be done by keeping a journal or notebook handy and noting when, under what circumstances or conditions, how often, and your feelings when you engage in this behavior. If you know that you overeat at social events or that you become depressed when you get overly tired, it becomes easier to plan alternative actions or avoid the situation(s).

3. **Identify the behaviors that will lead to the goals you want to achieve and the rewards associated with those behaviors.** When you become aware of what actions, situations, and conditions contribute to you engaging in a negative behavior, you can then begin to find other behaviors to engage in during those periods of time. If you know you overeat in social situations, you can choose to avoid them, but this may make you feel deprived and lonely. Since the ability to interact socially is important to one's total well-being, this may not be the most advisable suggestion for this situation. What you may want to do is substitute drinking a diet drink, eating a low-calorie alternative, stay away from the food as much as possible, or have a "buddy" encourage you to not overeat and who will be there to patrol your eating behaviors in this situation. Also, spend as much time as possible interacting with the people at the gathering since this is the purpose of social events. The positive rewards associated with not overeating include preventing you from gaining weight, a sense of control over making conscious decisions and following them, and not feeling depressed because you did overeat.

4. **Commit yourself to change; envision your change in your mind.** Making a change of any kind is not easy. It takes conscious effort and some degree of sacrifice to change. You must be committed to some amount of discomfort to improve any aspect of your life. It might be of benefit to seriously consider how much sacrifice you are willing to really make before writing your contract. That contract *is* your commitment to change and should not be taken lightly. Meanwhile, it is of benefit to picture the "new you". Mentally *see* yourself in situations that have previously resulted in a negative behavior and *see*

 Making a change

Behavior change is only possible when there is a *recognized* need to make a change. Recognizing that there is a need is vital, but it is only the first step in an overall process. To make changes in lifestyle requires at least five distinct elements:
Awareness: I realize that I can choose to change.
Cognition: I know how to make a change in my life.
Emotion: I really want to make a change in my life.
Decision: I am committing myself to making a change.
Action: I am changing.

yourself not engaging in that behavior. Envision yourself successful. If you do not want to overeat at social events any more, picture yourself at an event not overeating but still talking and having a good time. Do this consistently, but especially *before* you will be in a tempting situation.

5. **Divide your wellness change into achievable goals and plan rewards for yourself.** One of the major problems people encounter when planning behavioral change is trying to do too much or making the goal so long range that discouragement sets in before the goal can be reached. Perhaps your goal is to become president of your own company. This is a worthy goal, but as a student at a university the probability of accomplishing this in the next few months is rather remote. It may be just about as difficult for you to change your eating habits overnight or exercise an hour a day, 7 days a week when you have never exercised in your life. While a few people may be able to make this type of wholesale change, planning such large-scale goals with no intermediate steps is almost surely setting yourself up for failure and a great deal of misery. The initial step of establishing an exercise program would be to realistically decide what you can do. Ideas you could consider for this type of program would be to walk 30 minutes a day every other day for the next 2 to 3 weeks and then gradually pick up either the intensity of the workout (perhaps alternating running with walking until you can run for 30 minutes at a time) or increasing the amount of time spent walking (attempting 45 minutes and then an hour) or walking more days a week. Each time a goal is accomplished, reward yourself. The first week you successfully complete what you planned to do, do something special for yourself; get a manicure or a massage or buy a new CD or whatever you would like to use to reward yourself. Each time you are successful at some new phase of your behavioral change, continue to treat yourself to something special. For instance, your next goal may be to continue this program for 6 weeks at the end of which time you may want to give yourself a bigger reward, such as new workout clothes. This will fa-

cilitate making a change and alleviate any sense of being deprived that you may experience.

6. **Try out your plan and make changes in it if necessary.** If you find that you have "bitten off more than you can chew" or if you need to make the changes in smaller increments or if you find that the change is easier than you first realized, adjust your plan accordingly. It is better to alter your schedule than to abandon your plan for change. Any steps in the right direction are better than remaining stagnant. You are the only one who knows your particular needs, but keep in mind that the purpose of making these changes is to improve your life and keep working towards your goals.

7. **Evaluate your progress periodically.** When you are doing good, stop and give yourself a pat on the back. When you are not accomplishing what you would like to, regroup and try again. The most important thing is to keep moving forward and never quit. You can do anything if you just keep working at it.

With the above guidelines in mind, begin to develop your wellness contract. (If you need help in formulating your contract, see Figure 2-4 in Chapter 2.)

A Final Word

From all the possible health and wellness changes you have identified in your life, you should choose the one that should be easiest for you to master first. Nothing breeds success like success; therefore, it is wise to select areas in your life where you *can* experience success and then use that success as a basis for your next change. Keep working on and practicing your plan until it is automatic in your life. Then target another behavior that is negatively influencing your life and write another contract.

If you experience failure in any of your attempts or if you become discouraged, complete Assessment Activity 12-5 and answer those questions honestly. Then, resume your original plan or modify it if necessary and continue.

Assessing Your Medical/Health History

I. Physical assessments

Directions: Some of the following assessments can easily be done. A lipid profile must be done by a blood analysis through a doctor's office, health clinic, or similar situation. Physical assessments can be done through a physical education department that has the appropriate equipment or through many wellness centers. If all the information that is asked for is not available to you, fill in all that you can. If you cannot provide or do not know all the information that is requested, it may indicate a need for additional screening and assessment. Fill in all the information that you can.

Name_____

Height_____Weight_____Blood type_____

Rh_____

Blood pressure_____Systolic_____

Diastolic_____

Lipid profile: Total cholesterol_____LDLs_____

HDLs_____

Triglycerides_____

Body composition_____% Spirometry_____

Strength Test (Grip Strength)_____Abdominal strength

(Sit-up test)_____

Flexibility test ("Sit and reach" test)_____

Aerobic Fitness Assessment_____

Alcohol use: None_____Moderate_____Heavy_____

Smoke:_____How Long:_____

Amount per day_____

II. Disease history

Directions: The list of diseases are fairly common conditions. If you have experienced any of these conditions, mark "yes" and fill out the information as to when (date) and the treatment you received. If you have never had certain conditions, such as German measles, but you have received the immunization for them, also mark "yes" and specify when and what. Any other diseases that you may have had and are a significant condition (you would not mention a cold but would want to mention if you had serious or chronic tonsillitis) should also be listed. If you have never received treatment for these conditions or not experienced them, simply mark "no".

Disease	No	Yes	Date	Immunization or Treatment
Arthritis	—	—	—	_____
Anemia	—	—	—	_____
Cancer	—	—	—	_____
Cardiovascular disease	—	—	—	_____
Chicken pox	—	—	—	_____
Diabetes	—	—	—	_____
Diphtheria	—	—	—	_____
Diverticulitis	—	—	—	_____
Ear infections/injury	—	—	—	_____
Epilepsy	—	—	—	_____
Eye disease/injury	—	—	—	_____
German measles	—	—	—	_____
Heart murmur	—	—	—	_____
Jaundice or hepatitis	—	—	—	_____
Low back pain	—	—	—	_____
Kidney or bladder disease	—	—	—	_____
Migraines	—	—	—	_____
Mononucleosis	—	—	—	_____
Mumps	—	—	—	_____
Pneumonia/bronchitis/asthma	—	—	—	_____
Rheumatic fever	—	—	—	_____
Scarlet fever	—	—	—	_____
Skin disease	—	—	—	_____
Ulcers/colitis	—	—	—	_____
Varicose veins	—	—	—	_____
Other diseases:	—	—	—	_____
_____	—	—	—	_____
_____	—	—	—	_____
_____	—	—	—	_____
_____	—	—	—	_____
_____	—	—	—	_____

III. Surgical history

Directions: List and provide the pertinent information if you have had any surgery.

What kind	When	Age	Physician
_____	_____	_____	_____
_____	_____	_____	_____
_____	_____	_____	_____

IV. Allergies

Directions: List any allergies that you may have or have had as a child. These can be to drugs or living things (for example, dogs, pollen, etc.) or foods.

Drug   **Other**

_____   _____
_____   _____
_____   _____
_____   _____

V. Medical evaluations

Directions: List any medical evaluations that you have had. Some of these tests are age related and will not necessarily apply.

Test	Date	Results
ECG	_____	_____
Pap smear	_____	_____
Glucose	_____	_____
TB skin test	_____	_____
Hemoccult	_____	_____
Tonometry	_____	_____
Sigmoidoscopy	_____	_____
Urinalysis	_____	_____
Chest X-ray	_____	_____
Blood pressure	_____	_____
Lipid profile (cholesterol)	_____	_____
Multiple blood screening (blood sugar, anemia, etc.)	_____	_____
Mammogram	_____	_____
Prostate	_____	_____

VI. Family history

Directions: Family history is an important component of a personal assessment. Although there is a lot of controversy as to the hereditary nature of diseases, there is a tendency for some conditions to run in families. This might be a good opportunity for you to investigate your family and find out if your relatives have or had any of those listed. If so, these are areas of particular concern to you and should be recognized when planning your behavioral changes.

	Arthritis	Cancer	Diabetes	Heart disease	Hypertension	Stroke	Other	Age of death	Cause
Father	___	___	___	___	___	___	___	___	___
Mother	___	___	___	___	___	___	___	___	___
Grandfather	___	___	___	___	___	___	___	___	___
Grandmother	___	___	___	___	___	___	___	___	___
Brother	___	___	___	___	___	___	___	___	___
Sister	___	___	___	___	___	___	___	___	___

ASSESSMENT ACTIVITY

Assessing Your Spiritual, Social, Emotional, and Intellectual Wellness

Your assessment of each of the components of your life should relate back to the descriptors that are given. For instance, the statement "I am at ease with myself" should have a specific response such as "most of the time". These should be responses to each of the sentences as well as specific aspects that may apply to you personally and are not listed here. These statements provide a basis or starting point for determining your wellness in each of the categories listed. Complete the assessment by writing out your assessment of where you are personally in relation to these statements and their importance or relevance to you.

Spiritual

Descriptors:
I am at ease with myself.
I have a philosophy of life that encompasses a sense of purpose, direction, and meaning.
I maintain a positive outlook.
I have a strong value system that I follow.
I have faith in a higher force guiding my life.
I use private time daily in prayer and/or meditation.

Personal assessment:_____

_____

_____

_____

Social

Descriptors:
I feel comfortable with others.
I am comfortable with my sexuality.
I have several close friends.
I am able to love without being dominating or being dominated.
I enjoy interacting with others.
I have a variety of interests.
I communicate well with others.
I regularly find humor in daily challenges.
I frequently find positive traits in the people I around me.
I take time to help or serve someone else.

Personal assessment:_____

_____

_____

_____

Emotional

Descriptors:
I am self-confident.
I display self-confidence around others.
I have a positive body image.

I can appropriately express my feelings, emotions, and love towards others.
I know how to make my needs known in a way that enhances communication.
I can confront my problems and deal with them realistically.
I deal with my problems and control my life.
I can laugh at myself.
I am able to ask for help without feeling ashamed or fearful.

Personal assessment:_____
_____
_____
_____

Intellectual

Descriptors:
I stay informed of community problems and changes.
I keep up with national and international events.
I lead a productive lifestyle.
I contribute to my community and civilization.
I find it easy to concentrate.
My attitudes are positive and life-affirming.
I use creativity to solve problems.
I am not afraid to change or bend, if necessary, to accomplish the tasks that need doing.
I am continuing to grow as an individual.
I enjoy expanding my knowledge and understanding about the world in which I live.
My grades (or job) are satisfying.
I take time each day to study or learn something not required of me.

Personal assessment:_____
_____
_____

Physical

Descriptors:
My body fat is appropriate for my age and sex.
I have a relatively high fitness level.
I engage in regular, aerobic exercise.
I keep my eating habits within recommended guidelines to assure I get adequate nutrition.
My lipid profile is within recommended ranges.
I take time each week to work on the components of muscular strength, flexibility, and endurance.
I have enough energy to meet the daily requirements of living.
I use alcoholic beverages moderately or not at all.
I get adequate sleep and rest each day.
My body is free from the effects of illicit drugs and tobacco.

Personal assessment:_____
_____
_____

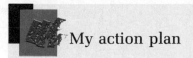My action plan

Throughout the term you have completed Assessment Activities and an Action Plan at the end of each chapter. In addition, you have just completed a current assessment of your spiritual, emotional, intellectual, social, and physical functioning. It is now time to synthesize the information you have gathered while doing these tasks and use that knowledge to formulate an action plan that demonstrates what you have learned about yourself. While completing this action plan it is important to be as specific as possible. The purpose of this activity is to hone in on those areas in your life that are primary for change.

1 Based on the assessments I have done, the health issues that I need to be most concerned about are:_____

_____

_____

2 Of those health concerns listed in no. 1, the one I most need to act on is:_____

_____

_____

3 Possible actions that I can take to improve my level of wellness are (try to be as specific as possible):_____

_____

_____

4 Of the actions listed in no. 3, the one that I most need to include in a behavioral contract is:___

_____

_____

_____

5 Factors I need to keep in mind in order to be successful in my action plan are:_____

_____

_____

ASSESSMENT ACTIVITY   12-3

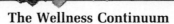

The Wellness Continuum

Directions: There are many ways to analyze the information you have gathered in the wellness assessment. A continuum scale can be used to clarify your areas of greatest concern. A continuum for each of the wellness areas follows. Place an "X" on each of the scales in the range that most closely reflects your feelings and attitudes toward this area in your life. Your responses should be based on your interpretations in Assessment Activity 12-2.

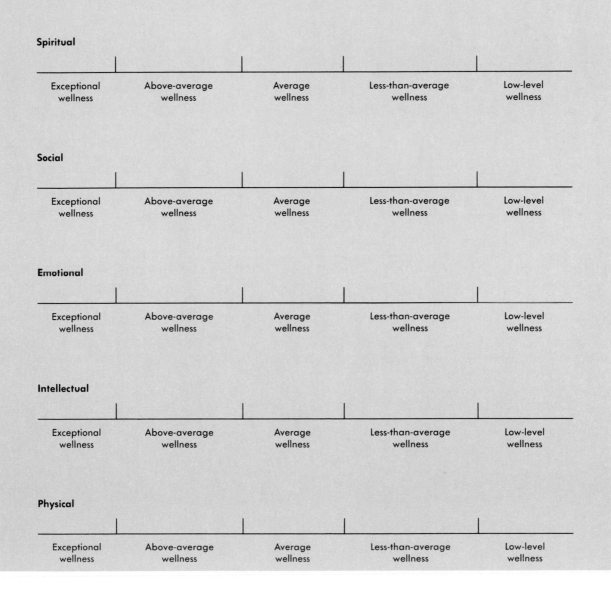

ASSESSMENT ACTIVITY   12-4

Lifestyle Change Wellness Contract

I, _____, pledge that within the next

_____, beginning _____ and ending _____,

I will accomplish the goals listed below.

_____   _____
(Signature)   *(Witness)*

My health goal:_____

_____

_____

My intermediate goals are:

1._____

2._____

3._____

4._____

5._____

Intervention strategies:

1._____

2._____

3._____

4._____

Rewards:

1._____

2._____

3._____

4._____

Penalties:

1._____

2._____

3._____

ASSESSMENT ACTIVITY

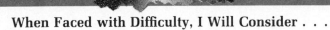

12-5

When Faced with Difficulty, I Will Consider . . .

Directions: Review your original contract and answer the following questions:

_____

Y   N   Did I persist long enough to experience the rewards associated with making my change?

Y   N   Did I practice the change as often or as long as I originally planned?

Y   N   Did I keep in mind where I started from and what improvements I made from where I started?

Y   N   Have I considered exactly what my old behavior was costing me in terms of money, physical health, or emotional well-being?

Y   N   Did I enlist support from significant others in my life and did they provide it?

Y   N   Did I set realistic goals for myself?

Y   N   Have I really been *committed* to my goals and making this change?

What do I want to do now?_____

_____

_____

How am I going to change my contract so that I can make it work?_____

_____

_____

Appendix A

Food
Composition
Tables

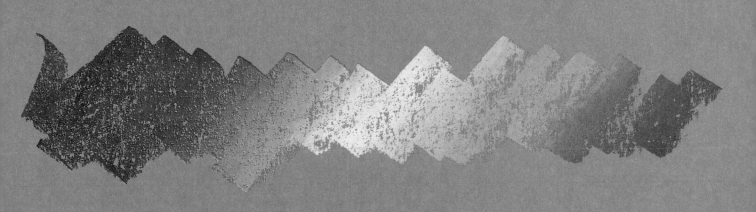

Composition Key

Abbreviation	Definition
KCAL	Calories
PROT	Protein
CARB	Carbohydrates
FAT	Fat
CHOL	Cholesterol
SAFA	Saturated fats
SOD	Sodium
POT	Potasium
MAG	Magnesium
IRON	Iron
ZINC	Zinc
V-A	Vitamin A
V-ET	Vitamin E
V-C	Vitamin C

■ Nutritive Components for Beverages

Food name	Serving	Gm wt	KCAL	PROT Gm	CARB Gm	FAT Gm	CHOL Mg	SAFA Gm	SOD Mg	POT Mg	MAG Mg
BEER-LIGHT	1 fl oz	29.5	8.000	0.100	0.400	0.000	0.000	0.000	1.000	5.000	1.000
BEER-REGULAR	1 fl oz	29.7	12.00	0.100	1.100	0.000	0.000	0.000	2.000	7.000	2.000
CHAMPAGNE-DOMESTIC-GLASS	1 item	120.0	84.00	0.200	3.000	—	—	—	—	—	—
CLUB SODA	1 fl oz	29.6	0.000	0.000	0.000	0.000	0.000	0.000	6.000	0.000	0.000
COFFEE-BREWED	1 fl oz	30.0	1.000	0.000	0.100	0.000	0.000	0.000	1.000	16.00	2.000
COLA-TYPE-SODA	1 fl oz	30.8	13.30	0.000	3.200	0.000	0.000	0.000	1.000	0.000	0.000
DIET SOFT DRINK	1 fl oz	29.6	0.000	0.000	0.000	0.000	0.000	0.000	2.000	0.000	0.000
LEMON LIME SODA-7UP	1 fl oz	30.7	12.00	0.000	3.200	0.000	0.000	0.000	3.000	0.000	0.000
TEA-BREWED	1 fl oz	29.6	0.000	0.000	0.100	0.000	0.000	0.000	1.000	11.00	1.000
WATER	1 cup	237.0	0.000	0.000	0.000	0.000	0.000	0.000	7.000	1.000	2.000
WHIS/GIN/RUM/VOD-80 PROOF	1 fl oz	27.8	64.00	0.000	0.000	0.000	0.000	0.000	0.000	1.000	0.000
WINE-WHITE-TABLE	1 fl oz	29.5	20.00	0.000	0.200	0.000	0.000	0.000	18.00	33.30	3.000
WINE COOLER-WHITE WINE/7UP	1 srvg	102.0	54.90	0.050	5.720	0.000	0.000	0.000	7.480	41.00	5.000
GATORADE-THIRST QUENCHER	1 fl oz	30.1	7.000	0.000	1.900	0.000	0.000	0.000	12.00	3.000	0.000

Abbreviation	Definition
THIA	Thiamin
RIBO	Riboflavin
NIAC	Niacin
V-B6	Vitamin B-6
FOL	Folic acid
VB-12	Vitamin B-12
CALC	Calcium
PHOS	Phosphorus
SEL	Selenuim
FIBD	Dietary fiber
Gm	gram
Mg	milligram
IU	International Units
μg	microgram

Nutritive Components for Beverages—cont'd

IRON Mg	ZINC Mg	V-A IU	V-ET Mg	V-C Mg	THIA Mg	RIBO Mg	NIAC Mg	V-B6 Mg	FOL μg	VB12 μg	CALC Mg	PHOS Mg	SEL Mg	FIBD Gm
0.010	0.010	0.000	—	0.000	0.003	0.009	0.116	0.010	1.200	0.000	1.000	4.000	0.000	—
0.010	0.000	0.000	—	0.000	0.002	0.008	0.135	0.015	1.800	0.010	1.000	4.000	—	—
—	—	—	—	—	—	—	—	—	—	—	—	—	—	—
—	0.030	0.000	—	0.000	0.000	0.000	0.000	0.000	0.000	0.000	1.000	0.000	—	0.000
0.120	0.000	0.000	—	0.000	0.000	0.000	0.066	0.000	0.000	0.000	1.000	0.000	0.000	0.000
0.010	0.000	0.000	—	0.000	0.000	0.000	0.000	0.000	0.000	0.000	1.000	4.000	—	0.000
0.010	0.020	0.000	—	0.000	0.001	0.007	0.000	0.000	0.000	0.000	1.000	3.000	—	0.000
0.020	0.020	0.000	0.000	0.000	0.000	0.000	0.005	0.000	0.000	0.000	1.000	0.000	—	0.000
0.010	0.010	0.000	—	0.000	0.000	0.004	0.000	0.000	1.500	0.000	0.000	0.000	0.000	0.000
0.010	0.060	0.000	—	0.000	0.000	0.000	0.000	0.000	0.000	0.000	5.000	0.000	—	0.000
0.030	0.020	0.000	0.000	0.000	0.002	0.000	0.000	0.000	0.000	0.000	0.000	1.000	0.000	0.000
0.090	0.020	0.000	—	0.000	0.001	0.001	0.020	0.004	0.100	0.000	3.000	4.000	—	0.000
0.193	0.063	—	—	—	0.002	0.043	0.003	0.007	0.100	0.000	6.110	6.950	—	—
0.020	0.010	0.000	0.000	0.000	0.002	0.000	0.000	0.000	0.000	0.000	0.000	3.000	—	0.000

Nutritive Components for Breads

Food name	Serving	Gm wt	KCAL	PROT Gm	CARB Gm	FAT Gm	CHOL Mg	SAFA Gm	SOD Mg	POT Mg	MAG Mg
BAGEL-EGG	1 item	55.0	163.0	6.020	30.90	1.410	8.000	0.500	198.0	40.70	11.00
BISCUITS-PREPARED/ MIX	1 item	28.0	93.20	2.070	13.60	3.320	—	0.600	262.0	56.00	6.720
BREAD-FRENCH-ENRICHED	1 slice	35.0	98.00	3.330	17.70	1.360	0.000	0.200	193.0	30.10	7.000
BREAD-WHITE-FIRM	1 slice	23.0	61.40	1.900	11.20	0.902	0.000	0.200	118.0	25.80	4.830
BREAD-WHOLE WHEAT-FIRM	1 slice	25.0	61.30	2.410	11.30	1.090	0.000	0.100	159.0	44.00	23.30
MUFFIN-ENGLISH-PLAIN	1 item	56.0	133.0	4.430	25.70	1.090	—	—	358.0	314.0	10.60
ROLL-BROWN & SERVE-ENR	1 item	26.0	85.00	2.000	14.00	2.000	—	0.400	144.0	25.00	5.460
CROISSANT-ROLL-SARA LEE	1 item	26.0	109.0	2.300	11.20	6.100	—	—	140.0	40.00	7.000
ROLL-HAMBURGER/ HOTDOG	1 item	40.0	114.0	3.430	20.10	2.090	—	0.500	241.0	36.80	7.600

Nutritive Components for Breakfast Cereals

Food name	Serving	Gm wt	KCAL	PROT Gm	CARB Gm	FAT Gm	CHOL Mg	SAFA Gm	SOD Mg	POT Mg	MAG Mg
CEREAL-ALPHA BITS	1 cup	28.4	111.0	2.200	24.60	0.600	—	—	219.0	110.0	17.00
CEREAL-CHEERIOS	1 cup	22.7	88.80	3.420	15.70	1.450	0.000	0.270	246.0	81.00	31.30
CEREAL-CORN CHEX	1 cup	28.4	111.0	2.000	24.90	0.100	—	—	271.0	23.00	4.000
CEREAL-CORN FLAKES-KELLOGG	1 cup	22.7	88.30	1.840	19.50	0.068	0.000	0.000	281.0	20.90	2.720
CEREAL-FRUIT LOOPS	1 cup	28.4	111.0	1.700	25.00	0.500	0.000	0.000	145.0	26.00	7.000
CEREAL-GRAPE NUTS	1 cup	114.0	407.0	13.30	93.50	0.456	0.000	0.000	792.0	381.0	76.30
CEREAL-LIFE-PLAIN/ CINNAMON	1 cup	44.0	162.0	8.100	31.50	0.800	0.000	0.000	229.0	197.0	14.00
CEREAL-GRANOLA-NATURE VAL	1 cup	113.0	503.0	11.50	75.50	19.60	0.000	13.00	232.0	389.0	116.0
CEREAL-RAISIN BRAN-KELLOGG	1 cup	49.2	154.0	5.300	37.10	0.984	0.000	—	359.0	256.0	63.50
CEREAL-RICE-PUFFED-SUGAR	1 cup	28.0	115.0	1.000	26.00	0.000	0.000	—	21.00	43.00	7.560
CEREAL-RICE KRISPIES	1 cup	28.4	112.0	1.900	24.80	0.200	0.000	0.000	340.0	30.00	10.00
CEREAL-WHEAT GERM-TOASTED	1 cup	113.0	431.0	32.90	56.10	12.10	0.000	2.090	4.000	1070	362.0
CEREAL-WHEATIES	1 cup	29.0	101.0	2.800	23.10	0.500	0.000	0.070	363.0	108.0	32.00
CEREAL-CREAM/ WHEAT-REG-HOT	1 cup	251.0	134.0	3.800	27.70	0.500	0.000	0.000	2.000	43.00	10.00
CEREAL-OATMEAL-INST-PACKET	1 item	177.0	104.0	4.400	18.10	1.700	0.000	—	286.0	100.0	—
CEREAL-FROST FLAKE-KELLOGG	1 cup	35.0	133.0	1.800	31.70	0.100	0.000	0.000	284.0	22.00	3.000
CEREAL-WHEAT-SHRED-BISCUIT	1 item	23.6	83.00	2.600	18.80	0.300	0.000	0.000	0.472	77.00	40.00

■ Nutritive Components for Breads—cont'd

IRON Mg	ZINC Mg	V-A IU	V-ET Mg	V-C Mg	THIA Mg	RIBO Mg	NIAC Mg	V-B6 Mg	FOL μg	VB12 μg	CALC Mg	PHOS Mg	SEL Mg	FIBD Gm
1.460	0.286	17.60	—	0.000	0.209	0.160	1.940	0.024	13.20	0.052	23.10	36.90	—	0.506
0.574	0.176	15.70	0.694	0.000	0.120	0.106	0.840	0.013	1.680	0.045	58.20	128.0	—	—
1.080	0.221	0.000	0.417	0.000	0.161	0.123	1.400	0.019	13.00	0.000	38.50	28.40	0.010	0.546
0.653	0.143	0.000	0.274	0.000	0.108	0.071	0.863	0.008	8.050	0.000	29.00	24.80	0.006	0.621
0.855	0.420	0.000	0.225	0.000	0.088	0.053	0.958	0.047	13.80	0.000	18.00	65.00	0.011	2.830
1.580	0.403	0.000	—	0.000	0.258	0.179	2.100	0.022	17.90	0.000	90.70	62.70	0.015	—
0.800	0.190	0.000	1.730	0.000	0.100	0.060	0.900	0.016	9.880	—	20.00	23.00	0.008	—
1.040	—	41.00	—	0.000	0.280	0.100	1.200	—	—	—	12.00	32.00	—	—
1.190	0.248	0.000	0.212	0.000	0.196	0.132	1.580	0.014	14.80	—	53.60	32.80	0.012	—

■ Nutritive Components for Breakfast Cereals—cont'd

IRON Mg	ZINC Mg	V-A IU	V-ET Mg	V-C Mg	THIA Mg	RIBO Mg	NIAC Mg	V-B6 Mg	FOL μg	VB12 μg	CALC Mg	PHOS Mg	SEL Mg	FIBD Gm
1.800	1.500	1250	—	—	0.400	0.400	5.000	0.500	100.0	1.500	8.000	51.00	—	0.300
3.610	0.629	1001	—	12.00	0.295	0.341	4.000	0.409	4.990	1.200	38.80	107.0	0.010	0.863
1.800	0.100	143.0	—	15.00	0.400	0.070	5.000	0.500	100.0	1.500	3.000	11.00	0.002	0.500
1.430	0.064	1001	—	12.00	0.295	0.341	4.000	0.409	80.10	—	0.681	14.30	0.001	0.250
4.500	3.700	1250	—	15.00	0.400	0.400	5.000	0.500	100.0	—	3.000	24.00	—	0.200
4.950	2.510	5026	—	—	1.480	1.710	20.10	2.050	402.0	6.040	43.30	286.0	0.034	5.470
11.60	1.450	—	—	—	0.950	1.000	11.60	—	37.00	—	154.0	238.0	—	1.400
3.780	2.190	—	—	—	0.390	0.190	0.830	—	85.00	—	71.00	354.0	0.037	4.200
6.000	5.020	1667	—	—	0.492	0.590	6.690	0.689	133.0	2.020	17.20	183.0	0.005	5.310
0.000	1.480	1240	—	15.00	0.000	0.000	0.000	0.504	98.80	1.480	3.000	14.00	0.002	0.200
1.800	0.480	1250	0.080	15.00	0.400	0.400	5.000	0.500	100.0	—	4.000	34.00	0.004	0.100
10.30	18.80	188.0	31.10	7.000	1.890	0.930	6.310	1.110	398.0	—	50.00	1294	—	7.800
4.600	0.650	1279	0.612	15.00	0.400	0.400	5.100	0.500	9.000	1.500	44.00	100.0	0.003	2.000
10.30	0.330	—	—	—	0.200	0.100	1.500	—	9.000	—	51.00	42.00	—	—
6.320	—	1514	2.710	—	0.530	0.290	5.490	0.742	150.0	—	163.0	133.0	—	1.620
2.200	0.050	1543	—	19.00	0.500	0.500	6.200	0.600	124.0	—	1.000	26.00	—	2.200
0.740	0.590	0.000	0.508	0.000	0.070	0.060	1.080	0.060	12.00	—	10.00	86.00	—	2.200

Nutritive Components for Combination Foods

Food name	Serving	Gm wt	KGAL	PROT Gm	CARB Gm	FAT Gm	CHOL Mg	SAFA Gm	SOD Mg	POT Mg	MAG Mg
BEEF-RAVIOLIOS-CANNED	1 srvg	28.4	27.50	1.140	4.260	0.568	—	—	131.0	45.70	—
CHICKEN POTPIE-BAKED-HOME	1 slice	232.0	545.0	23.00	42.00	31.00	72.00	11.00	593.0	343.0	—
MACARONI & CHEESE-ENR-HOME	1 cup	200.0	430.0	17.00	40.00	22.00	42.00	8.900	1086	240.0	52.00
MEAT LOAF-CELERY/ONIONS	1 serv	87.6	213.0	15.80	5.230	13.90	107.0	5.290	103.0	182.0	13.60
PIZZA-PEPPERONI-BAKED	1 slice	120.0	306.0	13.00	36.70	11.50	—	—	817.0	216.0	—
BEANS/PORK/TOM SAUCE-CAN	1 cup	253.0	247.0	13.00	49.00	2.600	17.00	1.000	1113	759.0	88.00
SALAD-CHICKEN	1 cup	205.0	502.0	26.00	17.40	36.20	—	—	1395	521.0	—
SALAD-POTATO	1 cup	250.0	358.0	6.700	27.90	20.50	171.0	3.570	1323	635.0	39.00
SALAD-TUNA	1 cup	205.0	350.0	30.00	7.000	22.00	68.00	4.300	434.0	—	—
SPAGHETTI/TOM/MEAT-CAN	1 cup	250.0	260.0	12.00	29.00	10.00	39.00	2.200	1220	245.0	28.00
TACO	1 item	81.0	187.0	10.60	12.70	10.40	21.10	—	456.0	263.0	36.50

Nutritive Components for Dairy Products

Food name	Serving	Gm wt	KCAL	PROT Gm	CARB Gm	FAT Gm	CHOL Mg	SAFA Gm	SOD Mg	POT Mg	MAG Mg
CHEESE-AMERICAN-PROCESSED	1 piece	28.0	106.0	6.280	0.450	8.860	27.00	5.580	406.0	46.00	6.000
CHEESE-CHEDDAR-SHREDDED	1 cup	113.0	455.0	28.10	1.450	37.50	119.0	23.80	701.0	111.0	31.00
CHEESE-COTTAGE-4% LAR CURD	1 cup	225.0	232.0	28.10	6.030	10.10	33.80	6.410	911.0	189.0	11.30
CHEESE-CREAM	1 srvg	28.0	99.00	2.140	0.750	9.890	31.00	6.230	84.00	34.00	2.000
CHEESE-SWISS	1 piece	28.0	107.0	8.060	0.960	7.780	26.00	5.040	74.00	31.00	10.10
CHEESE FOOD-AMERICAN-PROC	1 srvg	28.0	93.00	5.560	2.070	6.970	18.00	4.380	337.0	79.00	9.000
CREAM-HALF & HALF-FLUID	1 cup	242.0	315.0	7.160	10.40	27.80	89.00	17.30	98.00	314.0	25.00
CREAM-SOUR-CULTURED	1 cup	230.0	493.0	7.270	9.820	48.20	102.0	30.00	123.0	331.0	26.00
CREAM-WHIP-IMIT-FROZ	1 cup	75.0	239.0	0.940	17.30	19.00	0.000	16.30	19.00	14.00	1.000
MILK-CHOCOLATE-WHOLE	1 cup	250.0	208.0	7.920	25.90	8.480	30.00	5.260	149.0	417.0	33.00
MILK-HUMAN-WHOLE-MATURE	1 cup	246.0	171.0	2.530	17.00	10.80	34.00	4.940	42.00	126.0	8.000

Nutritive Components for Combination Foods—cont'd

IRON Mg	ZINC Mg	V-A IU	V-ET Mg	V-C Mg	THIA Mg	RIBO Mg	NIAC Mg	V-B6 Mg	FOL μg	VB12 μg	CALC Mg	PHOS Mg	SEL Mg	FIBD Gm
0.312	—	262.0	0.136	0.426	0.026	0.023	0.398	—	—	—	4.540	—	—	0.230
3.000	—	3090	—	5.000	0.340	0.310	5.500	—	—	—	70.00	232.0	—	—
1.800	—	860.0	—	0.000	0.200	0.400	1.800	—	—	—	362.0	322.0	—	1.200
1.910	3.080	61.50	0.068	0.725	0.052	0.148	3.160	0.162	10.90	1.520	22.80	112.0	0.001	0.110
2.520	—	532.0	—	2.400	0.324	0.288	5.150	0.096	78.00	0.360	196.0	—	—	2.160
8.300	14.80	313.0	2.750	7.800	0.132	0.116	1.260	0.175	56.80	0.030	141.0	297.0	—	13.80
—	—	—	—	—	—	—	—	—	—	—	—	—	—	—
1.630	0.780	523.0	—	24.90	0.193	0.150	2.230	0.353	16.80	0.385	48.00	130.0	—	5.250
2.700	—	590.0	3.050	2.000	0.080	0.230	10.30	—	—	—	41.00	291.0	—	1.030
3.300	—	1000	—	5.000	0.150	0.180	2.300	—	—	—	53.00	113.0	—	2.750
1.150	1.560	420.0	—	0.810	0.089	0.065	1.410	0.122	11.30	0.405	109.0	134.0	—	—

Nutritive Components for Dairy Products—cont'd

IRON Mg	ZINC Mg	V-A IU	V-ET Mg	V-C Mg	THIA Mg	RIBO Mg	NIAC Mg	V-B6 Mg	FOL μg	VB12 μg	CALC Mg	PHOS Mg	SEL Mg	FIBD Gm
0.110	0.850	343.0	0.280	0.000	0.008	0.100	0.020	0.020	2.000	0.197	174.0	211.0	0.003	0.000
0.770	3.510	1197	—	0.000	0.031	0.424	0.090	0.084	21.00	0.935	815.0	579.0	0.018	0.000
0.315	0.833	367.0	—	0.000	0.047	0.367	0.284	0.151	27.00	1.400	135.0	297.0	0.052	0.000
0.340	0.150	405.0	—	0.000	0.005	0.056	0.029	0.013	4.000	0.120	23.00	30.00	0.001	0.000
0.050	1.110	240.0	0.200	0.000	0.006	0.103	0.026	0.024	2.000	0.475	272.0	171.0	0.003	0.000
0.240	0.850	259.0	—	0.000	0.008	0.125	0.040	—	—	0.317	163.0	130.0	0.006	0.000
0.170	1.230	1050	1.520	2.080	0.085	0.361	0.189	0.094	6.000	0.796	254.0	230.0	0.001	0.000
0.140	0.620	1817	—	1.980	0.081	0.343	0.154	0.037	25.00	0.690	268.0	195.0	—	0.000
0.090	0.020	646.0	—	0.000	0.000	0.000	0.000	0.000	0.000	0.000	5.000	6.000	—	0.000
0.600	1.020	302.0	—	2.280	0.092	0.405	0.313	0.100	12.00	0.835	280.0	251.0	0.003	0.300
0.070	0.420	593.0	2.440	12.30	0.034	0.089	0.435	0.027	13.00	0.111	79.00	34.00	0.004	0.000

Nutritive Components for Dairy Products—cont'd

Food name	Serving	Gm wt	KCAL	PROT Gm	CARB Gm	FAT Gm	CHOL Mg	SAFA Gm	SOD Mg	POT Mg	MAG Mg
MILK-2% FAT-LOWFAT-FLUID	1 cup	244.0	121.0	8.120	11.70	4.680	18.00	2.920	122.0	377.0	33.00
MILK-NONFAT-INSTANT-DRIED	1 cup	68.0	244.0	23.90	33.50	0.490	12.00	0.320	373.0	1160	80.00
MILKSHAKE-CHOCOLATE-THICK	1 item	300.0	356.0	9.150	63.50	8.100	32.00	5.040	333.0	672.0	48.00
YOGURT-FRUIT FLAVOR-LOWFAT	1 cup	227.0	231.0	9.920	43.20	2.450	10.00	1.580	133.0	442.0	33.00
YOGURT-PLAIN-LOWFAT	1 cup	227.0	144.0	11.90	16.00	3.520	14.00	2.270	159.0	531.0	40.00

Nutritive Components for Desserts

Food name	Serving	Gm wt	KCAL	PROT Gm	CARB Gm	FAT Gm	CHOL Mg	SAFA Gm	SOD Mg	POT Mg	MAG Mg
BROWNIES/NUTS-MIX/PREP	1 item	20.0	85.00	1.000	13.00	4.000	0.000	0.900	50.00	34.00	—
CAKE-YELLOW/ICING-HOME REC	1 slice	69.0	268.0	2.900	40.30	11.40	36.00	3.000	191.0	72.50	13.10
COOKIE-CHOC CHIP-HOME REC	1 item	10.0	46.30	0.500	6.410	2.680	5.250	0.600	20.60	20.50	3.500
COOKIE-OATMEAL/RAISIN/MIX	1 item	13.0	61.50	0.732	8.930	2.600	0.000	0.500	37.10	22.60	3.640
DOUGHNUTS-YEAST-GLAZED	1 item	50.0	205.0	3.000	22.00	11.20	13.00	3.000	117.0	34.00	9.500
FROZ YOGURT-FRUIT VARIETY	1 cup	226.0	216.0	7.000	41.80	2.000	—	—	—	—	24.00
GRANOLA BAR	1 item	24.0	109.0	2.350	16.00	4.230	—	—	66.70	78.20	—
ICE CREAM-VAN-SOFT SERVE	1 cup	173.0	377.0	7.040	38.30	22.50	153.0	13.50	153.0	338.0	25.00
ICE CREAM SUNDAE-HOT FUDGE	1 item	165.0	312.0	7.260	46.50	10.90	18.20	—	177.0	413.0	34.70
PIE-APPLE-HOME REC	1 slice	135.0	323.0	2.750	49.10	13.60	0.000	3.900	207.0	115.0	10.80
PUDD-CHOC-COOKED-MIX/MILK	1 cup	260.0	320.0	9.000	59.00	8.000	32.00	4.300	335.0	354.0	—
TOASTER PASTRIES	1 item	50.0	196.0	1.930	35.20	5.750	0.000	—	230.0	84.50	9.000
TWINKIE-HOSTESS	1 item	42.0	143.0	1.250	25.60	4.200	21.00	—	189.0	—	—

Nutritive Components for Dairy Products—cont'd

IRON Mg	ZINC Mg	V-A IU	V-ET Mg	V-C Mg	THIA Mg	RIBO Mg	NIAC Mg	V-B6 Mg	FOL µg	VB12 µg	CALC Mg	PHOS Mg	SEL Mg	FIBD Gm
0.120	0.950	500.0	0.220	2.320	0.095	0.403	0.210	0.105	12.00	0.888	297.0	232.0	0.003	0.000
0.210	3.000	1612	—	3.790	0.281	1.190	0.606	0.235	34.00	2.720	837.0	670.0	—	0.000
0.930	1.440	258.0	—	0.000	0.141	0.666	0.372	0.075	15.00	0.945	396.0	378.0	0.005	0.900
0.160	1.680	104.0	—	1.500	0.084	0.404	0.216	0.091	21.00	1.060	345.0	271.0	—	0.800
0.180	2.020	150.0	—	1.820	0.100	0.486	0.259	0.111	25.00	1.280	415.0	326.0	—	0.000

Nutritive Components for Desserts—cont'd

IRON Mg	ZINC Mg	V-A IR	V-ET Mg	V-C Mg	THIA Mg	RIBO Mg	NIAC Mg	V-B6 Mg	FOL µg	VB12 µg	CALC Mg	PHOS Mg	SEL Mg	FIBD Gm
0.400	—	20.00	1.090	0.000	0.030	0.020	0.200	—	—	—	9.000	27.00	0.001	—
0.787	0.338	47.60	5.860	0.000	0.076	0.097	0.656	0.023	5.520	0.123	57.30	60.70	0.004	—
0.249	0.044	4.300	0.545	0.000	0.015	0.015	0.146	0.002	0.900	0.010	3.300	8.400	0.001	0.080
0.285	0.085	10.40	0.708	0.000	0.022	0.021	0.241	0.006	1.560	—	4.420	14.40	0.001	—
0.600	—	25.00	2.030	0.000	0.100	0.100	0.800	—	11.00	—	16.00	33.00	—	0.300
0.000	—	0.000	—	0.000	0.010	0.260	0.000	—	—	—	200.0	200.0	—	—
0.763	—	—	—	—	0.067	0.026	—	—	—	0.000	14.40	66.50	—	—
0.430	1.990	794.0	0.606	0.920	0.080	0.448	0.178	0.095	9.000	0.996	236.0	199.0	0.003	0.000
0.611	0.990	231.0	0.577	3.300	0.066	0.314	1.120	0.132	9.900	0.660	216.0	238.0	—	—
1.220	0.230	25.70	9.840	2.000	0.149	0.108	1.240	0.035	6.750	0.000	12.20	31.10	0.015	—
0.800	—	340.0	—	2.000	0.050	0.390	0.300	—	—	—	265.0	247.0	—	0.000
2.000	0.290	482.0	—	0.000	0.160	0.170	2.100	0.190	40.00	0.000	96.50	96.50	—	—
0.545	—	40.50	—	0.000	0.055	0.060	0.500	—	—	—	19.00	—	—	—

▊ Nutritive Components for Eggs

Food Name	Serving	Gm wt	KCAL	PROT Gm	CARB Gm	FAT Gm	CHOL Mg	SAFA Gm	SOD Mg	POT Mg	MAG Mg
EGG-FRIED IN BUTTER-LARGE	1 item	46.0	83.00	5.370	0.530	6.410	246.0	2.410	144.0	58.00	5.000
EGG-HARD-LARGE-NO SHELL	1 item	50.0	79.00	6.070	0.600	5.580	274.0	1.670	69.00	65.00	6.000
EGG-SCRAMBLED-MILK/BUTTER	1 item	64.0	95.00	5.960	1.370	7.080	248.0	2.820	155.0	85.00	8.000
EGG-SUBSTITUTE-LIQUID	1 cup	251.0	211.0	30.10	1.610	8.310	3.000	1.660	444.0	828.0	—

▊ Nutritive Components for Fast Foods

Food name	Serving	Gm wt	KCAL	PROT Gm	CARB Gm	FAT Gm	CHOL Mg	SAFA Gm	SOD Mg	POT Mg	MAG Mg
ARBYS-ROAST BEEF SANDWICH	1 item	140.0	350.0	22.00	32.00	15.00	45.00	—	880.0	—	—
BURGER KING-WHOP HAMBURGER	1 item	261.0	630.0	26.00	50.00	36.00	—	—	990.0	520.0	—
CHURCHS CHICK-WHITE MEAT	1 item	100.0	327.0	21.00	10.00	23.00	—	—	498.0	186.0	—
DAIRY QUEEN-CONE-REGULAR	1 item	142.0	230.0	6.000	35.00	7.000	20.00		—	—	—
JACK/BOX-JUMBO JACK HAMBUR	1 item	246.0	551.0	28.00	45.00	29.00	80.00	—	1134	492.0	44.00
KENTUCKY FRIED-EXTRA CRISP	1 srvg	375.0	765.0	38.30	54.70	44.00	183.0	10.50	1480	776.0	70.00
MCDONALD-BIG MAC HAMBURGER	1 item	204.0	563.0	26.00	41.00	33.00	86.00	—	1010	237.0	38.00
MCDONALDS-EGG MCMUFFIN	1 item	138.0	327.0	19.00	31.00	15.00	229.0	—	885.0	168.0	26.00
MCDONALDS-FILET O FISH	1 item	139.0	432.0	14.00	37.00	25.00	47.00	—	781.0	150.0	27.00
MCDONALDS-FRENCH FRIES	1 srvg	68.0	220.0	3.000	26.10	11.50	9.000	—	109.0	564.0	27.00
TACO BELL-BURRITO SUPREME	1 item	255.0	457.0	21.00	43.00	22.00	—	—	367.0	350.0	—
TACO BELL-TACO-REGULAR	1 item	83.0	186.0	15.00	14.00	8.000	—	—	79.00	143.0	40.70
WENDYS-SINGLE HAMBURGER	1 item	200.0	470.0	26.00	34.00	26.00	70.00	—	774.0	—	—

Nutritive Components for Eggs—cont'd

IRON Mg	ZINC Mg	V-A IU	V-ET Mg	V-C Mg	THIA Mg	RIBO Mg	NIAC Mg	V-B6 Mg	FOL µg	VB12 µg	CALC Mg	PHOS Mg	SEL Mg	FIBD Gm
0.920	0.640	286.0	—	0.000	0.033	0.126	0.026	0.050	22.00	0.581	26.00	80.00	—	0.000
1.040	0.720	260.0	—	0.000	0.037	0.143	0.030	0.057	24.00	0.657	28.00	90.00	—	0.000
0.930	0.700	311.0	—	0.130	0.039	0.156	0.042	0.058	22.00	0.638	47.00	97.00	—	0.000
5.270	3.260	5422	—	0.000	0.276	0.753	0.276	—	—	0.748	133.0	304.0	—	0.000

Nutritive Components for Fast Foods—cont'd

IRON Mg	ZINC Mg	V-A IU	V-ET Mg	V-C Mg	THIA Mg	RIBO Mg	NIAC Mg	V-B6 Mg	FOL µg	VB12 µg	CALC Mg	PHOS Mg	SEL Mg	FIBD Gm
3.600	—	—	—	—	0.300	0.340	5.000	—	—	—	80.00	—	—	—
6.000	—	641.0	—	13.00	0.020	0.030	5.200	—	—	—	37.00	—	—	—
1.000	—	160.0	—	1.000	0.100	0.180	7.200	—	—	—	94.00	—	—	—
0.000	—	300.0	—	0.000	0.090	0.260	0.000	—	—	0.600	200.0	150.0	—	—
4.500	4.200	246.0	—	3.700	0.470	0.340	11.60	0.300	—	2.680	134.0	261.0	—	—
4.090	3.580	255.0	—	37.00	0.320	0.380	10.40	0.540	46.00	1.560	130.0	383.0	—	—
4.000	4.700	530.0	—	2.200	0.390	0.370	6.500	0.270	21.00	1.800	157.0	314.0	—	—
2.900	1.900	97.00	—	1.400	0.470	0.440	3.800	0.210	29.00	0.750	226.0	322.0	—	—
1.700	0.900	42.00	—	1.400	0.260	0.200	2.600	0.100	20.00	0.820	93.00	229.0	—	1.110
0.600	0.300	17.00	—	13.00	0.120	0.020	2.300	0.220	19.00	0.030	9.000	101.0	—	—
3.800	—	3462	—	16.00	0.330	0.350	4.700	—	—	—	121.0	245.0	—	—
2.500	2.200	120.0	—	0.200	0.090	0.160	2.900	—	—	—	120.0	175.0	—	—
5.300	4.800	94.00	—	0.600	0.240	0.360	5.800	—	—	—	84.00	239.0	—	—

Nutritive Components for Fats & Oils

Food name	Serving	Gm wt	KCAL	PROT Gm	CARB Gm	FAT Gm	CHOL Mg	SAFA Gm	SOD Mg	POT Mg	MAG Mg
BUTTER-REGULAR-TABLESPOON	1 tbsp	14.0	100.0	0.119	0.008	11.40	30.70	7.070	116.0	3.640	0.280
MARGARINE-DIET-MAZOLA	1 tbsp	14.0	50.00	0.000	0.000	5.700	0.000	1.000	130.0	—	—
MARGARINE-CORN-REG-SOFT	1 tsp	4.7	33.70	0.000	0.000	3.800	0.000	0.700	50.70	1.770	0.110
MARGARINE-REG-HARD-STICK	1 item	113.0	815.0	1.000	1.000	91.30	0.000	17.90	1070	48.10	2.950
MAYONNAISE-LIGHT-LOW CAL	1 tbsp	14.0	40.00	0.000	1.000	4.000	5.000	—	—	—	—
SAL DRESS-BLUE CHEESE	1 tbsp	15.3	77.10	0.700	1.100	8.000	9.000	1.500	167.0	6.120	—
SAL DRESS-FRENCH	1 tbsp	15.6	67.00	0.100	2.700	6.400	1.950	1.500	214.0	12.30	—
SAL DRESS-ITALIAN	1 tbsp	14.7	68.70	0.000	1.500	7.100	0.000	1.000	116.0	2.000	—
SAL DRESS-ITALIAN-LOW CAL	1 tbsp	15.0	15.80	0.000	0.700	1.500	1.000	0.200	118.0	2.000	—
SAL DRESS-MAYONNAISE TYPE	1 tbsp	14.7	57.30	0.000	3.500	4.900	4.000	0.700	104.0	1.000	0.290
SAL DRESS-RANCH STYLE	1 tbsp	15.0	54.00	0.400	0.600	5.700	—	—	97.00	—	—
SAL DRESS-THOUSAND IS-LAND	1 tbsp	15.6	58.90	0.000	2.400	5.600	4.900	0.900	109.0	18.00	—
SHORTENING-VEGETABLE-SOY	1 cup	205.0	1812	0.000	0.000	205.0	0.000	51.20	—	—	—
VEGETABLE OIL-CORN	1 cup	218.0	1927	0.000	0.000	218.0	0.000	27.70	0.000	0.000	0.000

Nutritive Components for Fish

Food name	Serving	Gm wt	KCAL	PROT Gm	CARB Gm	FAT Gm	CHOL Mg	SAFA Gm	SOD Mg	POT Mg	MAG Mg
FISH-CLAMS-BREADED-FRIED	1 srvg	85.0	171.0	12.10	8.780	9.480	52.00	2.280	309.0	277.0	12.00
FISH-COD-COOKED-DRY HEAT	1 piece	180.0	189.0	41.10	0.000	1.550	99.00	0.302	141.0	440.0	76.00
FISH-CRAB-STEAMED-PIECES	1 cup	155.0	150.0	30.00	0.000	2.390	82.20	0.206	1662	406..0	52.70
FISH-STICK-BREAD-FROZ-COOK	1 item	28.0	76.00	4.380	6.650	3.420	31.00	0.882	163.0	73.00	7.000
FISH-LOBSTER-CKD-MOIST	1 cup	145.0	142.0	29.70	1.860	0.860	104.0	1.155	551.0	510.0	51.00
FISH-OYSTERS-RAW-MEAT ONLY	1 cup	248.0	170.0	17.50	9.700	6.140	136.0	1.570	277.0	568.0	135.0

Nutritive Components for Fats & Oils—cont'd

IRON Mg	ZINC Mg	V-A IU	V-ET Mg	V-C Mg	THIA Mg	RIBO Mg	NIAC Mg	V-B6 Mg	Fol µg	VB12 µg	CALC Mg	PHOS Mg	Sel Mg	FIBD Gm
0.022	0.007	428.0	0.221	0.000	0.001	0.005	0.006	0.000	0.420	—	3.360	3.220	—	0.000
0.000	—	500.0	1.350	0.000	0.000	0.000	0.000	—	—	—	0.000	—	—	0.000
—	—	155.0	2.000	0.007	0.000	0.002	0.001	0.000	0.050	0.004	1.250	0.950	—	0.000
0.070	—	3750	65.10	0.181	0.011	0.042	0.026	0.010	1.340	0.108	33.90	26.00	—	0.000
—	—	—	8.120	—	—	—	—	—	—	—	—	—	—	9,999
0.000	—	32.10	7.260	0.300	0.000	0.020	0.000	—	—	—	12.40	11.30	—	0.050
0.100	0.010	—	7.410	—	—	—	—	—	—	—	1.700	2.200	—	0.000
0.000	0.020	—	6.990	—	0.000	0.000	0.000	—	—	—	1.000	1.000	—	0.050
0.000	—	—	7.130	—	0.000	0.000	0.000	—	—	—	0.000	1.000	—	0.090
0.000	—	32.00	4.400	—	0.000	0.000	0.000	—	—	—	2.000	4.000	—	0.000
—	—	—	4.500	—	—	—	—	—	—	—	—	—	—	0.000
0.100	0.020	50.00	7.450	0.000	0.000	0.000	0.000	—	—	—	2.000	3.000	—	0.600
—	—	—	197.0	—	—	—	—	—	—	—	—	—	—	0.000
0.000	0.000	—	181.0	0.000	0.000	0.000	0.000	0.000	0.000	0.000	0.000	0.000	—	0.000

Nutritive Components for Fish—cont'd

IRON Mg	ZINC Mg	V-A IU	V-ET Mg	V-C Mg	THIA Mg	RIBO Mg	NIAC Mg	V-B6 Mg	Fol µg	VB12 µg	CALC Mg	PHOS Mg	Sel Mg	FIBD Gm
11.80	1.240	257.0	—	—	—	0.207	1.750	—	—	34.20	54.00	160.0	—	0.320
0.880	1.040	83.00	—	1.800	0.158	0.142	4.520	0.509	—	1.890	25.00	248.0	—	—
1.180	11.80	45.00	1.890	—	0.082	0.085	2.080	—	—	—	91.50	434.0	0.076	0.000
0.210	0.190	30.00	—	—	0.036	0.050	0.596	0.017	5.100	0.503	6.000	51.00	0.003	0.300
0.570	4.230	126.0	—	—	0.010	0.096	1.550	0.112	16.10	4.510	88.00	268.0	—	0.000
16.60	226.0	740.0	—	—	0.340	0.412	3.250	0.124	24.60	47.50	111.0	344.0	0.156	0.000

■ Nutritive Components for Fish—cont'd

Food name	Serving	Gm wt	KCAL	PROT Gm	CARB Gm	FAT Gm	CHOL Mg	SAFA Gm	SOD Mg	POT Mg	MAG Mg
FISH-SCALLOPS-STEAMED	1 srvg	28.4	31.80	6.590	0.511	0.398	15.10	—	75.20	135.0	—
FISH-SHRIMP-CKD-MOIST HEAT	1 srvg	85.0	84.00	17.80	0.000	0.920	166.0	0.246	190.0	154.0	29.00
FISH-SHRIMP-FRENCH FRIED	1 srvg	85.0	206.0	18.20	9.750	10.40	150.0	1.770	292.0	191.0	34.00
FISH-SOLE/FLOUNDER-BAKED	1 srvg	127.0	148.0	30.70	0.000	1.940	86.00	0.461	133.0	436.0	74.00
FISH-TROUT-RANBOW-CKD-DRY	1 srvg	85.0	129.0	22.40	0.000	3.660	62.00	0.707	29.00	539.0	33.00
FISH-TUNA-CAN/OIL-DRAINED	1 srvg	85.0	169.0	24.80	0.000	6.980	15.00	1.300	301.0	176.0	26.00

■ Nutritive Components for Frozen Dinners

Food name	Serving	Gm wt	KCAL	PROT Gm	CARB Gm	FAT Gm	CHOL Mg	SAFA Gm	SOD Mg	POT Mg	MAG Mg
BEEF DINNER-SWANSON	1 item	326.0	320.0	25.00	34.00	9.000	—	—	1085	—	—
CHE CANNELLONI-LEAN CUIS	1 item	259.0	270.0	22.00	24.00	10.00	45.00	—	900.0	270.0	—
FETTUCINI ALFREDO-STOUFFER	1 item	142.0	270.0	8.000	19.00	18.00	—	—	1195	240.0	—
FISH DIVAN-LEAN CUISINE	1 item	351.0	270.0	31.00	16.00	10.00	85.00	—	780.0	850.0	—
SALISBURY STEAK DIN-BANQ	1 item	312.0	390.0	18.10	24.00	24.60	—	—	2059	387.0	—
LASAGNA-STOUFFER	1 item	298.0	385.0	28.00	36.00	14.00	—	—	1200	580.0	—
CHICKEN KIEV-LE MENU	1 item	234.0	500.0	21.00	35.00	30.00	—	—	745.0	—	—
VEAL PARMIGIANA-FROZ DIN	1 item	213.0	296.0	24.00	17.00	14.00	—	—	973.0	466.0	—

Nutritive Components for Fats & Oils—cont'd

IRON Mg	ZINC Mg	V-A IU	V-ET Mg	V-C Mg	THIA Mg	RIBO Mg	NIAC Mg	V-B6 Mg	Fol μg	VB12 μg	CALC Mg	PHOS Mg	Sel Mg	FIBD Gm
0.852	—	—	—	—	—	—	—	—	—	—	32.70	96.00	0.015	0.000
2.620	1.330	—	—	—	0.026	0.027	2.200	0.108	2.900	1.270	33.00	116.0	—	0.000
1.070	1.170	—	—	—	0.110	0.116	2.610	0.083	6.900	1.590	57.00	185.0	0.027	0.480
0.430	0.800	48.00	—	—	0.102	0.145	2.770	0.305	—	3.190	23.00	368.0	—	0.000
2.070	1.180	63.00	—	3.100	0.072	0.191	—	—	—	—	73.00	272.0	—	0.000
1.180	0.770	66.00	—	—	0.032	—	—	0.094	4.500	—	11.00	265.0	—	0.000

Nutritive Components for Frozen Dinners—cont'd

IRON Mg	ZINC Mg	V-A IU	V-ET Mg	V-C Mg	THIA Mg	RIBO Mg	NIAC Mg	V-B6 Mg	Fol μg	VB12 μg	CALC Mg	PHOS Mg	Sel Mg	FIBD Gm
—	—	—	—	—	—	—	—	—	—	—	—	—	—	—
—	—	—	—	—	—	—	—	—	—	—	—	—	—	—
—	—	—	—	—	—	—	—	—	—	—	—	—	—	—
—	—	—	—	—	—	—	—	—	—	—	—	—	—	—
3.500	—	3956	—	7.000	0.160	0.190	3.600	—	—	—	90.00	206.0	—	—
3.150	—	1239	—	0.000	0.210	0.420	4.200	—	—	—	410.0	—	—	—
—	—	—	—	—	—	—	—	—	—	—	—	—	—	—
2.300	—	617.0	—	6.400	0.300	0.380	6.800	—	—	—	97.00	—	—	—

Nutritive Components for Fruits

Food name	Serving	Gm wt	KCAL	PROT Gm	CARB Gm	FAT Gm	CHOL Mg	SAFA Gm	SOD Mg	POT Mg	MAG Mg
APPLES-RAW-UNPEELED	1 item	138.0	81.00	0.270	21.10	0.490	0.000	0.080	1.000	159.0	6.000
APPLE JUICE-CANNED/BOTTLED	1 cup	248.0	116.0	0.150	29.00	0.280	0.000	0.047	7.000	296.0	8.000
APPLESAUCE-CAN-SWEETENED	1 cup	255.0	194.0	0.470	50.80	0.470	0.000	0.077	8.000	156.0	7.000
APRICOT-RAW-WITHOUT PIT	1 item	35.3	16.90	0.494	3.930	0.138	0.000	0.010	0.353	104.0	2.820
AVOCADO-RAW-CALIFORNIA	1 item	173.0	306.0	3.640	12.00	30.00	0.000	4.480	21.00	1097	70.00
BANANAS-RAW-PEELED	1 item	114.0	105.0	1.180	26.70	0.550	0.000	0.211	1.000	451.0	33.00
BLUEBERRIES-RAW	1 cup	145.0	82.00	0.970	20.50	0.550	0.000	0.000	9.000	129.0	7.000
CHERRIES-SWEET-RAW	1 item	6.8	4.900	0.082	1.130	0.065	0.000	0.015	0.000	15.20	0.800
FRUIT ROLL UP-CHERRY	1 item	14.4	50.00	0.000	12.00	1.000	—	—	5.000	45.00	—
GRAPEFRUIT-RAW-WHITE	1 item	236.0	78.00	1.620	19.80	0.240	0.000	0.034	0.000	350.0	22.00
GRAPEFRUIT JUICE-CAN-SWEET	1 cup	250.0	116.0	1.450	27.80	0.230	0.000	0.030	4.000	405.0	24.00
GRAPES-RAW-AMERICAN TYPE	1 cup	92.0	58.00	0.580	15.80	0.320	0.000	0.027	2.000	176.0	5.000
GRAPE JUICE-FROZ-DILUTED	1 cup	250.0	128.0	0.470	31.90	0.230	0.000	0.073	5.000	53.00	11.00
MELONS-CANTALOUPE-RAW	1 cup	160.0	57.00	1.400	13.40	0.440	0.000	0.000	14.00	494.0	17.00
MELONS-HONEYDEW-RAW	1 cup	170.0	60.00	0.770	15.60	0.170	0.000	0.000	17.00	461.0	12.00
NECTARINES-RAW	1 item	136.0	67.00	1.280	16.00	0.620	0.000	—	0.000	288.0	11.00
ORANGES-RAW-ALL VARIETIES	1 item	131.0	62.00	1.230	15.40	0.160	0.000	0.020	0.000	237.0	13.00
ORANGE JUICE-FROZ-DILUTED	1 cup	249.0	112.0	1.680	26.80	0.140	0.000	0.017	2.000	474.0	24.00
PEACHES-RAW-WHOLE	1 item	87.0	37.00	0.610	9.650	0.080	0.000	0.009	0.000	171.0	6.000
PEARS-RAW-BARTLET-UNPEELED	1 item	166.0	98.00	0.650	25.10	0.660	0.000	0.037	1.000	208.0	9.000
PINEAPPLE-RAW-DICED	1 cup	155.0	77.00	0.600	19.20	0.660	0.000	0.050	1.000	175.0	21.00
RAISINS-SEEDLESS	1 cup	145.0	434.0	4.670	115.0	0.670	0.000	0.218	17.00	1089	48.00
STRAWBERRIES-RAW-WHOLE	1 cup	149.0	45.00	0.910	10.50	0.550	0.000	0.030	2.000	247.0	16.00
WATERMELON-RAW	1 cup	160.0	50.00	0.990	11.50	0.680	0.000	0.000	3.000	186.0	17.00
PLUMS-RAW-PRUNE TYPE	1 item	28.0	20.00	0.000	6.000	0.000	0.000	0.000	0.000	48.00	1.960

Nutritive Components for Fruits—cont'd

IRON Mg	ZINC Mg	V-A IU	V-ET Mg	V-C Mg	THIA Mg	RIBO Mg	NIAC Mg	V-B6 Mg	Fol μg	VB12 μg	CALC Mg	PHOS Mg	Sel Mg	FIBD Gm
0.250	0.050	74.00	0.911	7.800	0.023	0.019	0.106	0.066	3.900	0.000	10.00	10.00	0.001	3.200
0.920	0.070	2.000	—	2.300	0.052	0.042	0.248	0.074	0.200	0.000	16.00	18.00	0.002	0.520
0.890	0.100	28.00	—	4.400	0.033	0.071	0.479	0.066	1.500	0.000	9.000	17.00	0.001	4.340
0.191	0.092	922.0	—	3.530	0.011	0.014	0.212	0.019	3.040	0.000	4.940	6.710	—	0.670
2.040	0.730	1059	—	13.70	0.187	0.211	3.320	0.484	113.0	0.000	19.00	73.00	—	6.130
0.350	0.190	92.00	0.365	10.30	0.051	0.114	0.616	0.659	21.80	0.000	7.000	22.00	0.001	2.650
0.240	0.160	145.0	—	18.90	0.070	0.073	0.521	0.052	9.300	0.000	9.000	15.00	0.001	3.920
0.026	0.004	14.60	—	0.480	0.003	0.004	0.027	0.002	0.286	0.000	1.000	1.300	0.000	0.100
—	—	—	—	—	—	—	—	—	—	—	—	—	—	—
0.070	0.160	24.00	0.614	78.60	0.088	0.048	0.634	0.102	23.60	0.000	28.00	18.00	0.001	2.500
0.890	0.150	0.000	0.450	67.30	0.100	0.058	0.798	0.050	25.90	0.000	20.00	27.00	0.001	0.000
0.270	0.040	92.00	—	3.700	0.085	0.052	0.276	0.101	3.600	0.000	13.00	9.000	0.001	1.500
0.260	0.100	19.00	—	59.70	0.038	0.065	0.310	0.105	3.100	0.000	9.000	11.00	0.001	0.000
0.340	0.250	5158	0.496	67.50	0.058	0.034	0.918	0.184	27.30	0.000	17.00	27.00	0.001	1.400
0.120	—	68.00	0.527	42.10	0.131	0.031	1.020	0.100	—	0.000	10.00	17.00	0.001	1.530
0.210	0.120	1001	—	7.300	0.023	0.056	1.350	0.034	5.100	0.000	6.000	22.00	0.001	2.990
0.130	0.090	269.0	0.314	69.70	0.114	0.052	0.369	0.079	39.70	0.000	52.00	18.00	0.002	2.620
0.240	0.130	194.0	0.498	96.90	0.197	0.045	0.503	0.110	109.0	0.000	22.00	40.00	0.001	0.700
0.100	0.120	465.0	—	5.700	0.015	0.036	0.861	0.016	3.000	0.000	5.000	11.00	0.001	2.000
0.410	0.200	33.00	—	6.600	0.033	0.066	0.166	0.030	12.10	0.000	19.00	18.00	0.001	4.650
0.570	0.120	35.00	0.155	23.90	0.143	0.056	0.651	0.135	16.40	0.000	11.00	11.00	0.001	2.390
3.020	0.380	11.00	—	4.800	0.226	0.128	1.190	0.361	4.800	0.000	71.00	140.0	0.001	12.60
0.570	0.190	41.00	0.387	84.50	0.030	0.098	0.343	0.088	26.40	0.000	21.00	28.00	0.001	3.200
0.280	0.110	585.0	—	15.40	0.138	0.032	0.320	0.230	3.400	0.000	13.00	14.00	0.001	0.300
0.100	0.028	80.00	—	1.000	0.010	0.010	0.100	0.023	0.161	0.000	3.000	5.000	0.000	0.588

Nutritive Components for Grains

Food name	Serving	Gm wt	KCAL	PROT Gm	CARB Gm	FAT Gm	CHOL Mg	SAFA Gm	SOD Mg	POT Mg	MAG Mg
CORN CHIPS	1 srvg	28.4	155.0	1.700	16.90	9.140	0.000	1.500	164.0	43.30	21.90
CRACKERS-GRAHAM-PLAIN	1 item	7.0	27.50	0.500	5.000	0.500	0.000	0.100	33.00	27.50	3.570
CRACKERS-SALTINES	1 item	2.8	12.50	0.250	2.000	0.250	0.750	0.100	36.80	3.250	0.770
CRACKERS-TRISCUITS	1 item	4.5	21.00	0.400	3.100	0.750	—	—	—	—	—
CROUTONS-HERB SEASONED	1 cup	30.0	100.0	4.290	20.00	0.000	—	0.000	372.0	38.60	11.40
MACARONI-COOKED-FIRM-HOT	1 cup	130.0	190.0	7.000	39.00	1.000	0.000	—	1.000	103.0	26.00
NOODLES-EGG-ENR-COOKED	1 cup	160.0	200.0	7.000	37.00	2.000	50.00	—	3.000	70.00	43.20
PANCAKES-PLAIN-MIX	1 item	27.0	58.90	1.850	19.00	2.170	20.00	0.700	160.0	43.20	51.30
POPCORN-POPPED-PLAIN	1 cup	6.0	25.00	1.000	5.000	0.000	0.000	0.000	0.000	—	—
PRETZEL-THIN-STICK	1 item	0.3	1.190	0.028	0.242	0.011	0.000	—	4.830	0.303	0.072
RICE-WHITE-INSTANT-HOT	1 cup	165.0	180.0	4.000	40.00	0.000	0.000	0.000	13.00	—	13.20
RICE-WHITE-PARBOIL-COOKED	1 cup	175.0	185.0	4.000	41.00	0.000	0.000	0.000	4.000	75.00	—
SPAGHETTI-COOK-TENDER-HOT	1 cup	140.0	155.0	5.000	32.00	1.000	0.000	—	1.000	85.00	23.80
TORTILLA CHIPS-DORITOS	1 srvg	28.4	139.0	2.000	18.60	6.600	0.000	1.430	180.0	51.00	21.00
WAFFLES-FROZEN	1 item	37.0	103.0	2.150	15.90	3.520	—	—	256.0	77.70	7.770

Nutritive Components for Meats

Food name	Serving	Gm wt	KCAL	PROT Gm	CARB Gm	FAT Gm	CHOL Mg	SAFA Gm	SOD Mg	POT Mg	MAG Mg
BACON-PORK-BROILED/FRIED	1 slice	6.3	36.30	1.930	0.036	3.120	5.330	1.100	101.0	30.70	1.670
BEEF-LIVER-FRIED/MARG	1 slice	85.0	184.0	22.70	6.680	6.800	410.0	2.400	90.00	309.0	20.00
BOLOGNA-PORK	1 slice	23.0	57.00	3.520	0.170	4.570	14.00	1.580	272.0	65.00	3.000
FRANKFURTER-HOT DOG-NO BUN	1 item	57.0	183.0	6.430	1.460	16.60	29.00	6.130	639.0	95.00	6.000
HAM-REG-ROASTED-PORK	1 cup	140.0	249.0	31.70	0.000	12.60	83.00	4.360	2100	573.0	30.00
HAMBURGER-GROUND-REG-FRIED	1 srvg	85.0	260.0	20.30	0.000	19.20	75.00	7.530	71.00	255.0	17.00
HAMB PATTY-BEEF-21% FAT	1 item	85.0	231.0	21.00	0.000	15.70	74.00	6.160	65.00	256.0	18.00

Nutritive Components for Grains—cont'd

IRON Mg	ZINC Mg	V-A IU	V-ET Mg	V-C Mg	THIA Mg	RIBO Mg	NIAC Mg	V-B6 Mg	FOL µg	VB12 µg	CALC Mg	PHOS Mg	SEL Mg	FIBD Gm
0.376	0.435	—	—	—	0.048	0.026	0.554	0.054	—	0.000	37.10	54.60	—	1.660
0.250	0.053	0.000	0.128	0.000	0.010	0.040	0.250	0.006	0.910	0.000	3.000	10.50	0.001	0.200
0.125	0.017	0.000	0.050	0.000	0.125	0.013	0.100	0.001	0.495	0.000	0.500	2.500	0.004	0.039
—	—	—	0.082	—	—	—	—	—	—	—	—	—	0.001	—
1.540	0.300	0.000	—	—	0.129	0.200	1.720	0.000	0.000	—	—	—	—	—
1.400	0.700	0.000	0.351	0.000	0.230	0.130	1.800	0.083	15.60	0.000	14.00	85.00	0.032	1.040
1.400	—	110.0	—	0.000	0.220	0.130	1.900	0.141	19.20	0.000	16.00	94.00	0.094	1.440
0.265	0.192	38.30	—	0.000	0.038	0.059	0.254	0.057	2.970	0.355	35.60	70.70	0.003	—
0.200	0.500	—	—	0.000	—	0.010	0.100	0.012	—	0.000	1.000	17.00	0.001	0.400
0.006	0.003	0.000	0.002	0.000	0.001	0.001	0.013	0.000	0.048	0.000	0.078	0.273	—	—
1.300	0.700	0.000	0.644	0.000	0.210	0.000	1.700	0.056	16.50	0.000	5.000	31.00	0.033	1.710
1.400	0.700	0.000	0.683	0.000	0.190	0.020	2.100	0.744	19.30	0.000	33.00	100.0	0.035	1.820
1.300	0.700	0.000	1.680	0.000	0.200	0.110	1.500	0.090	16.80	0.000	11.00	70.00	0.085	0.980
0.500	0.240	52.00	—	0.000	0.030	0.030	0.040	0.100	4.000	—	30.00	59.00	—	1.850
1.800	0.303	474.0	—	0.000	0.167	0.200	1.930	0.098	0.740	—	30.00	141.0	—	—

Nutritive Components for Meats—cont'd

IRON Mg	ZINC Mg	V-A IU	V-ET Mg	V-C Mg	THIA Mg	RIBO Mg	NIAC Mg	V-B6 Mg	FOL µg	VB12 µg	CALC Mg	PHOS Mg	SEL Mg	FIBD Gm
0.103	0.206	0.000	0.037	2.130	0.044	0.018	0.464	0.017	0.333	0.110	0.667	21.30	0.002	0.000
5.340	4.630	30690	1.380	19.40	0.179	3.520	12.30	1.220	187.0	95.00	9.000	392.0	0.042	0.000
0.180	0.470	—	0.112	8.100	0.120	0.036	0.897	0.060	1.000	0.210	3.000	32.00	0.003	0.000
0.660	1.050	—	0.080	15.00	0.113	0.068	1.500	0.080	2.000	0.740	6.000	49.00	0.013	0.000
1.880	3.460	0.000	0.728	31.70	1.020	0.462	8.610	0.430	—	0.980	12.00	393.0	0.066	0.000
2.080	4.310	—	—	0.000	0.026	0.170	4.960	0.200	8.000	2.300	10.00	145.0	—	0.000
1.790	4.560	30.00	0.517	0.000	0.043	0.179	4.390	0.220	8.000	2.000	9.000	134.0	0.020	0.000

Nutritive Components for Meats—cont'd

Food name	Serving	Gm wt	KCAL	PROT Gm	CARB Gm	FAT Gm	CHOL Mg	SAFA Gm	SOD Mg	POT Mg	MAG Mg
ITALIAN SAUSAGE-PORK-LINK	1 item	67.0	217.0	13.40	1.010	17.20	52.00	6.050	618.0	204.0	12.00
PORK-CHOP-LEAN/FAT-BROILED	1 item	82.0	284.0	19.30	0.000	22.30	77.00	8.060	54.00	287.0	20.00
POT ROAST-ARM-BEEF-COOKED	1 slice	100.0	231.0	33.00	0.000	9.980	101.0	3.790	66.00	289.0	24.00
ROAST BEEF-RIB-LEAN/FAT	1 slice	85.0	308.0	18.30	0.000	25.50	73.00	10.80	52.00	257.0	17.00
SALAMI-COOKED-BEEF	1 slice	23.0	58.00	3.380	0.570	4.620	14.00	1.940	266.0	52.00	3.000
SAUSAGE-LINK-PORK-COOKED	1 item	13.0	48.00	2.550	0.130	4.050	11.00	1.400	168.0	47.00	2.000
SPARERIBS-PORK-BRAISED	1 srvg	28.4	113.0	8.230	0.000	8.580	34.30	3.330	26.30	90.70	7.000
STEAK-ROUND-LEAN/FAT	1 srvg	85.0	179.0	26.20	0.000	7.490	72.00	2.800	51.00	365.0	26.00
STEAK-SIRLOIN-LEAN/FAT	1 item	85.0	271.0	22.70	0.000	19.40	77.00	8.070	52.00	297.0	23.00
VEAL-RIB-ROASTED-NO-BONE	1 srvg	85.0	230.0	23.00	0.000	14.00	87.00	6.100	68.00	259.0	17.00

Nutritive Components for Miscellaneous

Food name	Serving	Gm wt	KCAL	PROT Gm	CARB Gm	FAT Gm	CHOL Mg	SAFA Gm	SOD Mg	POT Mg	MAG Mg
BAKING POWDER-HOME USE	1 tsp	3.0	5.000	0.000	1.000	0.000	0.000	0.000	339.0	5.000	—
BAKING SODA	1 tsp	3.0	0.000	0.000	0.000	0.000	0.000	0.000	821.0	—	—
CHEWING GUM-WRIGLEYS	1 item	3.0	10.00	0.000	2.300	—	0.000	—	0.000	0.000	0.000
GELATIN DESSERT-PREP	1 cup	240.0	140.0	4.000	34.00	0.000	0.000	0.000	0.000	—	—
OLIVES-GREEN-PICKLED-CAN	1 item	4.0	3.750	0.100	0.100	0.500	0.000	0.050	80.80	1.750	—
PICKLE-DILL-CUCUMBER-MED	1 item	65.0	5.000	0.000	1.000	0.000	0.000	0.000	928.0	130.0	7.800
VINEGAR-CIDER	1 tbsp	15.0	0.000	0.000	1.000	0.000	0.000	0.000	0.125	15.00	—

Nutritive Components for Meats—cont'd

IRON Mg	ZINC Mg	V-A IU	V-ET Mg	V-C Mg	THIA Mg	RIBO Mg	NIAC Mg	V-B6 Mg	FOL µg	VB12 µg	CALC Mg	PHOS Mg	SEL Mg	FIBD Gm
1.010	1.590	—	—	1.300	0.417	0.156	2.790	0.220	—	0.870	16.00	114.0	0.022	0.000
0.660	2.010	7.000	0.492	0.200	0.690	0.294	4.320	0.310	4.000	0.810	5.000	193.0	0.014	0.000
3.790	8.660	—	—	0.000	0.081	0.289	3.720	0.330	11.00	3.400	9.000	268.0	0.006	0.000
1.770	4.270	69.90	—	0.000	0.065	0.146	2.650	0.250	5.000	2.370	10.00	140.0	0.020	0.000
0.460	0.490	—	0.156	3.000	0.029	0.059	0.785	0.050	0.000	1.110	2.000	23.00	0.004	0.000
0.160	0.330	—	0.042	0.000	0.096	0.033	0.587	0.040	—	0.220	4.000	24.00	0.004	0.000
0.527	1.300	3.000	0.170	—	0.116	0.108	1.550	0.100	1.330	0.307	13.30	74.00	0.005	0.000
2.390	4.590	20.00	0.468	0.000	0.097	0.221	4.980	0.460	10.00	2.080	5.000	203.0	0.029	0.000
2.490	4.730	50.00	0.468	0.000	0.092	0.218	3.210	0.330	7.000	2.220	9.000	180.0	0.029	0.000
2.900	3.500	—	0.204	—	0.110	0.260	6.600	—	—	1.400	10.00	211.0	—	0.000

Nutritive Components for Miscellaneous—cont'd

IRON Mg	ZINC Mg	V-A IU	V-ET Mg	V-C Mg	THIA Mg	RIBO Mg	NIAC Mg	V-B6 Mg	FOL µg	VB12 µg	CALC Mg	PHOS Mg	SEL Mg	FIBD Gm
—	—	0.000	—	0.000	0.000	0.000	0.000	—	—	—	58.00	87.00	0.000	0.000
—	—	—	0.000	0.000	0.000	0.000	0.000	0.000	0.000	0.000	—	—	—	0.000
0.000	0.000	0.000	—	0.000	0.000	0.000	0.000	0.000	0.000	0.000	3.000	0.000	—	—
—	—	—	—	—	—	—	—	—	—	—	—	—	—	0.000
0.050	—	10.00	—	—	—	—	—	—	0.040	0.000	2.000	0.500	0.000	0.080
0.700	0.176	70.00	—	4.000	0.000	0.010	0.000	0.005	0.650	0.000	17.00	14.00	0.000	—
0.100	0.020	—	—	—	—	—	—	0.000	—	—	1.000	1.000	—	0.000

Nutritive Components for Nuts & Seeds

Food name	Serving	Gm wt	KCAL	PROT Gm	CARB Gm	FAT Gm	CHOL Mg	SAFA Gm	SOD Mg	POT Mg	MAG Mg
NUTS-CASHEWS-DRY ROASTED	1 cup	137.0	787.0	21.00	44.80	63.50	0.000	12.50	21.00	774.0	356.0
NUTS-COCONUT-DRIED-SHRED	1 cup	93.0	466.0	2.680	44.30	33.00	0.000	29.30	244.0	313.0	47.00
NUTS-MIXED-DRY ROASTED	1 cup	137.0	814.0	23.70	34.70	70.50	0.000	9.450	16.00	817.0	308.0
NUTS-PEANUTS-OIL ROASTED	1 cup	145.0	840.0	38.80	26.70	71.30	0.000	9.900	22.00	1020	273.0
NUTS-PECANS-DRIED-HALVES	1 cup	108.0	721.0	8.370	19.70	73.10	0.000	5.850	1.000	423.0	138.0
NUTS-PISTACHIO-DRY ROASTED	1 cup	128.0	776.0	19.10	35.20	67.60	0.000	8.560	8.000	1242	166.0
PEANUT BUTTER-CHUNK STYLE	1 cup	258.0	1520	62.00	55.70	129.0	0.000	24.70	1255	1928	409.0
PEANUT BUTTER-SMOOTH TYPE	1 tbsp	16.0	95.00	4.560	2.530	8.180	0.000	1.360	75.00	110.0	28.00
SEEDS-PUMPKIN/SQUASH-ROAST	1 cup	64.0	285.0	11.90	34.40	12.40	0.000	2.350	12.00	588.0	168.0
SEEDS-SUNFLOWER-OIL ROAST	1 cup	135.0	830.0	28.80	19.90	77.60	0.000	8.130	4.000	652.0	171.0

Nutritive Components for Poultry

Food name	Serving	Gm wt	KCAL	PROT Gm	CARB Gm	FAT Gm	CHOL Mg	SAFA Gm	SPD Mg	POT Mg	MAG Mg
CHICKEN-BREAST-FRI/BATTER	1 item	280.0	728.0	69.60	25.20	36.90	238.0	9.860	770.0	564.0	68.00
CHECKEN-BREAST-FRIED/FLOUR	1 item	196.0	436.0	62.40	3.220	17.40	176.0	4.800	150.0	506.0	58.00
CHICKEN-BREAST-ROASTED	1 item	196.0	386.0	58.40	0.000	15.30	166.0	4.300	138.0	480.0	54.00
CHICKEN-BREAST-NO SKIN-FRI	1 item	172.0	322.0	57.50	0.880	8.100	156.0	2.220	136.0	474.0	54.00
CHICK-BREAST-NO SKIN-ROAST	1 item	172.0	284.0	53.40	0.000	6.140	146.0	1.740	126.0	440.0	50.00
CHICKEN-DRUMSTICK-FRIED	1 item	49.0	120.0	13.20	0.800	6.720	44.00	1.790	44.00	112.0	11.00
CHICKEN-LEG-ROASTED	1 item	114.0	265.0	29.60	0.000	15.40	105.0	4.240	99.00	256.0	26.00
CHICKEN-THIGH-FRIED/FLOUR	1 item	62.0	162.0	16.60	1.970	9.290	60.00	2.540	55.00	147.0	15.00
CHICKEN-WING-FRIED/FLOUR	1 item	32.0	103.0	8.360	0.760	7.090	26.00	1.940	25.00	57.00	6.000
DUCK-FLESH & SKIN-ROASTED	1 item	764.0	2574	145.0	0.000	217.0	640.0	73.90	454.0	1560	124.0
TURK-BREAST-NO SKIN-ROAST	1 item	612.0	826.0	184.0	0.000	4.500	510.0	1.440	318.0	1784	178.0

■ Nutritive Components for Nuts & Seeds—cont'd

IRON Mg	ZINC Mg	V-A IU	V-ET Mg	V-C Mg	THIA Mg	RIBO Mg	NIAC Mg	V-B6 Mg	FOL µg	VB12 µg	CALC Mg	PHOS Mg	SEL Mg	FIBD Gm
8.220	7.670	0.000	15.00	0.000	0.274	0.274	1.920	0.351	94.80	0.000	62.00	671.0	0.007	10.00
1.780	1.690	0.000	—	0.600	0.029	0.019	0.441	—	—	0.000	14.00	99.00	0.016	3.900
5.070	5.210	21.00	16.40	0.600	0.274	0.274	6.440	0.406	69.00	0.000	96.00	596.0	0.007	11.60
2.780	9.600	0.000	16.70	0.000	0.425	0.146	21.50	0.576	153.0	0.000	125.0	733.0	0.055	11.10
2.300	5.910	138.0	21.40	2.100	0.916	0.138	0.958	0.203	42.30	0.000	39.00	314.0	0.003	8.300
4.060	1.740	—	—	—	0.541	0.315	1.800	—	—	0.000	90.00	609.0	0.007	9.900
4.900	7.170	0.000	—	0.000	0.323	0.289	35.30	1.160	237.0	0.000	105.0	817.0	—	9.800
0.290	0.470	—	3.200	0.000	0.024	0.017	2.150	0.062	13.10	0.000	5.000	60.00	0.002	1.400
2.120	6.590	—	—	—	—	—	—	—	—	0.000	35.00	59.00	—	—
9.050	7.040	—	70.40	1.900	0.432	0.378	5.580	—	316.0	0.000	76.00	1538	—	—

■ Nutritive Components for Poultry—cont'd

IRON Mg	ZINC Mg	V-A IU	V-ET Mg	V-C Mg	THIA Mg	RIBO Mg	NIAC Mg	V-B6 Mg	FOL µg	VB12 µg	CALC Mg	PHOS Mg	SEL Mg	FIBD Gm
3.500	2.660	188.0	1.540	0.000	0.322	0.408	29.50	1.200	16.00	0.820	56.00	516.0	0.030	—
2.340	2.140	98.00	1.080	0.000	0.160	0.256	26.90	1.140	8.000	0.680	32.00	456.0	0.021	—
2.080	2.000	182.0	1.080	0.000	0.130	0.234	24.90	1.080	6.000	0.640	28.00	420.0	0.053	0.000
1.960	1.860	40.00	0.946	0.000	0.136	0.216	25.40	1.100	8.000	0.620	28.00	424.0	0.031	0.000
1.780	1.720	36.00	0.946	0.000	0.120	0.196	23.60	1.020	6.000	0.580	26.00	392.0	0.046	0.000
0.660	1.420	41.00	0.270	0.000	0.040	0.110	2.960	0.170	4.000	0.160	6.000	86.00	0.005	—
1.520	2.960	154.0	0.627	0.000	0.078	0.243	7.060	0.370	8.000	0.350	14.00	199.0	0.016	0.000
0.930	1.560	61.00	0.341	0.000	0.058	0.151	4.310	0.210	5.000	0.190	8.000	116.0	0.011	0.040
0.400	0.560	40.00	0.176	0.000	0.019	0.044	2.140	0.130	1.000	0.090	5.000	48.00	0.006	0.000
20.60	14.20	1608	5.350	0.000	1.330	2.060	36.90	1.400	50.00	2.260	86.00	1190	—	0.000
9.360	10.60	0.000	—	0.000	0.264	0.802	45.90	3.420	38.00	2.360	76.00	1370	—	0.000

▮ Nutritive Components for Sauces & Dips

Food name	Serving	Gm wt	KCAL	PROT Gm	CARB Gm	FAT Gm	CHOL Mg	SAFA Gm	SOD Mg	POT Mg	MAG Mg
DIP-FRENCH ONION-KRAFT	1 tbsp	15.0	30.00	0.500	1.500	2.000	0.000	—	120.0	—	—
DIP-GUACAMOLE-KRAFT	1 tbsp	15.0	25.00	0.500	1.500	2.000	0.000	—	108.0	—	—
MUSTARD-YELLOW-PREPARED	1 tsp	5.0	5.000	0.100	0.100	0.100	0.000	0.000	65.00	7.000	2.000
SAUCE-BARBECUE	1 cup	250.0	188.0	4.500	32.00	4.500	0.000	0.670	2032	435.0	—
SAUCE-SALSA/CHILIES-CANNED	1 fl oz	16.0	10.00	0.400	2.000	0.700	0.000	0.000	111.0	87.00	—
SAUCE-SPAGHETTI-CANNED	1 cup	249.0	272.0	4.530	39.70	11.90	0.000	1.700	1236	957.0	60.00
SAUCE-SOY	1 tbsp	18.0	11.00	1.560	1.500	0.000	0.000	0.000	1029	64.00	8.000
SAUCE-WORCHESTER-SHIRE	1 tbsp	15.0	12.00	0.300	2.700	0.000	—	0.000	147.0	120.0	—
TOMATO CATSUP	1 tbsp	15.0	15.00	0.000	4.000	0.000	0.000	0.000	156.0	54.00	3.600

▮ Nutritive Components for Soups

Food name	Serving	Gm wt	KCAL	PROT Gm	CARB Gm	FAT Gm	CHOL Mg	SAFA Gm	SOD Mg	POT Mg	MAG Mg
SOUP-VEGETABLE BEEF-CAN	1 cup	245.0	79.00	5.580	10.20	1.900	5.000	0.850	957.0	173.0	6.000
SOUP-CHICKEN NOODLE-CAN	1 cup	241.0	75.00	4.040	9.350	2.450	7.000	0.650	1107	55.00	5.000
SOUP-CLAM-NEW ENGLAND-MILK	1 cup	248.0	163.0	9.460	16.60	6.600	22.00	2.950	992.0	300.0	23.00
SOUP-ONION-DEHY-PACKET	1 srvg	39.0	115.0	4.520	20.90	2.330	2.000	0.540	3493	260.0	25.00
SOUP-CREAM/MUSHROOM-MILK	1 cup	248.0	203.0	6.050	15.00	13.60	20.00	5.120	1076	270.0	20.00
SOUP-VEGETARIAN-CAN-WATER	1 cup	241.0	72.00	2.100	12.00	1.930	0.000	0.290	823.0	209.0	7.000

Nutritive Components for Sauces & Dips—cont'd

IRON Mg	ZINC Mg	V-A IU	V-ET Mg	V-C Mg	THIA Mg	RIBO Mg	NIAC Mg	V-b6 Mg	FOL μg	VB12 μg	CALC Mg	PHOS Mg	SEL Mg	FIBD Gm
—	—	—	—	—	—	—	—	—	—	—	—	—	—	—
—	—	—	—	—	—	—	—	—	—	—	—	—	—	—
0.100	—	—	0.208	—	—	—	—	—	—	—	4.000	4.000	0.000	0.060
2.250	—	2170	—	17.50	0.075	0.050	2.250	0.188	—	0.000	48.00	50.00	—	2.300
0.280	—	395.0	—	9.100	0.020	0.010	0.290	—	—	—	4.200	9.300	—	—
1.620	0.530	3055	—	27.90	0.137	0.147	3.750	—	—	0.000	70.00	90.00	—	—
0.490	0.036	0.000	—	0.000	0.009	0.023	0.605	0.031	1.900	0.000	3.000	38.00	—	—
0.900	—	51.00	—	27.00	0.000	0.030	0.000	—	—	—	15.00	9.000	—	—
0.100	0.034	210.0	—	2.000	0.010	0.010	0.200	0.016	0.750	0.000	3.000	8.000	0.000	—

Nutritive Components for Soups—cont'd

IRON Mg	ZINC Mg	V-A IV	V-ET Mg	V-C Mg	THIA Mg	RIBO Mg	NIAC Mg	V-B6 Mg	FOL μg	VB12 μg	CALC Mg	PHOS Mg	SEL Mg	FIBD Gm
1.110	1.550	1891	—	2.400	0.037	0.049	1.030	0.076	10.60	0.310	17.00	40.00	0.008	0.980
0.780	0.395	711.0	—	0.200	0.053	0.060	1.390	0.027	2.200	—	17.00	36.00	0.008	—
1.480	0.799	164.0	—	3.500	0.067	0.236	1.030	0.126	9.700	10.30	187.0	157.0	0.008	—
0.580	0.231	8.000	—	0.900	0.111	0.238	1.990	—	6.300	—	55.00	126.0	0.000	2.200
0.590	0.640	154.0	—	2.300	0.077	0.280	0.913	0.064	—	—	178.0	156.0	0.008	—
1.080	0.460	3005	—	1.400	0.053	0.046	0.916	0.055	10.60	0.000	21.00	35.00	0.008	1.210

▌ Nutritive Components for Sugars & Sweets

Food name	Serving	Gm wt	KCAL	PROT Gm	CARB Gm	FAT Gm	CHOL Mg	SAFA Gm	SOD Mg	POT Mg	MAG Mg
CANDY-MILK CHOCOLATE-PLAIN	1 srvg	28.0	145.0	2.000	16.00	9.000	0.000	5.500	28.00	109.0	16.00
CANDY-JELLY BEANS	1 item	2.8	6.600	0.000	1.670	0.000	—	0.000	0.300	0.000	—
CANDY-KIT KAT BAR	1 item	43.0	210.0	3.000	25.00	11.00	—	—	38.00	129.0	19.00
CANDY-M & M'S-PACKAGE	1 item	45.0	220.0	3.000	31.00	10.00	—	—	—	—	—
CANDY-MILKY WAY BAR	1 item	60.0	260.0	3.000	43.00	9.000	—	—	—	—	—
CANDY-PEANUT BUTTER CUP	1 piece	17.0	92.00	2.200	8.700	5.350	2.500	3.000	54.50	68.00	14.50
CANDY-SNICKERS BAR	1 item	57.0	270.0	6.000	33.00	13.00	—	—	—	—	—
ICING-CAKE-WHITE-UNCOOKED	1 cup	319.0	1200	2.000	260.0	21.00	0.000	12.70	156.0	57.00	—
JAMS/PRESERVES-REGULAR	1 tbsp	20.0	55.00	0.000	14.00	0.000	0.000	0.000	2.000	18.00	—
SYRUP-CHOC FLAVORED-FUDGE	1 fl oz	38.0	125.0	2.000	20.00	5.000	0.000	3.100	26.60	107.0	—
SYRUP-PANCAKE-KARO	1 tbsp	20.5	60.00	0.000	14.90	0.000	—	0.000	35.00	1.000	—
SUGAR-BROWN-PRESSED DOWN	1 cup	220.0	820.0	0.000	212.0	0.000	0.000	0.000	66.00	757.0	—
SUGAR-WHITE-GRANULATED	1 tbsp	12.0	45.00	0.000	12.00	0.000	0.000	0.000	0.120	0.000	—
SUGAR-WHITE-POWDER-SIFTED	1 cup	100.0	385.0	0.000	100.0	0.000	0.000	0.000	0.830	3.000	—

▌ Nutritive Components for Vegetables

Food name	Serving	Gm wt	KCAL	PROT Gm	CARB Gm	FAT Gm	CHOL Mg	SAFA Gm	SOD Mg	POT Mg	MAG Mg
ARTICHOKES-BOIL-DRAIN	1 item	120.0	53.00	2.760	12.40	0.200	0.000	0.048	79.00	316.0	47.00
ASPARAGUS-FROZ-BOIL-SPEARS	1 cup	180.0	50.40	5.310	8.770	0.756	0.000	0.171	7.200	392.0	23.40
BEANS-BAKED BEANS-CANNED	1 cup	254.0	235.0	12.20	52.10	1.140	0.000	0.295	1008	752.0	82.00
BEANS-REFRIED BEANS	1 cup	253.0	270.0	15.80	46.80	2.700	—	1.040	1071	994.0	99.00
BEANS SNAP GREEN CAN CUTS	1 cup	135.0	27.00	1.550	6.000	0.135	0.000	0.030	339.0	147.0	17.50
BEETS-CAN-SLICED-DRAIN	1 cup	170.0	54.00	1.560	12.20	0.240	0.000	0.040	479.0	284.0	22.10
BROCCOLI-RAW-BOIL-DRAIN	1 cup	155.0	46.00	4.640	8.680	0.440	0.000	0.068	16.00	254.0	94.00

Appendix

Nutritive Components for Sugars & Sweets—cont'd

IRON Mg	ZINC Mg	V-A IV	V-ET Mg	V-C Mg	THIA Mg	RIBO Mg	NIAC Mg	V-B6 Mg	FOL µg	VB12 µg	CALC Mg	PHOS Mg	SEL Mg	FIBD Gm
0.300	—	80.00	1.570	0.000	0.020	0.100	0.100	—	1.960	—	65.00	65.00	0.001	—
0.030	—	0.000	—	0.000	0.000	—	—	—	—	—	0.300	0.100	0.000	0.000
0.560	0.430	30.00	—	—	0.030	0.110	0.100	—	—	—	65.00	78.00	0.002	—
—	—	—	1.890	—	—	—	—	—	—	—	—	—	0.002	—
—	—	—	2.520	—	—	—	—	—	—	—	—	—	0.002	—
0.240	0.240	3.500	0.714	—	0.050	0.030	0.800	—	—	—	14.50	41.00	0.001	—
—	—	—	2.390	—	—	—	—	—	—	—	—	—	0.002	—
0.000	—	860.0	—	0.000	0.000	0.060	0.000	—	—	—	48.00	38.00	0.003	0.000
0.200	—	0.000	—	0.000	0.000	0.010	0.000	0.004	1.600	0.000	4.000	2.000	0.000	—
0.500	0.300	60.00	—	0.000	0.020	0.080	0.200	—	—	—	48.00	60.00	—	—
0.800	—	0.000	—	0.000	0.000	0.000	0.000	—	—	—	9.000	3.000	0.000	0.000
7.500	—	0.000	—	0.000	0.020	0.070	0.400	—	—	—	187.0	42.00	0.003	0.000
0.000	0.006	0.000	—	0.000	0.000	0.000	0.000	—	—	—	0.000	0.000	0.000	0.000
0.100	—	0.000	—	0.000	0.000	0.000	0.000	—	—	—	0.000	0.000	0.001	0.000

Nutritive Components for Vegetables—cont'd

IRON Mg	ZINC Mg	V-A IV	V-ET Mg	V-C Mg	THIA Mg	RIBO Mg	NIAC Mg	V-B6 Mg	FOL µg	VB12 µg	CALC Mg	PHOS Mg	SEL Mg	FIBD Gm
1.620	0.430	172.0	—	8.900	0.068	0.059	0.709	0.104	53.40	0.000	47.00	72.00	—	4.000
1.150	1.000	1472	2.860	43.90	0.117	0.185	1.870	0.036	242.0	0.000	41.40	99.00	0.007	2.160
0.740	3.550	434.0	—	—	0.389	0.152	1.090	0.340	60.70	0.000	128.0	264.0	—	6.600
4.470	3.450	—	—	15.20	0.124	0.139	1.230	—	—	—	118.0	214.0	—	—
1.200	0.390	471.0	0.068	6.500	0.020	0.075	0.270	0.054	43.00	0.000	35.00	34.00	0.001	1.760
3.100	0.360	30.00	—	5.000	0.020	0.050	0.200	0.085	40.80	0.000	32.00	31.00	0.001	3.200
1.780	0.240	2198	0.992	98.00	0.128	0.322	1.180	0.308	107.0	0.000	178.0	74.00	—	6.400

▉ Nutritive Components for Vegetables—cont'd

Food name	Serving	Gm wt	KCAL	PROT Gm	CARB Gm	FAT Gm	CHOL Mg	SAFA Gm	SOD Mg	POT Mg	MAG Mg
BRUSSEL SPROUTS-RAW-BOIL	1 cup	156.0	60.00	3.980	13.50	0.800	0.000	0.164	34.00	494.0	32.00
CABBAGE COMMON RAW SHRED	1 cup	90.0	21.60	1.090	4.830	0.162	0.000	0.021	16.20	221.0	13.50
CARROTS-BOIL-DRAIN-SLICED	1 cup	156.0	70.00	1.700	16.30	0.280	0.000	0.054	104.0	354.0	20.00
CAULIFLOWER-RAW-BOIL-DRAIN	1 cup	124.0	30.00	2.320	5.740	0.220	0.000	0.046	8.000	400.0	14.00
CELERY-PASCAL-RAW-STALK	1 item	40.0	6.000	0.260	1.450	0.050	0.000	0.013	35.00	114.0	5.000
CORN-KERNELS FROM 1 EAR	1 item	77.0	83.00	2.560	19.30	0.980	0.000	0.152	13.00	192.0	24.00
CORN-SWEET-CAN-DRAINED	1 cup	165.0	132.0	4.300	30.50	1.640	0.000	0.254	470.0	160.0	28.00
CUCUMBER-RAW-SLICED	1 cup	104.0	14.00	0.560	3.020	0.140	0.000	0.034	2.000	156.0	12.00
LETTUCE-ICEBERG-RAW-CHOP	1 cup	55.0	7.150	0.556	1.150	0.105	0.000	0.014	4.950	86.90	4.950
LETTUCE-ROMAINE-RAW-SHRED	1 cup	56.0	8.000	0.900	1.320	0.120	0.000	0.014	4.000	162.0	4.000
MUSHROOMS-RAW-CHOPPED	1 cup	70.0	18.00	1.460	3.260	0.300	0.000	0.040	2.000	260.0	8.000
ONIONS-MATURE-RAW-CHOPPED	1 cup	160.0	54.00	1.880	11.70	0.420	0.000	0.070	4.000	248.0	16.00
PEAS-GREEN-FROZ-BOIL-DRAIN	1 cup	160.0	126.0	8.240	22.80	0.440	0.000	0.078	140.0	268.0	46.00
POTATO-FLESH & SKIN-BAKE	1 item	202.0	220.0	4.650	51.00	0.200	0.000	0.052	16.00	844.0	55.00
POTATO-FRENCH FRIED-FROZ	1 item	5.0	11.10	0.173	1.700	0.438	0.000	0.208	1.500	22.90	1.100
POTATO-MASHED-MILK/BUTTER	1 cup	210.0	222.0	3.950	35.10	8.870	4.000	2.170	619.0	607.0	37.00
POTATO CHIPS-SALT ADDED	1 item	2.0	10.50	0.128	1.040	0.708	0.000	0.181	9.400	26.00	1.200
SPINACH-RAW-CHOPPED	1 cup	56.0	12.00	1.600	1.960	0.200	0.000	0.032	44.00	312.0	44.00
SQUASH-ACORN-BAKED	1 cup	205.0	115.0	2.290	29.90	0.290	0.000	0.059	9.000	896.0	87.00
SQUASH-ZUCCHINI-RAW-BOIL	1 cup	180.0	28.00	1.140	7.080	0.100	0.000	0.018	4.000	456.0	38.00
SWEET POTATO-CANDIED	1 piece	105.0	144.0	0.910	29.30	3.410	0.000	1.420	73.00	198.0	12.00
TOFU-SOYBEAN CURD	1 piece	120.0	86.00	9.400	2.900	5.000	0.000	—	8.000	50.00	—
TOMATO-RAW-RED-RIPE	1 item	135.0	24.00	1.090	5.340	0.260	0.000	0.037	10.00	254.0	14.00
TOMATO JUICE-CAN	1 cup	244.0	42.00	1.860	10.30	0.140	0.000	0.020	882.0	536.0	28.00
TOMATO PASTE-CAN-SALT ADD	1 cup	262.0	220.0	9.900	49.30	2.330	0.000	0.332	2070	2442	134.0
VEGETABLE JUICE-CAN	1 cup	242.0	44.00	1.520	11.00	0.220	0.000	0.032	884.0	468.0	26.00

Nutritive Components for Vegetables—cont'd

IRON Mg	ZINC Mg	V-A IV	V-ET Mg	V-C Mg	THIA Mg	RIBO Mg	NIAC Mg	V-B6 Mg	FOL µg	VB12 µg	CALC Mg	PHOS Mg	SEL Mg	FIBD Gm
1.880	0.500	1122	1.320	96.80	0.166	0.124	0.946	0.278	93.60	0.000	56.00	88.00	0.001	4.520
0.504	0.162	113.0	1.500	42.60	0.045	0.027	0.270	0.086	51.00	0.000	42.30	20.70	0.002	1.800
0.960	0.460	38300	0.713	3.600	0.054	0.088	0.790	0.384	21.60	0.000	48.00	48.00	0.002	5.770
0.520	0.300	18.00	0.113	68.60	0.078	0.064	0.684	0.250	63.40	0.000	34.00	44.00	0.001	2.230
0.190	0.070	51.00	0.292	2.500	0.012	0.012	0.120	0.012	3.600	0.000	14.00	10.00	0.000	0.400
0.470	0.370	167.0	0.868	4.800	0.166	0.055	1.240	0.046	35.70	0.000	2.000	79.00	0.001	6.600
1.400	0.640	256.0	1.020	7.000	0.050	0.080	1.500	0.330	59.40	0.000	8.000	81.00	0.001	2.150
0.280	0.240	46.00	0.322	4.800	0.032	0.020	0.312	0.054	14.40	0.000	14.00	18.00	0.001	1.460
0.275	0.121	182.0	0.413	2.150	0.025	0.017	0.103	0.022	30.80	0.000	10.50	11.00	0.000	0.600
0.620	—	1456	0.420	13.40	0.056	0.056	0.280	—	76.00	0.000	20.00	26.00	0.000	0.773
0.860	0.344	0.000	0.203	2.400	0.072	0.314	2.880	0.068	14.80	0.000	4.000	72.00	0.009	1.260
0.580	0.280	0.000	0.496	13.40	0.096	0.016	0.160	0.252	31.80	0.000	40.00	46.00	0.003	2.640
2.520	1.500	1068	1.040	15.80	0.452	0.160	2.370	0.180	93.80	0.000	38.00	144.0	0.001	6.080
2.750	0.650	—	0.121	26.10	0.216	0.067	3.320	0.701	22.20	0.000	20.00	115.0	0.001	4.850
0.067	0.021	0.000	—	0.550	0.006	0.002	0.115	0.012	0.830	0.000	0.400	4.300	0.000	0.160
0.550	0.580	355.0	0.126	12.90	0.176	0.084	2.270	0.470	16.70	0.000	54.00	97.00	0.001	—
0.024	0.021	0.000	0.146	0.830	0.003	0.000	0.084	0.010	0.900	0.000	0.500	3.100	0.000	0.029
1.520	0.300	3760	1.650	15.80	0.044	0.106	0.406	0.110	108.0	0.000	56.00	28.00	0.001	1.760
1.910	0.350	878.0	—	22.10	0.342	0.027	1.810	0.398	38.40	0.000	90.00	93.00	0.002	4.300
0.640	0.320	432.0	—	8.400	0.074	0.074	0.770	0.140	30.20	0.000	24.00	72.00	0.006	2.300
1.190	0.160	4399	—	7.000	0.019	0.044	0.414	0.043	12.00	0.032	27.00	27.00	0.001	1.100
2.300	—	0.000	—	0.000	0.070	0.040	0.100	—	—	—	154.0	151.0	—	—
0.590	0.130	1394	0.603	21.60	0.074	0.062	0.738	0.059	11.50	0.000	8.000	29.00	0.001	2.100
1.420	0.360	1356	1.730	44.60	0.114	0.076	1.640	0.270	48.40	0.000	20.00	46.00	0.001	2.900
7.830	2.100	6468	—	111.0	0.406	0.498	8.440	0.996	—	0.000	91.70	207.0	0.003	—
1.020	0.480	2832	—	67.00	0.104	0.068	1.760	0.339	—	0.000	26.00	40.00	0.001	2.700

Appendix *B*

The Lifestyle Inventory:
Wellness for Life

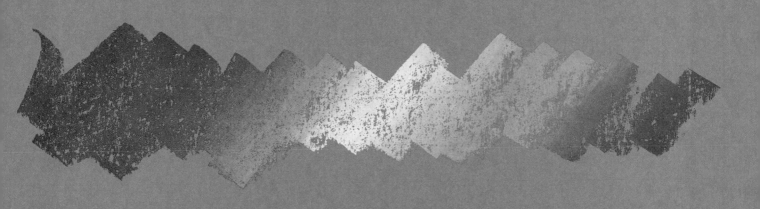

Introduction

Over time, you are either strengthened or weakened by what you do with yourself on a regular basis. Your present state of wellness and your life-long well-being are largely determined by your accustomed patterns of thought and behavior. The way you eat, your level of physical activity, how you handle stress and your avoidance of chemical dependencies all affect your ability to function effectively and to enthusiastically partake of the good life. To a large extent, these aspects of your lifestyle determine the mileage you're likely to get out of your natural gifts. They either squander or preserve your basic genetic endowment.

What does it mean to enjoy a high level of wellness? Beyond the absence of illness and pain, wellness means feeling really alive, with a genuine gusto for life, and having plenty of energy to enjoy it fully. It's a trim, flexible, well-toned body, a twinkle in your eye, and a warm, friendly smile on your face. In short, wellness is the capacity to live your life to its fullest.

On the other hand, a lack of wellness is often at the root of common problems, such as:

a lack of energy and vitality
looking and feeling out of shape
difficulty coping with daily pressures
nagging aches and pains
over- or under-weight
shortness of breath
frequent minor illnesses
loss of muscle tone
persistent lower back pain
diminished work performance
difficulty concentrating
more frequent emotional upsets
lowered endurance
limited flexibility

And over the long term a lack of wellness can lead not only to a loss of trim appearance and vitality, but also to a heightened susceptibility to injury and to many of the major health problems of our time: among them heart and arterial disease, stroke, cancer, diabetes, cirrhosis, emphysema and bronchitis.

The lifestyle inventory quickly gives you a clear picture of how your current lifestyle patterns are shaping your future well-being. In completing it, bear in mind that there are no right or wrong answers. The correct answer—indeed, the only useful answer—is the one which best reflects your real-life practices today.

How You See Yourself

The term "wellness" is of relatively recent vintage. It came into being primarily because the notion of "health" has so often referred simply to an absence of illness. It is easy to see, however, that even in the absence of obvious symptoms of illness, great variations can exist in one's level of health and vitality. In other words, your vast potential for experiencing physical, mental and emotional well-being cannot be adequately described simply as an absence of illness. The term "wellness" refers to this great positive potential.

The graph shown at the top of p. A-33 can help to illustrate the idea of wellness. In it, the midpoint—represented by zero—symbolizes the borderline between illness and the absence of illness. Above this seemingly neutral point rises a broad range of positive potential for enhanced well-being; below it looms the gruesome spectre of creeping illness and gradual loss of ability.

From top to bottom, the scale ranges from what you might consider to be your ideal state of health, fitness and well-being, at +10, to a minimum state of wellness at −10.

Mark the point on the right side of the scale that you feel best represents your overall condition today—that is, your present state of wellness and vitality.

Next, think back in time to a period about five years ago. Get an image of your condition at that time. Now mark the point on the scale to the left which you feel best represents your overall condition as of five years ago.

Connect these two points with an arrow directed from your past to your present condition. This arrow indicates the direction of your recent health history as you have experienced it.

Your ideal physical, mental and emotional condition

5 Y E A R S A G O	Exceptional wellness	+10 / +8 / +6	+10 / +8 / +6	Exceptional wellness	**T O D A Y**
	Above average wellness	+4 / +2	+4 / +2	Above average wellness	
	Average wellness	0 / −2	0 / −2	Average wellness	
	Less than average wellness	−4 / −6	−4 / −6	Less than average wellness	
	Low level wellness	−8 / −10	−8 / −10	Low level wellness	

Minimal state of well-being

Measure Your Present Condition

Your Body Composition

You may use these guidelines to determine your ideal weight:

Adult male: Allow 106 pounds for the first five feet of height, and add 6 pounds for each additional inch.

Adult female: Allow 100 pounds for the first five feet of height, and add 5 pounds for each additional inch.

Adjustment for Frame Size: Subtract 10% from these results if you have a light frame; add 10% for a heavy frame.

Your Present Weight _____

Divided By Your Ideal Weight ÷_____

Equals =_____

Minus − 1.00

Equals Percent Overweight =_____

Enter the score from the table that matches your percent overweight. _____ Your Score from the table

Your Resting Heart Rate

How fast your heart beats when you are at rest indicates how hard your heart has to work simply to maintain your basic body functions. This, in turn, is a useful indicator of the fitness of your heart, lungs, blood and blood vessels.

Percent overweight	Your score	Your weight tends to support
0	50	Exceptional wellness
1 to 2	47	
3 to 4	44	Above average wellness
5 to 6	41	
7 to 9	38	Average wellness
10 to 13	35	
14 to 19	32	Less than average wellness
20 to 26	29	
27 to 33	26	Low level wellness
34 to 50	23	
over 75	20	

Resting heart rate	Your score	Your rate tends to support
under 50	50	Exceptional wellness
50 to 54	47	
55 to 59	44	Above average wellness
60 to 64	41	
65 to 68	38	Average wellness
69 to 72	35	
73 to 76	32	Less than average wellness
77 to 80	29	
81 to 84	26	Low level wellness
85 to 88	23	
over 88	20	

Summarize Your Present Condition

Summarize your Present Condition by adding up the three scores you've developed so far.

		Mark your score here	Your patterns tend to support
Your Body Composition Score	+ _____		Exceptional wellness
		86	Above average wellness
plus: Your Resting Heart Rate Score	+ _____	72	
			Average wellness
equals: Subtotal	= _____	58	
			Less than average wellness
minus: Your Smoking History Score	− _____	44	
			Low level wellness
Your Present Condition Score	= _____		

The sections to follow explore a number of ways in which your Present Condition is being shaped by your lifestyle.

Your resting heart rate may be measured after you have been sitting or lying in a relaxed state for five minutes or so. To determine your heart rate, place the second and third fingers along the thumb side of the opposite wrist, and count the pulsations for one minute.

Your Resting Heart Rate _____

Enter the score from the table that matches your resting heart rate. _____
Your Score from the table

Your Smoking History

Circle the score beside the one statement that best describes your experience with smoking.

 0 I have never smoked, or I quit smoking more than 15 years ago.
−1 I quit smoking 10 to 15 years ago.
−2 I quit smoking 5 to 10 years ago.
−3 I quit smoking less than 5 years ago.
−20 I presently smoke 1 to 7 cigarettes per day.
−23 I presently smoke 8 to 14 cigarettes per day or I smoke cigars or a pipe.
−26 I presently smoke 15 to 25 cigarettes per day.
−30 I presently smoke more than 25 cigarettes per day.

Circle the score beside *each* statement that is true for you.

−2 I have lived with a person who smokes during 2 or more of the past 4 years.
−2 I have worked in a smoky area during 2 or more of the past 4 years.
−1 I have lived in a high smog area during 2 or more of the past 4 years.

Add up your smoking history scores and enter the total here. −_____
Your Score

Measure Your Lifestyle

For each of the following questions, mark one of the squares beside the single answer that is most correct for you at this time. (Two columns of squares are provided so that you can note your responses on two separate occasions. On each such occasion, be sure to mark all of your answers in the same column.)

Your Stress Management Patterns
Clarity and personal organization

In my present life situation:

- ☐ ☐ **3** I feel confined and unable to express myself as I would like.
- ☐ ☐ **6** I feel somewhat limited.
- ☐ ☐ **9** I am able to be the person I choose to be, and to do the things I enjoy most.

In areas where I have expectations:

- ☐ ☐ **3** In one or more key matters, I frequently fear undesired outcomes.
- ☐ ☐ **6** My expectations are sometimes clouded with doubt regarding my ability to be, do or have as I would like.
- ☐ ☐ **9** In general, I clearly see myself thinking, feeling and behaving just as I most truly choose to be.

When I feel that I have been slighted, offended or somehow harmed by the actions of another:

- ☐ ☐ **3** I tend to remain angry, resentful and bitter, hoping that somehow the score can be evened.
- ☐ ☐ **6** I generally excuse others for their errors and omissions, chalking it up to their ignorance or incompetence.
- ☐ ☐ **9** I consistently choose to unconditionally forgive any harmful words or actions by others, thus freeing myself for fully effective action, unburdened by blameful thoughts or destructive emotions.

When working on tasks which demand concentration:

- ☐ ☐ **3** I am frequently distracted by other matters.
- ☐ ☐ **6** I have some difficulty staying focused on what I'm doing.
- ☐ ☐ **9** I can usually stay focused on what I'm doing without undue distraction.

Regarding my sense of responsibility:

- ☐ ☐ **3** I generally feel responsible for everything that is going on.
- ☐ ☐ **6** I often feel responsible for situations and events that are beyond my control.
- ☐ ☐ **9** I feel responsible for assuring that my thoughts, feelings and behavior represent me at my very best, and that my conduct is fully harmonized with my values, intuitions and most noble intentions.

Attitude control

Regarding personal achievement, I am:

- ☐ ☐ **3** constantly driven to work harder in order to measure up to my own high standards.
- ☐ ☐ **6** somewhat pressured to work harder in order to prove myself.
- ☐ ☐ **9** relaxed, confident that I am responding appropriately to my circumstances.

When I am working against a tight schedule:

- ☐ ☐ **3** I am often nervous, and frequently become impatient with delays.
- ☐ ☐ **6** I am sometimes nervous, and occasionally become impatient with delays.
- ☐ ☐ **9** I generally remain calm, responding to delays with patience and renewed determination.

Regarding my need for information:

- ☐ ☐ **3** I become very uncomfortable when I don't know exactly what is going on.
- ☐ ☐ **6** I feel somewhat uncomfortable with uncertainty and try hard to eliminate the unknowns.
- ☐ ☐ **9** I can live with uncertainty, even enjoying the adventure of facing the unknown.

When the assistance of others could aid me in getting my needs met:

- ☐ ☐ **3** I often expect them to be unresponsive to me, and may not even bother to request their help.
- ☐ ☐ **6** I often expect others to be at least somewhat reluctant to assist me, and plan to get what I want through pleading, trickery, intimidation or force.
- ☐ ☐ **9** I generally expect others to be supportive and cooperative once I have brought my needs to their attention.

My satisfaction and sense of accomplishment are derived from:

- ☐ ☐ **3** mainly the rewards and recognition I receive from others.
- ☐ ☐ **6** sometimes my own appreciation; more often the recognition I receive from others.
- ☐ ☐ **9** mainly the personal knowledge that I have performed to be best of my ability.

My interests are:

☐ ☐ **3** mostly confined to matters which are related to my work.

☐ ☐ **6** somewhat varied.

☐ ☐ **9** numerous and varied, including areas that are quite unrelated to my work.

With regard to expressing my feelings:

☐ ☐ **3** I keep my true feelings to myself in most situations.

☐ ☐ **6** I find it somewhat difficult to express my real feelings.

☐ ☐ **9** I find it easy to express my feelings in most situations.

In dealing with my deepest personal concerns.

☐ ☐ **3** I feel unable to discuss my most difficult problems with anyone.

☐ ☐ **6** sometimes I feel I have no one to talk with about what's really bothering me.

☐ ☐ **9** I have trusted persons with whom I can usually discuss whatever is on my mind.

When others are speaking to me:

☐ ☐ **3** I'm often thinking of what I'm going to say next, and frequently interrupt the speaker.

☐ ☐ **6** I listen intermittently, sometimes interrupting the speaker with my own thoughts.

☐ ☐ **9** I usually listen attentively, rarely interrupting the speaker.

The quality of my sleep is:

☐ ☐ **3** often disturbed by anxious thoughts or distressing dreams.

☐ ☐ **6** sometimes sound; other times disturbed.

☐ ☐ **9** sound, peaceful and refreshing: undisturbed by the concerns of the day.

Conscious relaxation

I reduce the effect of stress in my life by engaging in some method of conscious relaxation:

☐ ☐ **25** infrequently—once a week or less.

☐ ☐ **50** occasionally—every few days.

☐ ☐ **75** almost every day.

Mark your score here	Your patterns tend to support:
168	Exceptional wellness
140	Above average wellness
112	Average wellness
84	Less than average wellness
	Low level wellness

Add up your stress management scores for your current set of responses and enter the total here.

Your stress management score _____ _____

Your Physical Activity Patterns

Full-body stretches

I perform full-body stretches to maintain my flexibility and range of motion:

☐ ☐ **20** once a week or less.

☐ ☐ **40** every few days.

☐ ☐ **60** almost every day.

Cardiorespiratory activity

An "aerobic workout" consists of five essential parts: first, a brief pre-exercise stretch; second, a short warm-up period; third, at least 12 minutes of continuous activity which is sufficiently vigorous to maintain your heart rate at 80 percent of its maximum for your age; fourth, a short cool-down period; and fifth, a brief post-exercise stretch.

I provide my body with a complete, five-part aerobic workout:

☐ ☐ **40** once a week or less.

☐ ☐ **80** two or three times a week.

☐ ☐ **120** more than three times a week.

Body-toning

I engage in activities which help me to maintain the tone and strength of my major muscles and bones:

☐ ☐ **10** once a week or less.

☐ ☐ **20** one or two times a week.

☐ ☐ **30** three or more times each week.

Mark your score here			Your patterns tend to support:
170	+	+	Exceptional wellness
			Above average wellness
140	+	+	
			Average wellness
110	+	+	
			Less than average wellness
80	+	+	
			Low level wellness

Add up your physical activity scores for your current set of responses and enter the total here: Your physical activity score _____ _____

Your Nutritional Patterns

Eating independence

I feel that the quantity of food I eat at meals is:

☐ ☐ 10 frequently excessive—I usually don't stop eating until I feel full.
☐ ☐ 20 occasionally excessive.
☐ ☐ 30 rarely excessive—I usually finish eating before feeling full.

I feel that the eating and drinking I do—*aside from meals*—is:

☐ ☐ 10 frequent; substantial; high fat or sugar.
☐ ☐ 20 occasional; moderate.
☐ ☐ 30 infrequent; insubstantial; unrefined carbohydrates.

Unrefined carbohydrates intake (vegetables, fruit, whole grains)

I eat fresh fruit:

☐ ☐ 5 infrequently—many days none at all.
☐ ☐ 10 occasionally—many days I get some.
☐ ☐ 15 once or twice almost every day.

I eat leafy green vegetables:

☐ ☐ 10 infrequently—many days none at all.
☐ ☐ 20 occasionally—many days I get some.
☐ ☐ 30 once or twice almost every day.

I eat other vegetables such as beans, potatoes, peas, lentils, squash and yams.

☐ ☐ 5 infrequently—many days none at all.
☐ ☐ 10 occasionally—many days I get some.
☐ ☐ 15 almost every day.

The wheat and other grains I eat are mostly:

☐ ☐ 5 highly processed, bleached white.
☐ ☐ 10 medium processed, enriched whole wheat.
☐ ☐ 15 coarse ground, whole grain.

Fat Intake

The meats that I eat are mostly:

☐ ☐ 10 high fat—pork, prime beef, hamburger, organ meats, duck, lamb, etc.
☐ ☐ 20 medium fat—lean beef, veal, chicken and turkey with skin.
☐ ☐ 30 lean—fish, chicken and turkey without skin, or no meat at all.

The dairy products that I consume are mostly:

☐ ☐ 5 high fat—whole milk, cream, cheddar and other full-fat cheeses.
☐ ☐ 10 low fat.
☐ ☐ 15 skim milk, low fat cheeses, or no dairy products at all.

I eat deep-fried foods, including most fast foods:

☐ ☐ 5 often—three or more times a week.
☐ ☐ 10 occasionally—about twice a week.
☐ ☐ 15 seldom—once a week or less.

Regarding fats such as butter, margarine, mayonnaise, salad dressings and oils:

☐ ☐ 5 I don't control my intake.
☐ ☐ 10 I eat 3 or 4 teaspoons per day.
☐ ☐ 15 I eat 2 teaspoons or less per day.

Mark your score here			Your patterns tend to support:
170	+	+	Exceptional wellness
			Above average wellness
140	+	+	
			Average wellness
110	+	+	
			Less than average wellness
80	+	+	
			Low level wellness

Add up your nutritional scores for your current set of responses and enter the total here: Your Nutritional Score _____ _____

Chemical Independence

Caffeine

My average daily consumption of caffeine drinks, including coffee, non-herbal tea, cocoa, cola and chocolate is:

- ☐ ☐ **0** one cup or less.
- ☐ ☐ **−5** two or three cups.
- ☐ ☐ **−10** four or more cups.

Alcohol

The amount of alcohol I consume averages (standard serving = 12 oz beer; 4 oz wine; 1-1/4 oz whiskey):

- ☐ ☐ **0** one standard serving per day or less of any alcoholic beverage.
- ☐ ☐ **−10** two standard servings per day.
- ☐ ☐ **−40** three or more standard servings per day.

Drug independence

I use other mood altering substances:

- ☐ ☐ **0** seldom or never.
- ☐ ☐ **−10** occasionally—less than once a week.
- ☐ ☐ **−20** frequently—once a week or more.

With regard to both prescription and over-the-counter medications:

- ☐ ☐ **0** I take as little as possible, and then only as directed.
- ☐ ☐ **−10** I take quite a bit, sometimes simply for "extra insurance."
- ☐ ☐ **−20** I take a lot, whether or not it is clearly necessary at the time; or, I take them in unapproved combinations.

Tobacco

With regard to tobacco:

- ☐ ☐ **0** I am a non-smoker.
- ☐ ☐ **−50** I use tobacco.

Mark your score here		Your patterns tend to support:
0		Exceptional wellness
		Above average wellness
0		Average wellness
−18		Less than average wellness
−25		Low level wellness

Add up your chemical independence scores for your current set of responses and enter the total here.

Your Chemical Independence Score _____   _____

Summarize Your Lifestyle

Summarize your Lifestyle Inventory by adding up your total scores from the preceding lifestyle measurements.

Your Stress Management Score (from page A-36) + _____   + _____

plus: Your Physical Activity Score (from page A-37)   + _____   + _____

plus: Your Nutritional Score (from page A-37)   + _____   + _____

equals: Subtotal   = _____   = _____

minus: Your chemical Independence Score (above)   − _____   − _____

Your Lifestyle Score   = _____   = _____

Then enter your **Present Condition Score** (from page A-34) _____

Your present condition score supports	Your present condition score				Your lifestyle score	Your lifestyle score supports
Exceptional wellness	93				547	Exceptional wellness
	86				503	
Above average wellness	79				464	Above average wellness
	72				419	
Average wellness	65				366	Average wellness
	58				336	
Less than average wellness	51				274	Less than average wellness
	44				225	
Low level wellness	37				67	Low level wellness

Your Wellness Direction

Place a mark representing your Present Condition Score on the scale to the left.

Place a second mark, representing your Lifestyle Score, on the scale to the right.

Connect these two points with an arrow pointing from your Present Condition mark to your Lifestyle mark.

This arrow gives a general indication of the influence your present lifestyle might be expected to exert on your level of wellness with the passage of time.

Your wellness can be maintained and improved by developing these key factors in your lifestyle:

Proper Physical Activity
Balanced Nutritional Intake
Effective Stress Management
Positive Weight Control
Chemical Independence

Now that you've had a look at the wellness-related factors in your lifestyle, make it a point to begin building these more healthful patterns of living into your own accustomed way of life.

Consult with your physician to develop an even more comprehensive picture of your present condition, and to obtain his or her assistance in establishing a safe and effective strategy for improving your overall state of health.

Glossary

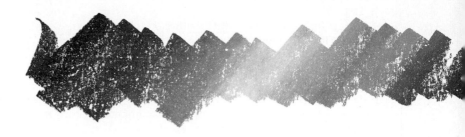

abstinence to refrain completely from engaging in a particular behavior. (p. 21)

Acquired Immunodeficiency Syndrome (AIDS) viral destruction of the immune system, causing loss of ability to fight infections. (p. 235)

adipose cells fat cells. (p. 79)

adrenocorticotropic hormone (ACTH) hormone released by the hypothalamus during periods of stress that initiates various physiological responses. (p. 188)

aerobic literally "with oxygen"; when applied to exercise, refers to activities whose oxygen demand can be supplied continuously by individuals during performance. (p. 141)

aerobic capacity maximum oxygen consumption. (p. 141)

AIDS related complex (ARC) condition in which an individual has tested positive for the AIDS virus but symptoms are either absent or less severe. (p. 236)

alcoholism disease in which an individual loses control over drinking; inability to refrain from drinking. (p. 217)

aldosterone hormone released from the adrenal cortex that increases blood pressure, facilitating the transportation of food and oxygen to the active parts of the body.

amino acid chemical structures that form protein. (p. 41)

anabolic steroids drugs closely related to testosterone that increase muscle mass in humans. (p. 150)

anaerobic literally "without oxygen"; when applied to exercise, refers to high-intensity physical activities whose oxygen demand is greater than that which can be supplied during performance. (p. 152)

android deposition of fat that is characteristic of males; fat tends to accumulate in the abdomen and upper body. (p. 107)

aneurysm weak spot in an artery that forms a balloon-like pouch that can rupture. (p. 116)

angina chest pain that is the result of ischemia (see ischemic). (p. 114)

anorexia nervosa serious illness of deliberate self-starvation with profound psychiatric and physical components. (p. 91)

arthritis inflammatory disease of the joints. (p. 255)

asymptomatic without symptoms. (p. 282)

atherosclerosis slow progressive disease of the arteries characterized by the deposition of plaque on the inner lining of arterial walls. (p. 115)

ATP adenosine triphosphate, the actual unit of energy used for muscular contraction. (p. 142)

autogenics form of suggestion that precipitates relaxation. (p. 194)

autoimmune disease disease in which the immune system fails to recognize its own body parts and produces antibodies against them to the point of causing injury. (p. 255)

autonomic nervous system part of the nervous system that is concerned with control of involuntary bodily functions. (p. 188)

balloon angioplasty surgical procedure that involves the insertion of a catheter with a balloon at the tip used to compress fatty deposits and plaque against the walls of the artery. (p. 128)

basal metabolic rate (BMR) number of calories needed to sustain life. (p. 81)

behavior assessment process of counting, recording, observing, measuring, and describing behavior. (p. 24)

behavior substitution lifestyle change technique in which an incompatible behavior is substituted for a behavior being altered. (p. 27)

behavioral contract a written agreement in a lifestyle-change program. (p. 25)

benign noncancerous. (p. 247)

biofeedback educational tool used to provide information about an individual's physiological actions. (p. 195)

blood alcohol concentration (BAC) percentage of alcohol content in the blood. (p. 216)

body composition amount of lean versus fat tissue in the body. (p. 160)

body mass index (BMI) measure of relative fatness. (p. 81)

bulimia eating disorder characterized by episodes of secretive binge eating and purging. (p. 92)

caffeine a stimulant that increases the heart rate. (p. 214)

calorie short for *kilocalorie,* which is the unit of measurement for food energy. A calorie is the amount of heat required to raise the temperature of 1 gram of water 1 degree centigrade. (p. 39)

cancer group of diseases characterized by uncontrolled, disorderly cell growth. (p. 246)

cannabinoids chemicals found only in marijuana. (p. 222)

cannabis sativa Indian hemp plant from which marijuana and hashish are derived. (p. 222)

carbon monoxide deadly gas emitted in the exhaust of cars and in burning tobacco. (p. 220)

carcinogens substances that cause cancer or enable the growth of cancer cells; cancer causing agents. (p. 247)

cardiac arrhythmia irregular heart rate that is sometimes intractable. (p. 82)

cardiac output amount of blood ejected by the heart in 1 minute. (p. 141)

cardiorespiratory endurance ability to take in, deliver, and extract oxygen for physical work. (p. 141)

catheterization in relation to heart disease, the passage of a catheter (slender plastic tube) into the heart through an arm vein and blood vessels leading into the heart to obtain cardiac blood samples, detect abnormalities, and determine intracardiac pressure. (p. 127)

cause and effect in medical research, the type of relationship in which one variable is scientifically proved to cause a certain effect. (p. 267)

cerebral hemorrhage bursting of a blood vessel in the brain. (p. 116)

Caesarean section delivery surgical removal of the fetus through the abdominal wall. (p. 233)

chemotherapy use of drugs and hormones to treat various cancers. (p. 250)

cholesterol steroid that is an essential structural component of neural tissue and cell walls and is required, for the manufacture of hormones and bile. (p. 49)

chronic effects of exercise the physiological changes that result from cardiorespiratory training. (p. 141)

complete protein protein that contains all of the essential amino acids. (p. 41)

complex carbohydrates polysacchrides, including starch and fiber. (p. 53)

condyloma warts on the genitalia. (p. 232)

constipation condition of having painful or difficult bowel movements. (p. 63)

contraindication reason for not prescribing a drug or treatment. (p. 278)

control group in health research, the group receiving no treatment. (p. 269)

coping effort(s) made to manage or deal with stress. (p. 192)

coronary artery bypass surgery procedure involving the removal of a leg vein that is used as a shunt around the blocked area in the coronary artery. (p. 128)

cortisol primary hormone that provides fuel to respond with the fight-or-flight reaction. (p. 188)

crack smokable form of cocaine that is extremely dangerous and very addictive. (p. 221)

crude fiber residue of plant food following chemical treatment in the laboratory. (p. 54)

deceptive advertising advertising that misleads consumers by overstating or exaggerating the performance of a product. (p. 269)

delta-9-tetrahydrocannabinol (THC) major psychoactive drug found in marijuana. (p. 222)

diarrhea condition of having frequent, loose, watery stools. (p. 64)

dietary fiber residue of plant food after digestion in the human body. One gram of crude fiber equals 2-3 grams of dietary fiber. (p. 54)

distress form of stress that results in negative responses. (p. 185)

diverticulitis infection of the diverticula of the intestines. (p. 66)

diverticulosis condition of having sac-like swellings (diverticula) in the walls of the intestines. (p. 66)

double blind study type of health research in which neither the researcher nor the subjects know who is receiving an experimental treatment. (p. 269)

drug chemical substance that has the potential to alter the structure and functioning of a living organism. (p. 210)

echocardiography noninvasive technique that uses sound waves to determine the shape, texture, and movement of the valves of the heart. (p. 127)

edema condition in which body tissues contain an excessive amount of fluid.

electrocardiograph (EKG) device for recording electrical variations in action of heart muscle. (p. 82)

embolus mass of undissolved matter in the blood or lymphatic vessels that detaches from the vessel walls. (p. 116)

endorphins mood-elevating, pain-killing substances produced by the brain. (p. 188)

energy nutrients nutrients such as carbohydrates, fat, and protein that provide a source of energy for the body. (p. 39)

epinephrine hormone produced by the adrenal medulla that speeds up body processes. (p. 188)

essential fat fat that is indispensable for individuals to function biologically and necessary to support life. (p. 93)

essential hypertension high blood pressure due to unknown reasons. (p. 122) essential nutrients nutrients that cannot be made by the body and must be supplied in the diet. (p. 39)

ethyl alcohol intoxicating agent in alcoholic drinks; colorless liquid with a sharp, burning taste. (p. 216)

eustress stress judged as "good"; positive stress or stress that contributes to positive outcomes. (p. 185)

experimental group in health research, the group receiving some form of experimental treatment. (p. 269)

false negative test results that incorrectly show a person is healthy when an abnormality actually exists. (p. 280)

false positive test results that incorrectly show an abnormality when a person is actually healthy. (p. 280)

family practice physician medical doctor who serves as a general practitioner for an individual or family. (p. 275)

fat mixture of triglycerides. (p. 47)

fiber substances in food that resist digestion; formerly called roughage. (p. 54)

fight-or-flight syndrome initial phase of the general adaptation syndrome (GAS); when a stressor is encountered, the body responds by preparing to stand and fight or to run away, depending on the situation; also called the alarm phase of the GAS. (p. 186)

flexibility range of motion at a joint. (p. 154)

fraternal twins twins who emanate from separate eggs and do not have identical genes. (p. 81)

freebasing smoking liquefied cocaine. (p. 221)

fructose fruit sugar. (p. 53)

General Adaptation Syndrome (GAS) series of physiological changes that occur when a stressor is encountered; the GAS is conceived of as having three phases: alarm, resistance, and exhaustion. (p. 186)

glucose primary source of energy utilized by the body; blood sugar. (p. 53)

glyceride general term for fat compounds, including triglyceride, monoglyceride, and diglyceride. (p. 47)

gonorrhea bacterial disease that is sexually transmitted and can lead to serious complications if left untreated, including sterility and scarring of the heart valves. (p. 234)

gynoid fat deposition characteristic of females, in whom fat tends to accumulate on the hips and thighs. (p. 107)

hardiness label used is describing a particular type of personality that tends to remain healthy even under extreme stress; the three components of hardiness are challenge, commitment, and control. (p. 192)

hashish resin from the cannabis sativa plant that can be smoked to alter mood; a frequently abused drug (p. 222)

health balancing of the physical, emotional, social, and spiritual components of personality in a manner that is conducive to optimal wellbeing and a higher quality of existence. (p. 2)

health behavior gap discrepancy between what people know and what they actually do regarding their health (p. 18)

health care providers people and facilities such as physicians and hospitals that provide health care services. (p. 266)

health fatalism in health information the view that new information cannot be believed or trusted because it will inevitably be refuted. (p. 266)

health hysteria refers to a reactionary cycle in which new health findings suggest a cause-and-effect relationship between some variable and health that leads to publicity, notoriety, fear, and sometimes legislation. (p. 266)

Health Maintenance Organization (HMO) prepaid group insurance program that provides a full range of medical services. (p. 282)

health-promoting behaviors things done to maintain and improve one's level of wellness. (p. 22)

health promotion art and science of helping people change their lifestyle to move toward a higher state of wellness. (p. 3)

health-related fitness components of fitness that include cardiorespiratory endurance, muscular strength, muscular endurance, flexibility, and body composition. (p. 140)

health risk appraisals questionnaires used to provide information about health habits, lifestyle, and medical history. (p. 279)

heat exhaustion serious, heat-related condition characterized by dizziness, fainting, rapid pulse, and cool skin. (p. 171)

heat stroke heat-related medical emergency characterized by high temperature (106° F or higher) and dry skin and accompanied by some or all of the following: delirium, convulsions, and loss of consciousness. (p. 171)

herpes simplex (HSV) virus responsible for herpes genitalis, a sexually transmitted disease. (p. 233)

heterogeneous group group of subjects that represents the social, religious, sexual, and cultural characteristics of the population at large.

hiatal hernia condition in which part of the stomach pushes through the opening (hiatus) of the diaphragm. (p. 65)

highly polyunsaturated fat fatty acid composed of triglycerides in which the carbon chain has room for many hydrogen atoms. (p. 48)

homeostasis state of balance or constancy; the body is continually attempting to maintain homeostasis. (p. 186)

homogeneous group group of subjects with similar characteristics. (p. 269)

human immunodeficiency virus (HIV) virus that is the source of AIDS. (p. 236)

human papilloma virus (HPV) causative agent of condyloma (genital warts). (p. 232)

hydrogenated process of adding hydrogen to unsaturated fatty acid to make it more saturated.

hyperglycemia high blood sugar. (p. 254)

hyperplasia increase in the number of cells. (p. 79)

hypertension high blood pressure. (p. 121)

hypertrophy increase in the size of a cell. (p. 79)

hypokinesis physical inactivity.

hypothalamus part of the limbic system that contains the center for many bodily functions; in stressful situations the hypothalamus releases specific hormones to elicit appropriate bodily responses. (p. 188)

hypothermia cold weather–related condition that results in abnormally low body temperature. (p. 173)

iatrogenic disease condition caused as a result of receiving medical care. (p. 271)

identical twins twins who emanate from the same egg. (p. 81)

immunization a vaccine or other preparation administered to prevent disease. (p. 282)

implied consent nonverbal authorization of a medical procedure such as cooperation during the administration of tests. (p. 273)

incomplete protein protein that doesn't contain all the essential amino acids in the proportions needed by the body. (p. 41)

informed consent legal provision requiring patient's authorization of any medical procedure, therapy, or treatment. (p. 273)

insoluble fiber fiber that does not dissolve in water; comes from wheat bran and vegetables. (p. 54)

insulin hormone secreted by the pancreas that increases the utilization of glucose by the tissues of the body. (p. 254)

intensity degree of vigorousness of a single bout of exercise. (p. 160)

internal bleeding bleeding that occurs anywhere inside the body.

internist medical doctor specializing in internal medicine and sometimes serving as a primary care physician. (p. 271)

ischemic diminished supply of blood to heart muscle. (p. 115)

isokinetic method for developing muscular strength that involves a constant rate of speed and changes in the amount of weight resistance. (p. 145)

isometric use of static contractions to develop strength. (p. 150)

isotonic method for developing muscular strength that involves a variable rate of speed and a constant weight resistance. (p. 145)

Kaposi's sarcoma (KS) rare form of cancer often acquired by people with AIDS. (p. 236)

lactic acid metabolite formed in muscles as a result of incomplete breakdown of sugar. (p. 164)

lactose simple sugar; milk sugar. (p. 53)

limbic system large, C-shaped area that contains the centers for emotions, memory storage, learning relay, and hormone production (the pituitary gland, thalamus, and hypothalamus). (p. 188)

lipid class of nutrients more commonly referred to as fat. (p. 47)

lipoprotein lipase enzyme that increases the body's ability to store fat. (p. 82)

locus-of-control perspective from which an individual views life. Individuals with an internal locus-of-control believe that their decisions make a difference and that they have control over their lives. People with external locus-of-control see themselves as "victims" and consider other people, situations, and conditions as being the controlling factor in their lives. (p. 9)

low-calorie diet diet that limits intake to 800 to 1,000 calories a day; results in atrophy of heart muscle. (p. 82)

major minerals those minerals required in large amounts (more than 5 grams a day). (p. 45)

malignant cancerous; harmful. (p. 247)

maltose maltose sugar. (p. 53)

mammography x-ray examination of the breast to detect cancer. (p. 281)

marijuana comes from the cannabis plant. (p. 222)

measurable on food labels means that a food contains at least 2% of the USRDA of a nutrient.

megadose large doses, usually in the form of supplements. (p. 44)

metabolism sum total of all chemical reactions that occur within the cells of the body. (p. 88)

metastasis process by which cancerous cells spread from their original location to another location in the body. (p. 247)

migraine headaches headaches characterized by throbbing pain that can last for hours or days, sometimes accompanied by nausea and vomiting. Migraines are thought to be the result of dilation of blood vessels in the head. (p. 257)

minerals inorganic compounds in food necessary for good health. (p. 45)

mitochondria the cell's "powerhouse." (p. 142)

moderate calorie diet diet that limits caloric intake to 1,300 to 1,600 calories a day. (p. 82)

monounsaturated fat fatty acid composed of triglycerides in which the carbon chain has room for one more hydrogen atom. (p. 48)

morbidity incidence of disease and/or sickness. (p. 18)

mortality incidence of death. (p. 18)

muscular endurance application of repeated muscular force developed by many repetitions against resistances considerably less than maximum. (p. 153)

muscular strength maximal force that a muscle or muscle group can exert in a single contraction. (p. 145)

myocardial infarction heart attack; death of heart muscle tissue. (p. 114)

myocardium heart muscle. (p. 82)

negative reinforcers penalties incurred in a lifestyle change program when goals are not achieved. (p. 26)

neoplasm abnormal mass of cells; also called a tumor and can be benign or malignant. (p. 247)

nicotine addictive substance and alkaloid poison found in tobacco. (p. 219)

nutrient substance found in food that is required by the body. (p. 36)

nutrient density ratio of nutrients to calories; also called index of nutritional quality. (p. 58)

nutrition science that deals with the study of nutrients and the way the body ingests, digests, absorbs, transports, metabolizes, and excretes these nutrients. (p. 36)

obesity excessive amount of storage fat. (p. 77)

omega-3 fatty acids type of fatty acid found in cold water seafood and thought to lower the risks of heart disease. (p. 49)

osteoarthritis most common form of arthritis characterized by the deterioration of articular cartilage that covers the gliding surfaces of the bones in certain joints. (p. 169)

osteoporosis progressive decrease in the mineral content of bone, making bones brittle. (p. 166)

overfat may or may not be within normal guidelines for weight but with an excessive ratio of fat compared to lean tissue. (p. 77)

overweight excessive weight for one's height without regard for body composition. (p. 77)

pathogen disease-producing organism. (p. 272)

pelvic inflammatory disease (PID) chronic condition of infection in the uterus, fallopian tubes, and upper reproductive areas; the leading cause of infertility in women. (p. 233)

performance-related fitness sports fitness; composed of speed, power, balance, coordination, agility, and reaction time. (p. 140)

peristalsis involuntary muscular contractions of the intestine. (p. 63)

placebo inactive substance, such as a fake drug. (p. 269)

pneumocystis carinii **pneumonia (PCP)** type of pneumonia caused by a protozoan infection of the lungs; rarely found in healthy people but quite common in AIDS patients. (p. 236)

polyunsaturated fat fatty acid composed of triglycerides in which the carbon chain has room for two or more hydrogen atoms. (p. 48)

positive reinforcers rewards earned for achieving goals in a lifestyle change program. (p. 26)

post natal after birth. (p. 79)

preventive health behaviors health practices associated with the promotion of wellness and the prevention of sickness and death. (p. 18)

primary care physician medical doctor who is responsible for an individual's overall health. (p. 273)

radiotherapy use of radiation to either destroy cancer cells or destroy their reproductive mechanism so they cannot replicate. (p. 250)

RDA acronym for Recommended Dietary Allowances. (p. 39)

reactance motivation theory maintaining that coercion causes an opposite effect in desired behavior. (p. 21)

recidivism in lifestyle change, refers to the tendency to revert to prior or original behavior.

Recommended Dietary Allowances (RDA) daily recommended intakes of nutrients for normal, healthy people in the United States. (p. 39)

relationship in health research, the association or correlation between two or more variables.

relaxation techniques techniques used in coping with and managing stress. (p. 194)

reliability extent to which health studies yield consistent results. (p. 269)

residual volume amount of air remaining in the lungs after expiration. (p. 142)

reticular activating system (RAS) reciprocal neural network between the brain and bodily reactions/actions; considered as serving as the mind-body connection.

rheumatoid arthritis most crippling form of arthritis, characterized by inflammation of the joints, pain, swelling, and deformity. (p. 255)

saccharides refers to sugars (general term). (p. 53)

saturated fat fatty acid composed of triglycerides in which all the fatty acids contain the maximum number of hydrogen atoms. (p. 48)

selective health examination specific test used in response to specific symptoms or for diagnosing a specific problem. (p. 279)

self-efficacy refers to people's belief in their ability to accomplish a specific task or behavior; that belief then affects the outcome of the task or behavior; the theory that individuals who expect to succeed tend to succeed and those who expect to fail tend to fail. (p. 9)

self-help approach to lifestyle change which assumes that an individual can plan and execute his/her own plan. (p. 21)

setpoint theory theory that the body has a preference for maintaining a certain amount of weight and defends that weight quite vigorously. (p. 81)

sexually transmitted diseases (STDs) diseases spread through sexual contact, such as AIDS, chlamydia, gonorrhea, and herpes. (p. 232)

sidestream smoke smoke inhaled by nonsmokers when they are around people who smoke. (p. 220)

skinfold measures method for determining the amount of body fat by using skin calipers. (p. 95)

soluble fiber fiber that dissolves in water; comes from fruit pectins and oat bran. (p. 54)

starch plant polysaccharides composed of glucose and digestible by humans. (p. 53)

stimulus control technique in lifestyle management involving the elimination and/or manipulation of stimuli related to a specific behavior. (p. 26)

stroke volume amount of blood that the heart can eject in one beat. (p. 141)

subliminal advertising technique in which sexual messages, words, and symbols are embedded in the pictures, sounds, or words in advertisements that can be perceived by the subconscious and thereby influence behavior. (p. 20)

sucrose table sugar. (p. 53)

stress nonspecific response of the body to any demands made upon it. (p. 184)

stressor any physical, psychological, or environmental event or condition that initiates the stress response. (p. 185)

tar black, sticky, dark fluid composed of thousands of chemicals and found in tobacco. (p. 220)

tension headaches most common kind of headaches, caused by involuntary contractions of the scalp, head, and neck muscles and may be precipitated by anxiety, stress, or allergic reactions. (p. 256)

thrombus stationary blood clot; can occlude an artery supplying the brain. (p. 116)

trace minerals those minerals required in small amounts. (p. 45)

transit time refers to the time it takes food to move through the body.

triglyceride compound composed of carbon, hydrogen, and oxygen with three fatty acids. (p. 48)

tropical oils oils that come from the fruit of coconut and palm trees. (p. 52)

ulcer sore or lesion of the top layer of cells that can occur outside or inside the body (such as the stomach). (p. 64)

unsaturated fat fatty acid composed of triglycerides in which the carbon chain has room for more hydrogen atoms. (p. 48)

validity extent to which the research design of a health study permits the assertion of certain health claims. (p. 268)

visualization a form of meditation that makes use of the imagination. (p. 195)

vital capacity amount of air that can be expired after a maximum inspiration. (p. 142)

vitamins organic compounds in food necessary for good health. (p. 43)

wellness engaging in activities and behaviors that enhance quality of life and maximize personal potential. (p. 2)

weight cycling potentially harmful pattern of repeated weight loss and weight gain. (p. 81)

Index

Fast-food eating, 61-62
Fast-food items
  calorie sources of, 62
  nutritive components for, A-10–A-11
Fat(s), 47-52
  dietary
    and cancer, 248
    comparison of, 53
    vs. dietary carbohydrate, 126
    guidelines for, 52
    sources of, 50-51
  distribution of, 79-80
  essential, 93
  estimated
    for men, 97
    for women, 98
  facts about, 47-49
  in food, 53
  food substitutions that reduce, 83
  health effects of, 49-50
  hidden, 51-52
  highly polyunsaturated, 48
  intake of, daily, assessment of, 69
  manufacture of, in body, 79
  monounsaturated, 48-49
  nutrition objectives about, 37
  nutritive components for, A-12–A-13
  polyunsaturated, 48-49
  saturated, 48-49, 50, 51
    dietary, sources of, 118
  stress and, 190
  unsaturated, 48-49
Fat cells, increase in, 79
Fat-soluble vitamins, 43, 44
Fat-weight loss, 78
Fatalism, health, 266
Fatigue, muscle, lactic acid and, 164
Fatty acids, omega-3, 49
Feces, 63
Fee-for-service insurance plan, 282
Feedback and lifestyle change, 28
Female physicians, 275
Fentanyl, analogs of, 213
Fever, 272
"Fever blisters," 233
Fiber, 54-56
  and cancer prevention, 248
  crude, 54
  dietary, 54
  insoluble, 54-55
  need for, 55-56
  nutrition objectives about, 37
  soluble, 54
"Fight-or-flight" syndrome, 186
Fish, nutritive components for, A-12–A-15
Fish oils, 49
Fit or Fat Target Diet, 84
Fit for Life, 85
Fitness
  exercise for, 139-181
  health-related, 140
  lack of, and low back pain, 169
  performance-related, 140
  physical, components of, 140-160
Fitness walking test, Rockport, 177-179

"Flashbacks," 224
Flavor enhancers, 59
Flexibility, 154-160
  aging and, 154
  exercises for, 154-157
  and wellness, 160
"Flu" and lifestyle, 256
Flucanazole for AIDS, 237
Fluid intake in hot weather, 172
Fluoride
  daily dietary intake of, 40
  nutrition objectives about, 37
Folate, stress and, 190
Food
  and disease, relationship between, 56
  fortified, 60
  "light," 60
  protein in, 43
  for wellness, choosing, 63
Food combination diets, 85
Food composition tables, A-1–A-29
Food groups and good nutrition, 38
Food labels, 58-60
Food substitutions that reduce fat, cholesterol, and
    calories, 83
Formula, Karvonen, to calculate exercise heart rate,
    161
Formula diets
  over-the-counter, 85
  prescription, 84
Fortified, meaning of word, 270
Fortified foods, 60
Framingham Heart Disease Study, 113
Fraternal twins, obesity studies in, 81
Freebasing of cocaine, 221
Frequency of exercise and conditioning, 162-163
Front of body, muscles of, 149
Frostbite, 173
Frozen dinners, 62-63
  nutritive components for, A-14–A-15
Fructose, 53
Fruits, nutritive components for, A-16–A-17

G

Gastric ulcers, 64-65
General adaptation syndrome, 186-187
  phases of, 186-187
General practitioners, 275
Genetic predisposition to disease, 4
Genetics and obesity, 80-81
Genital herpes, 233
Genital warts, 232-233
Geophagia, 92
Getting Thin, 84
Glucagon and diabetes, 254
Glucose, 53
Glycerides, 47, 49
Goals
  realistic, and lifestyle change, 24-25
  unrealistic, 23
Gonorrhea, 234-235
Government insurance, 283
Graft, coronary artery bypass, 128
Grains, nutritive components for, A-18–A-19
Groin stretch, 156

Primary-care physician, 273, 275
Primary syphilis, 235
Private insurance, 282
Proctoscope, 279
Professional, health-care, selection of, 273-279; *see also* Physician(s)
Progress, evaluation of, and lifestyle change, 28
Progression of exercise and conditioning, 163
Progressive muscle relaxation, 194
Proof of alcohol, 216
Proprioceptive neuromuscular facilitation, 159
Prostaglandins, stress and, 190
Prostate cancer, 249-250
Protein, 41
    complete, 41
    excess of, avoiding, 40-43
    in food, 43
    high-quality, 41
    incomplete, 41
    low-quality, 41
    RDA for, assessment for, 69
    recommended intake of, 41-43
    stress and, 190
    synthesis of, 41
Protein complement, 41
"Protein-sparing" diets, 82
Protein supplement, 42
Prudent Diet, 52
Psilocybin, 212
Psychoactive, definition of, 211
Psychoactives, 214
    common, 212
Psychological dependence, definition of, 211
Psychological needs determining behavior, 20
Psychotherapy, 21
Pulmonary disease, chronic obstructive, and smoking, 220
Pulse, taking, methods for, 161-162
Pulse rate, 281

Q

Quadriceps stretch, 157
Quality of life, 210
    activities enhancing, 6, 7
    personal environment and, 4

R

Race as risk factor for heart disease, 118
Radial artery, taking pulse at, 161-162
Radiotherapy for cancer, 250-251
RDA; *see* Recommended dietary allowances
Reactance motivation, 21
Readiness for lifestyle change, assessment of, 33
Rebellion, drug use as form of, 211
Rebound effect of nasal sprays, 256
Recidivism, 20
Recommended dietary allowances, 38, 39
    for protein, assessment for, 69
Recreational use of drugs, 210
Red blood cells, 114
Reduced sodium, meaning of word, 270
Reflex
    myotatic, 158
    stretch, 158
Reinforcers, positive and negative, 26-27

Relaxation, muscle, progressive, 194
Relaxation techniques, 194-196
Reliability of health information, 268
Religious reasons for using drugs, 210-211
Reproductive system
    effects of anabolic steroids on, 151
    marijuana and, 223
Reserve, heart rate, 161
Residual volume, decrease in, with exercise, 142
Resistance exercises, guidelines for, 153
Resistance phase of general adaptation syndrome, 186-187
Resistance/strength training, 140-141
Resistance training, 150
    guidelines for, 153
Respiratory responses and exercise, 142
Responses, metabolic, and exercise, 142-143
Resting heart rate, 113, 281
Rheumatic heart disease, 114
Rheumatoid arthritis, 255
Rhinoviruses, 255
Ribonucleic acid and cell growth, 247
Rice Diet Report, 85
Rights, patient's, 273
RNA and cell growth, 247
Rockport Fitness Walking Test, 177-179
Rotation Diet, 85
Roughage; *see* Fiber

S

SA node, 113
Saccharides, 53
Saccharin, 57
Safer sex, 238
Salt, 57-58
    and hypertension, 122
    intake of, in hot weather, 172-173
Sarcoma, 246
    common sites for, 246
    Kaposi's, 236
Saturated fat, 48-49, 50, 51
    dietary, sources of, 118
Sauces, nutritive components for, A-24—A-25
Screening, blood cholesterol, 281
Screening tests, blood, multiple, 280
Second opinions, 278
Secondary syphilis, 235
Seeds, nutritive components for, A-22—A-23
"Seesaw" weight loss, 81-82
Selective health examination, 279
Self-efficacy, 9-10
Self-esteem and stress, 191
Self-help approach to lifestyle change, 21
Self-help plan for lifestyle change, developing, 21-28
Self-responsibility in health-care market, 265-291
Selye, Hans, studies of stress of, 184-185
Sensation-seeking, use of drugs for, 210
Setpoint Diet, 84
Setpoint theory of weight control, 81
Sex, safer, 238
Sexual intercourse, decisions about, assessment of, 243
Sexuality, 232
Sexually transmitted diseases, 232
    preventing, 231-243

Credits

Chapter 1: p. 5 (Table 1-1), From the Monthly vital statistics report, Annual, Provisional Data for the National Center for Health Statistics, vol 37, no. 13, July 26, 1989; **pp. 13-14,** Adapted from Noland MP: The efficacy of a new model to explain leisure exercise behavior, PhD dissertation, University of Maryland, 1981, reprinted by permission of the author; **p. 15,** Source: The Society for Public Health Education, Berkeley, Calif.

Chapter 2: p. 19 (Fig. 2-1), From Survey highlights, the prevention index '89, summary report: a report card on the nation's health, Emmaus, Pa, Rodale Press, Inc, 1989; **p. 23 (Fig. 2-3),** Source: Louis Harris survey for *Prevention* magazine.

Chapter 3: pp. 37, 41 (Figs. 3-1, 3-2), From U.S. Department of Health and Human Services: The surgeon general's report on nutrition and health: summary and recommendations, Washington, DC, U.S. Government Printing Office, 1988; **p. 38 (Table 3-1),** Modified from Wardlaw G and Insel P: Perspectives in nutrition, St. Louis, Times Mirror/Mosby College Publishing, 1990; **pp. 38-40 (Table 3-2),** From National Research Council: Recommended dietary allowances, ed 10, Washington, DC, National Academy Press, 1989, reprinted by permission of National Academy Press; **p. 49 (Fig. 3-5),** From Lamb L: Fats and oils in food, The Health Letter 32(2):1-2, 1988, reprinted with special permission of North American Syndicate, Inc; **pp. 51, 53, 55 (Table 3-3, Fig. 3-6, Table 3-4),** Data from U.S. Department of Agriculture: Home and garden bulletin no. 72, nutritive value of foods, Washington, DC, U.S. Government Printing Office, 1988; **p. 53 (Fig. 3-7),** Source: Mayer J: What is a gram of fat and how much should you eat, Tufts University Diet and Nutrition Letter 7(8):3, 1989; **p. 59 (Fig. 3-8),** Modified from Klockenbrink M: How to read a food label, *The New York Times Magazine* 137(47,275):67-68, 1987; **p. 62 (Table 3-6),** Data from Williams SR: Nutrition and diet therapy, ed 6, St. Louis, Times Mirror/Mosby College Publishing, 1989.

Chapter 4: p. 82 (Table 4-1), Data from Zuti B and Golding L: Comparing diet and exercise as weight reduction tools, The Physician and Sportsmedicine 4:49-54, 1976; **pp. 84-85 (Table 4-3),** Reprinted by permission of **The Walking Magazine,** June 1989, © 1989, Raben Publishing Co, Boston, Mass: **p. 87 (Table 4-4),** Source: Physical fitness for practically everybody: the Consumers Union report on exercise, Mount Vernon, NY. The Consumers Union of the United States, 1983; **p. 90 (Table 4-6),** Adapted from the Surgeon General's Report on Nutrition and Health, Washington, DC., U.S. Department of Health and Human Services, 1988; **pp. 92, 93 (Figs. 4-3, 4-4),** Adapted from the American Psychiatric Association, Diagnostic and Statistical Manual of Mental Disorders, Washington, DC, 1987, American Psychiatric Association; **pp. 97-98 (Table 4-7, 4-8),** Source: Jackson AS and Pollack ML: Practical assessment of body composition, The Physician and Sportsmedicine 13 (5):86, May 1985; **p. 99 (Fig. 4-12),** From Evans LA, editor: Wake-up workouts, *Daily Pulse* 5(3):4, Jan/Feb, 1987.

Chapter 5: pp. 119, 120 (Tables 5-2, 5-3), Adapted from Report of the National Cholesterol Education Program Expert Panel in Detection, Evaluation, and Treatment of High Blood Cholesterol in Adults, Arch Intern Med 148:36, Jan 1988; **p. 120 (Table 5-4),** Adapted from National Institutes of Health Consensus Development Conference statement: lowering blood cholesterol, *JAMA* 253:2080, 1985; **p. 125 (Fig. 5-9),** Source: Trying to quit smoking? Drink less coffee, Tufts University Diet and Nutrition Letter 7(9):1, Nov 1989; **pp. 133-134,** Adapted from A self-test for smokers, U.S. Department of Health and Human Services, 1983; **pp. 135-136,** Arizona Heart Institute.

Chapter 6: p. 151 (Fig. 6-13), Reprinted with permission from Human physiology by L. Sherwood © St. Paul, 1989, by West Publishing Co, reprinted by permission; **p. 165 (Table 6-4),** From Conrad CC: How different sports rate in promoting physical fitness, Medical Times (reprint), May 1976, p. 4, used by permission; **p. 167 (Table 6-5),** Adapted from Rosato FD: Fitness and wellness: the physical connection, St. Paul, West Publishing Co, 1986; **p. 173 (Table 6-6),** Adapted from Sharkey BJ: Physiology of fitness, Champaign, Ill, 1979, Human Kinetics Publishers, p. 226; **pp. 177-179,** Reprinted by permission of The Rockport Company.

Chapter 7: p. 186 (Fig. 7-3), From Selye H: Stress without distress, Philadelphia, 1974, JB Lippincott Co; **p. 190 (Fig. 7-5),** Adapted from Williams SR: Nutrition and diet therapy, St. Louis, 1989, Times Mirror/Mosby College Publishing; **p. 199,** Holmes TH and Rahe RH: The social adjustment rating scale, J Psychosom Res, reprinted by permission of Pergamon Press, © 1967; **p. 201,** From What's your stress style? American Health, April 1986, pp. 41-45, reprinted by permission of The New York Times; **pp. 203-204,** *American Health Magazine* © Sept 1984, pp. 64-77.

Chapter 8: pp. 210-211, From Schlaadt RG and Shannon PT: Drugs of choice, ed 2, Englewood Cliffs, NJ, 1986, Prentice Hall; **pp. 212-213, (Table 8-1),** From What works: schools without drugs, U.S. Department of Education, 1988; **p. 215 (Table 8-2),** From the National Center for Drugs and Biologies, Food and Drug Administration, Washington, DC; **p. 221 (Fig. 8-6),** Adapted from the Mayo Clinic Health Letter; **p. 227,** Courtesy Alcoholics Anonymous.

Chapter 10: p. 248 (Fig. 10-1), Adapted from Take control of your health: five do's and five don'ts, American Cancer Society; **p. 250 (Fig. 10-3), pp. 261-262,** Adapted from the American Cancer Society.

Chapter 11: p. 270 (Fig. 11-1), Modified from Wardlaw G and Insel P. Perspectives in nutrition, St. Louis, 1990, Times Mirror/Mosby College Publishing, pp. 61-62; **p. 278 (Fig. 11-2),** Source: Lipman M: Office visit, Consumer Reports Health Letter 1(2):14, 1989; **p. 281 (Fig. 11-3),** Data source: Editors: The prevention index '89, summary report: a report card on the nation's health, Emmaus, Pa, 1989, Rodale Press, Inc, pp. 8-9.

Appendix B: © 1987 Fitness Publications, reprinted by permission.

Photo Credits

Chapter 1: p. 1, Frank Oberle, Photograhic Resources; **p. 2,** Superstock FourByFive; **p. 6,** Bob Daemmrich, Stock, Boston; **p. 9,** Superstock FourByFive; **p. 10,** Jeffry Myers, Stock, Boston.

Chapter 2: p. 16, Linsley Photographics; **p. 19,** Brownie Harris, The Stock market; **p. 20,** Jon Reis, The Stock Market; **p. 21,** Jeff Dunn, The Picture Cube; **p. 27,** Charles Gupton, Stock, Boston; **p. 28,** Superstock FourByFive.

Chapter 3: p. 34, Charles Gupton, Stock, Boston; **p. 40,** Stephen Pfusch, Stock, Boston; **p. 44,** Linsley Photographics; **p. 45,** Jeffry W. Myers, Stock, Boston; **p. 47,** Roy Morsch, The Stock Market; **p. 50,** NutraSweet, Monsanto; **p. 52,** Linsley Photographics; **p. 54,** Patricia Watson, The Stock Shop; **p. 57,** Linsley Photographics; **p. 60,** Linsley Photographics; **p. 61** (top), Linsley Photographics; **p. 61** (bottom), Superstock FourByFive.

Chapter 4: p. 74, Linsley Photographics; **p. 77,** Ellis Herwig, Stock, Boston; **p. 86,** Mike Mazzaschi, Stock, Boston; **p. 87,** Mike Mazzaschi, Stock, Boston; **p. 88,** Addison Geary, Stock, Boston; **pp. 95, 96** (Figs. 4-7, 4-8, 4-9, 4-10, 4-11), Sheri Seiser.

Chapter 5: p. 110, Charles Gupton, The Stock Market; **p. 122,** Blaine Harrington, The Stock Market; **p. 123,** Michael Keller, The Stock Market; **p. 124,** Bill Bachman, Photo Researchers; **p. 127,** Tony Schanuel, Photographic Resources; **p. 128** (Fig. 5-11), Tom Tracy, Medichrome; **p. 129,** Linsley Photographics.

Chapter 6: p. 138, Charles Gupton, Stock, Boston; **p. 141,** Charles Gupton, Stock, Boston; **p. 144,** Charles Gupton, Stock, Boston; **pp. 145-149, 150, 154-157, 162** (Figs. 6-2 through 6-9, 6-12, 6-15 through 6-22, 6-27), Sheri Seiser; **p. 166,** Bob Daemmrich, Stock, Boston; **p. 167,** Tom Tracy, Photographic Resources; **pp. 168, 170-171** (Figs. 6-29, 6-30), Sherry Seiser; **p. 172,** Gabe Palmer, Superstock FourByFive.

Chapter 7: p. 182, Bob Daemmrich, Stock, Boston; **p. 188,** Rene Sheret, The Stock Shop; **p. 191,** R. Huntzinger, The Stock Market; **p. 195,** David Pollack, The Stock Market; **p. 196** (top), Jon Riley, The Stock Shop; **p. 196** (bottom), R. Huntzinger, The Stock Market.

Chapter 8: p. 208, Elihu Blotnick, FPG; **p. 211,** Bob Daemmrich, Stock, Boston; **p. 216,** Superstock FourByFive; **p. 218,** Patrick Watson, Photographic Resources; **p. 223,** Dennis Oda, SIPA; **p. 224,** Gabe Palmer, The Stock Market.

Chapter 9: p. 230, Minardi, Photographic Resources; **p. 232,** Habif: Clinical Dermatology, ed 2, 1990, The C.V. Mosby Co; **p. 234,** Centers for Disease Control, Atlanta; **p. 236,** Wide World Photos; **p. 238,** Joseph Nettis, Stock, Boston.

Chapter 10: **p. 244,** Michael P. Cadomski, Photo Researchers; **p. 247,** Howard Sochurek, Medichrome; **p. 249,** MacDonald Photography, The Picture Cube; **p. 255,** Paul Manske, From Seeley/Stephens/Tate: Anatomy and physiology, 1988, Times Mirror/Mosby College Publishing; **p. 256,** Burkhart, Photographic Resources.

Chapter 11: **p. 264,** John Anderson, Photographic Resources; **p. 268,** Linsley Photographics; **p. 271,** David Stoecklein, The Stock Market; **p. 272,** Linsley Photographics; **p. 275,** Barbara Kirk, The Stock Market; **p. 279,** Grace Moore, Medichrome; **p. 281,** David Frazier, The Stock Market.

Chapter 12: **p. 292,** Superstock FourByFive.